Human Ecology
and Infectious Diseases

Edited by

NEIL A. CROLL

Institute of Parasitology
Macdonald College
McGill University
Montreal, Canada

JOHN H. CROSS

Scientific Director
United States Naval Medical Research Unit No. 2
Manila, Philippines

1983

ACADEMIC PRESS

A Subsidiary of Harcourt Brace Jovanovich, Publishers
New York   London
Paris   San Diego   San Francisco   São Paulo   Sydney   Tokyo   Toronto

ACADEMIC PRESS, INC.
111 Fifth Avenue, New York, New York 10003

United Kingdom Edition published by
ACADEMIC PRESS, INC. (LONDON) LTD.
24/28 Oval Road, London NW1 7DX

Library of Congress Cataloging in Publication Data

Main entry under title:

Human ecology and infectious diseases.

     Includes index.
     1. Parasitic diseases. 2. Host-parasite relation-
ships. 3. Human ecology. I. Croll, Neil Argo.
II. Cross, John H.
RA643.H79 1983   614.4'2   82-24466
ISBN 0-12-196880-4

PRINTED IN THE UNITED STATES OF AMERICA

83 84 85 86   9 8 7 6 5 4 3 2 1

In Memoriam

What began as a state-of-the-art presentation of a rapidly growing field under the editorship of its dynamic and innovative spokesman has become the Editor's epitaph.

Neil A. Croll, Ph.D., M.D., D.Sc., clearly established himself as a forceful, effective, and innovative scientist, teacher, and administrator during his 1974–1980 tenure as third director of the Institute of Parasitology at Macdonald College of McGill University, following a long period of leadership under its founder, T. W. M. Cameron, and the subsequent directorship of K. G. Davey. While continuing to extend his wide-ranging interests in host–parasite behavior, Croll showed increasing concern with international aspects of human health and human behavioral characteristics associated with parasitic disease. One of his earliest efforts at Macdonald College was to embrace the powerful new information-gathering tools of computer storage and access, extending the Institute's National Reference Center for Parasitology into a world repository for data from studies and surveys in India, Africa, and elsewhere in the Third World. These expanding parasitological interests did not dilute his scientific focus; continuing interest in the host–parasite interface caused him to raise new questions on host resistance and parasite selectivity. Why should one dog, one host, one human end up with the bulk of parasites equally available to others? Why is unequal distribution of parasites the common mode?

Croll's studies on factors responsible for parasite concentration in specific individual hosts were begun and programs for future experimental implementation laid out. It was to enter this little-studied arena of human ecology and its effect on disease that he undertook the extremely concentrated two-year medical curriculum at the University of Miami. Even during this period of intensive medical training, Croll's boundless energy and organizational talents were not contained. He continued to organize, supervise, and initiate new plans for data collection and analysis and to develop and direct new programs for ecological and behavioral research to be undertaken at home and abroad. Croll's return to

McGill in 1980 was marked by rapid implementation of his broadening views on international medicine—epidemiology on a global plane—and on the study of factors responsible for the highly focal nature of human infection and disease. "McGill International" was Croll's vehicle for these studies, for which he quickly provided the impetus of his leadership and organizational talents for raising funds despite a rapidly diminishing economy. His persuasive talents, soaring imagination, and scientific leadership were now focused and on track. Neil Croll's research potential and scientific leadership were only beginning to take their mature form when he died of a heart attack on June 23, 1981—four months short of his fortieth birthday. An unmeasurable curve of future accomplishment and leadership was cut off at its steepest angle of ascent.

Markers were laid out, however, and much of what Croll envisaged may yet be realized. Host–parasite behavioral interaction, the focus of Neil's ecologically based thinking for some years, led to a renewed interest in human ecology and factors affecting the human–parasite interaction complex. Many of the views stimulated by Croll are presented in this volume, studies and reviews by colleagues Neil selected and invited, each to write on a focus of man as host, whose behavior and ecology often determine factors responsible for the onset and expression of human disease. These authors, including Croll himself, have pooled their findings in this volume under the capable editoral leadership of John Cross, himself an outstanding student of the ecology and distribution of human parasitic disease in the Pacific basin and an important contributor to this book. The present volume is therefore a current statement on human disease ecology and a projection of patterns and directions for future work anticipated by Neil Croll, to whom this field will be indebted for much of its future progress.

DONALD HEYNEMAN

Contents

3. Human Behavior and Zoonotic Diseases in Malaysia

B. L. Lim and J. W. Mak

4. Filariasis in Southeast Asia

V. Zaman

5. Intestinal Capillariasis in the Philippines and Thailand

John H. Cross and Manoon Bhaibulaya

10. The Transmission of *Trypanosoma cruzi* Infection to Man and Its Control

P. D. Marsden

11. Paleoparasitology: On the Origins and Impact of Human–Helminth
Relationships

Michael McKinnon Kliks

12. Brucellosis in Nigeria: Epidemiology and Practical Problems of Control

Olanipekun K. Alausa

13. Epidemiology Patterns in Directly Transmitted Human Infections

A. D. M. Smith

Contributors

Numbers in parentheses indicate the pages on which the authors' contributions begin.

Olanipekun K. Alausa (315), Department of Epidemiology and Community Health, University of Ilorin, Ilorin, Kwara, Nigeria

Manoon Bhaibulaya (103), Faculty of Tropical Medicine, Mahidol University, Bangkok, Thailand

Neil A. Croll[1] (1), Institute of Parasitology, Macdonald College, McGill University, Montreal, Quebec H9X 1CO, Canada

John H. Cross (103), Medical Ecology Department, United States Naval Medical Research Unit No. 2, (Manila, Philippines,) APO San Francisco, California 96528

Michael McKinnon Kliks (291), Division of Comparative Medicine, John A. Burns School of Medicine, University of Hawaii, Honolulu, Hawaii 96816

Akio Kobayashi (137), Department of Parasitology, Jikei University School of Medicine, Tokyo 105, Japan

V. Kochar (187), Department of Sociology and Anthropology, University of Hyderabad, Hyderabad, India 500 001

Chojiro Kunii (169), Hoken Kaikan Bekkan, 1.1, Sadohara-Cho, Ichigaya, Shinjuku-Ku, Tokyo, Japan

B. L. Lim (49), Medical Ecology Division, Institute for Medical Research, Jalan Pahang, Kuala Lumpur, 02-14, Malaysia

J. W. Mak (49), Filariasis Division, Institute for Medical Research, Jalan Pahang, Kuala Lumpur, 02-14, Malaysia

P. D. Marsden (253), Nucleo de Medicina Tropical e Nutricao, University of Brasilia, Brasilia DF, Brasil

[1]Deceased.

T. A. Nawalinski (187), Division of Parasitology, SmithKline Animal Health Products, Philadelphia, Pennsylvania 19380

Alphonsus B. C. Nwosu (225), Biomedical Sciences Research Group, University of Technology, PMB 1660 Enugu, Nigeria

G. A. Schad (187), Department of Pathobiology, School of Veterinary Medicine, University of Pennsylvania, Philadelphia, Pennsylvania 19104

Peter M. Schantz (21), Helminthic Diseases Branch, Division of Parasitic Diseases, Center for Infectious Diseases, Centers for Disease Control, Public Health Service, Atlanta, Georgia 30333

A. D. M. Smith (333), Department of Zoology, University of Adelaide, Adelaide, South Australia, Australia

V. Zaman (73), Department of Microbiology, Faculty of Medicine, National University of Singapore, Singapore 0511

Preface

This book was conceived, organized, and developed by Neil Croll. Having traveled widely throughout the world, he came to the realization that human behavior and ecology provide the interaction between man and his infectious diseases. In his proposal for the book he stated that, at a time of growing political activism among the world's social philosophies and between the haves and have nots, there remains an intolerable burden of infectious disease. Advances have been made, but at times the problems seem to continue to be overwhelming. Some diseases are on the increase, not only because of the rapid growth in susceptible populations but also because of the breakdown in the continual vigilance required to combat biological systems that do not conform to short-term political expediency. It is people, not policies, models, or computers, who acquire diseases. It is individuals who decide whether to comply with medications or to use latrine pits. People and their communities establish their own attitudes to disease and create their own priorities in which disease is placed within the social hierarchy of needs.

This volume brings together contemporary thinking relative to current experiences and thoughts in the field of human ecology and transmissible diseases to focus attention on methodologic and specific studies. Although there are a number of excellent books on various aspects of human ecology and related subjects, there is none that has an approach comparable to this.

The contributors are multinational with proven authority in human behavior, ecology, and disease, who have studied intensively the cultural, behavioral, anthropological, and social factors in the transmission of infectious diseases. Some of the authors provide a contemporary account of methods used to make human ecology a more quantitative predictive science in the global challenge of infectious diseases, and others attempt to identify behavioral patterns which place man at risk to infections and to examine the nature of risk factors. Studies presented on hookworm include an analysis of human behavior and religions that affect transmission of the parasitoses. Human behavior and transmission of zoonotic diseases in North America and Malaysia are documented as are the habits, customs, and superstitions associated with the epidemic of intestinal capillariasis that occurred in the Philippines. There is a review of filarial diseases in Southeast Asia, and Japanese authors report the changing patterns of parasitic infections and describe the cooperation of government and private sources to lower infection rates in Japan. A study on human environment and intestinal helminthiasis and a review on brucellosis are presented from Nigeria; from Brazil comes an in-depth discussion on the transmission of *Trypanosoma cruzi* and details of the control of Chagas' disease. An essay on the development of host–parasite systems affecting paleolithic humans follows, and finally, the volume concludes with a study on the importance of behavioral and social–cultural factors in determining regional and national patterns in disease incidence and transmission.

Unfortunately, the book could neither cover all infectious diseases nor relate the influences that human ecology, agricultural practices, customs, beliefs, and religions may have upon them. Such a task would have been overwhelming. The emphasis, however, has been on parasitic and zoonotic diseases, because these seem to be influenced more by man's habits and ecological practices. The book should be valuable to students of tropical diseases and public health and to physicians, epidemiologists, anthropologists, and veterinarians as well as to parasitologists. It was the hope of Dr. Croll and myself that the book would add vigor and innovation to biomedical research and provide some direction to those who fail daily against the bewildering disease problems facing most of the world's population.

JOHN H. CROSS

Human Behavior, Parasites, and Infectious Diseases

*NEIL A. CROLL**
Institute of Parasitology
Macdonald College
McGill University
Montreal, Quebec, Canada

I. Introduction

Parasites are dispersed discontinuously within the individuals of a community and within communities; they are dispersed discontinuously over the globe. This pattern is consistent with other infectious diseases and is broadly due to the availability of vectors, the complexities of the environment, and factors that determine exposure and susceptibility. *What* man does, *when* he does it, and *where* he does it determine his exposure. Understanding *why* he does it is essential for effective prevention and control of parasitic infections. This chapter attempts to analyze some of the research into those aspects of human behavior that determine risk of helminth infection.

Infrequently, human behavioral analysis with respect to infection has been

*This chapter was unfinished at the time of the death of Neil A. Croll.

HUMAN ECOLOGY AND INFECTIOUS DISEASES
ISBN 0-12-196880-4

attempted by anthropologists, sociologists, and ethnologists. It is a subdiscipline in search of an identity, and although it has many cousins, and even some brothers and sisters, it is not legitimized by an intellectual pedigree. There have been a few specific attempts to review aspects of human behavior and infectious disease: "cultural epidemiology," "socioepidemiology," and recently "medical sociology." Some of these studies have introduced parasitic diseases: (May, 1950; Audy, 1958, 1972; Pavlovsky, 1963; Nnochiri, 1968; Chen Paul, 1970; Roundy, 1978; Petersdorff and Feinstein, 1981). Much of the information in this catalog of human experience, although fascinating and of considerable intrinsic interest, has rarely been quantified or placed in a workable unified conceptual framework.

People with a fever attract hematophagous diptera thus enhancing the spread of infection. Dysentery causes the constant excretion of many infective stages. Patients with dengue fever are relatively indifferent to sensory input and will tolerate mosquitoes on their bodies. Human trypanosomiasis in Africa, although more severe than dengue, allows patients to go to the fields and streams and transmit the disease to tse-tse flies; attacks of stupor under the blazing tropical sun are well known. The celebrated outbreak of trichinellosis in Kenya (Forrester *et al.*, 1961) was probably due to a lapse in the usual practice among the Kikuyu tribe of cooking the flesh of wild bush pig (Nelson, 1972). Dr. D. Carleton Gajdusek won the 1976 Nobel Prize for Medicine for his brilliant epidemiological and anthropological studies of Kuru, a "slow virus" transmitted when cannibals eat the brains of victims, in the Fore tribe of New Guinea. Such intriguing statements are widespread and similar anecdotes may regularly be encountered in the literature of geographic medicine.

There have been many reports of association between human behavior and hydatid disease caused by the larvae of the tapeworm *Echinococcus granulosus*. These include the use of "dog nurses" by the Turkana tribe of Northern Kenya which increases exposure to hydatid; this is not the case in another nomadic tribe, the Masai of East Africa, who are less intimate with their dogs (Schwabe, 1969). The risk of hydatid disease among Muslim Arabs in Lebanon is much lower than among Christian Arabs; this has been related to the Islamic teaching about the uncleanliness of dogs: "Angels do not enter a house where there is a dog (Abou Daoud and Schwabe, 1964)." The risk of hydatid infection in Beirut is more than 20 times greater among persons who own dogs than among those who do not (W.H.O., 1979). In New Zealand, the risk of hydatidosis is six times greater among the Maoris than among New Zealanders of European origin. Using multivariate analysis, this risk has been shown to be associated with the Maoris' intimacy with their dogs, rather than with their sheep-rearing practices (Burridge and Schwabe, 1977). Human activities, by supporting vector populations, may indirectly enhance man's infections. Reviewing his experiences in Africa, Gillett (1975, 1979) has described the "malariogenic behavior" of man, in which man's practices, cultivations, and impact on the environment encourage the mosquito vectors of malaria, encephalitis, other arboviruses, and filariasis.

The early epidemiologists, in their search for the causes of disease, were equally as concerned with human activities as with the physical and biological factors. The pioneering studies of Panum in 1846 on measles in the Faröes (Panum, 1940), of Holmes (1892) on puerperal fever, and of Baker on endemic colic (Maxcy, 1956) all preceded the "germ theory." Snow's classic investigation on the cholera outbreak in London in 1854 was carried out before the birth of modern epidemiology and microbiology. Jenner (1798) was one of the earliest European scientists to recognize the danger of zoonoses from pets. In his report on cowpox he wrote

> The deviation of man from the state in which he was placed by nature, seems to have proven to him a prolific source of diseases. From the love of splendour, from the indulgence of luxury and from his fondness for amusement (man) has familiarized himself with the great number of animals which may not usually have been intended for his amusement.

It was only after the discovery of bacteria that the vision of infectious diseases became more restricted and human behavior was overlooked in favor of microbiological investigation. After the Second World War, with postwar optimism, it was confidently hoped that with antibiotics, new antiparasitic agents, and DDT infections would be globally eradicated. Now, with a few important battles won and by using the same tools the war may be lost against malaria, filariasis, and schistosomiasis (W.H.O., 1980). Only 10% of the 85 million children born each year are immunized against diphtheria, whooping cough, measles, and tetanus (Zahra, 1980). Clearly, the technology and management of infectious disease control need to improve. This narrowness of vision in infectious diseases is not shared by epidemiologists studying cancer, automobile accidents, or coronary disease.

A minority of thinkers advocated a wider view. Fleck and Ianni (1958) provided evidence for the widely accepted view that infection with the tubercle bacillus of tuberculosis was not the major determining factor in the production of the disease. Pavlovsky (1963) placed emphasis on the human habitation within the wider landscape. Observations on the intimacy and frequency of human physical interactions were used to predict the risk of transmission of leprosy in New Guinea. In these studies, Hausfeld (1970) argued that "if leprosy is transmitted in a community by contact, then the social structure of the community will reflect the transmission and distribution of the disease." The beautifully illustrated report of Bang et al., (1975) related human activities and social conditions in Bengali villages and in Calcutta to infectious respiratory diseases.

Attempts to identify those behavioral patterns that place man at risk of infection are probably as old as culture itself. A large catalog of fascinating examples has been assembled which includes risk behaviors and health-promoting activities. To provide a context for these epidemiological pearls and to find effective methods of intervention which are socially, culturally, and environmentally acceptable is the contemporary state of the art. There has been a series of quantitative approaches that have stressed different factors and used quite distinct methodologies. Some of these will be discussed in the following sections.

II. The Measurement of Individual Behavioral Actions as Risk Factors of Infection

Infectious diseases may be approached as hazard systems rather than as individual and isolated medical problems. In applying this concept to the Amhara communities of rural highland Ethiopia, the behavioral repertoire of the villagers was related to disease transmission. The social unit (e.g., individual, household, or community) was related to sociocultural activities (e.g., religion, water use, and trade) and scored with respect to frequency and intimacy (Table I). From this analysis and other field observations, Roundy (1978) was able to equate each social unit with the relative hazards of exposure to selected communicable diseases (Table II). From this simple and inexpensive methodology, it was possible to suggest a series of key places for intervention, surveillance, and vector control.

Among the helminth studies, those on human behavior and schistosomiasis are

TABLE I

Associations between Systems of Behavior and Habitat Interactions[a,b]

	Degree of association					
Systems	Individual	Household	Compound	Settlement	Productive area	Further ranging
Family	0	3	2	2	2	2
Extrafamiliar socializing	0	2	1	2	0	2
Religious activities	2	2	1	3	1	2
Primary production	2	2	3	2	3	1
Trade	0	1	0	1	0	3
Water use	3	3	2	3	1	1
Animal contact	0	3	2	1	3	1
Defecation	0	1	3	1	3	2

[a]Adapted from Roundy, 1978.

[b]0 = negligible association, 1 = low association, 2 = moderate association, 3 = high association.

TABLE II

Selected Communicable Diseases in which Great Hazard Is Associated with Particular Levels
of Social Organization for Rural-Dwelling Ethiopians[a,b]

Social unit	Disease
Individual	Trachoma, scabies, ringworm, (smallpox)
Household	Tuberculosis, trachoma, scabies, ringworm, poliomyelitis, tapeworm, ascariasis, trichuriasis, infectious hepatitis, amebiasis, salmonellosis, shigellosis, malaria
Compound	Poliomyelitis, tapeworm, ascariasis, trichuriasis, infectious hepatitis, amebiasis
Settlement	Tuberculosis, trachoma, scabies, ringworm, tapeworm, ascariasis, trichuriasis, infectious hepatitis, amebiasis, salmonellosis, shigellosis
Production area	Tapeworm, infectious hepatitis, amebiasis, salmonellosis, shigellosis, schistosomiasis
Further ranging area of contact	Tuberculosis, trachoma, syphilis, gonorrhea, schistosomiasis, malaria

[a]Adapted from Roundy, 1978.
[b]Helminth and protozoal infections are underlined.

the most detailed. Observations on man in endemic areas are available from St. Lucia, Puerto Rico, Egypt, Zimbabwe and Ghana (reviewed by Jordan *et al.*, 1980). The results of human–water contact studies from these diverse countries are remarkably similar. It is a biological comment that, in Egypt "the human exposure pattern favours the transmission of bilharzia . . . the peak seasonal and diurnal cycles of infectivity of water coincide closely with the frequency of and duration of contact and with the period of maximum body exposures (Farooq and Mallah, 1966)."

The integration of behavior, belief, and culture is illustrated from water contact studies in Nigeria. Among the Hausa, Fulani, and Maguzowa, the tenets of Islam which prohibit public bathing by women cause *Schistosoma haematobium* to be an infection of the male population (Pugh and Gilles, 1978). The Hazda tribe of Tanzania is relatively free of schistosomiasis, whereas the Bantu in nearby Sukumuland are heavily infected. The Hazda apparently collect their water from predug holes in dry river beds, thereby avoiding cercariae (Bennett *et al.*, 1970).

Using data from P. R. Dalton, Jordan *et al.* (1980) published typical water contact data from water infected with *Schistosoma mansoni* in St. Lucia (Table III). These results show that exposure is greater in youth during bathing and swimming. Being a female, washing, and water carrying also account for a greater additional risk of exposure. Dalton (1976) accumulated many months of data gathered by observation and interview at a few key sites of extensive water usage. A socioanthropological approach was used to quantify the relationship

TABLE III

Frequency of Water Contacts Categorized by Age and Sex in Relation to Behavior[a]

Contact method	Age (years)							
	0–4	5–9	10–14	15–19	20–29	30–39	40–49	50+
Males								
Water carrying	2	57	78	17	6	4	2	5
Washing	0	10	22	2	3	4	2	1
Bathing	107	109	56	19	19	5	6	15
Swimming	120	145	64	9	2	1	0	1
Fording	6	69	48	29	43	37	19	57
Other	1	3	16	1	0	1	0	1
Total	236	393	284	77	73	52	29	80
% of total contacts	19.2	32.1	23.2	6.2	5.9	4.2	2.3	6.5
Females								
Water carrying	10	47	97	88	85	47	22	31
Washing	4	47	116	145	160	131	58	57
Bathing	98	113	73	67	49	26	18	16
Swimming	80	128	59	5	4	1	2	0
Fording	22	33	82	88	40	34	40	31
Other	3	4	28	13	17	7	3	1
Total	217	372	455	406	355	246	143	136
% of total contacts	9.3	15.9	19.5	17.4	15.2	10.5	6.1	5.8

[a]Data of P. R. Dalton in St. Lucia, adapted from Jordan et al., 1980.

between role allocation and patterns of water use. Sixty-nine households were observed over a 3-year period to monitor the changing roles of members in this community with respect to the type, frequency, and duration of water contact.

Results of water contact studies have led to intervention and subsequent evaluation of the prevalence of schistosomiasis. In Puerto Rico, for example, by using a multifactorial regression analysis it was concluded that the greatest reduction of *S. mansoni* followed an improved water supply, rather than an upgraded sewage disposal system or increased education (Bhajan *et al.*, 1978). It is likely that the improved water supply was more convenient and more acceptable. Several strategies of biological and sociological intervention are discussed by Jordan *et al.* (1980).

Although Roundy (1978) classified human activity as a function of social units and organization, there are other methods that may give other insights. One such inventory of epidemiologically significant actions or behaviors, enumerated in Table IV, recognizes metabolic, information gathering, reproductive, comfort, protective, and territorial behaviors. It is instructive that most risk factors of parasitic diseases fall within "metabolic behavior", that is, food gathering, eating, drinking, defecation, and urination—the activities of peoples from nonin-

TABLE IV

Inventory of Epidemiologically Significant Actions and Behaviors

Metabolic behavior: breathing, coughing, sneezing, food cultivation and gathering, drinking, eating, storage, defecation and urination
Reproductive behavior: sex, copulation, gestation, parturition, parental care, nursing, and ritual aggression
Protection and Defense: flight, attack, and argument
Comfort Actions: scratching, bathing, cleaning, and licking
Territorial Behavior: space allocation and organization, home and shelter, construction and core, group interactions, and community functions
Information Gathering and Ordering: orientation, exploring, reading, writing, travel, and metaphysical pursuits

dustrialized, rural populations. Conversely, information gathering and territorial behavior, which dominate the time of westernized and urbanized peoples, are not high-risk activities. Although this inventory is clearly incomplete, it illustrates another approach to human behavioral classification and its relationship to disease.

III. Overdispersion of Helminths as a Consequence of Exposure and Susceptibility

In the last decade it has been demonstrated repeatedly that helminths are not distributed at random, but are overdispersed[1] within populations of their hosts (Crofton, 1971, Anderson, 1976, Croll and Ghadirian, 1981, Croll *et al.* 1981a).

A frequency distribution approaching a truncated log-normal and best described as a negative binomial is approximated. This results in a few hosts carrying a disproportionate number of worms (Fig. 1); 20–30% of all worms can be harbored by 1–5% of those persons sampled. Those heavily infected "wormy persons" (Croll and Ghadirian, 1981) include individuals who are most in need of medical attention and who are contributing excessive numbers of infective stages to their communities. Identification of wormy persons enables limited medical resources to be directed to those most in need and may significantly reduce parasite transmission. Except in areas of very high prevalence and intensity, the phenomenon of overdispersion seriously challenges the effectiveness of mass chemotherapy programs in the pursuit of managing or controlling endemic

[1] An ecological term; also described as "clumped," "aggregated," "contagious."

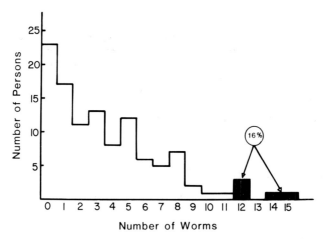

FIG. 1. The frequency distribution of *Ascaris lumbricoides* in Jazin, near Esfahan, Iran. Five persons (shaded) carry 16% of all the worms.

helminths. Attempts to explain the phenomenon of overdispersion have stressed the role of "exposure" and "susceptibility". Although these are not the only explanations, they are intuitively important; there is evidence that each is critical in several disease etiologies (Croll and Ghadirian, 1981).

The extensive studies on water contact and schistosomiasis (Table III) are examples of the role of exposure in determining helminth burden. Similar studies on hydatid disease (Chapter 2; Sections III and IV), or the association of visceral larval migrans with pet dogs (Woodruff *et al.*, 1966), or clonorchiasis and anisakiasis with the habit of consuming undercooked fish (Croll *et al.*, 1982) underline the association of habit and exposure.

The mechanism of *susceptibility,* less well documented in helminthic disease, is widely integrated into the thinking of microbiologists: lepromatous leprosy is manifested in individuals with a specific cell-mediated defect, *Klebsiella* pneumonia is high in alcoholics, *Candida albicans* in diabetics, cryptococcal meningitis in lymphoma patients, and *Pneumocystis carinii* in leukemic or marasmic patients. High-susceptibility groups are now being identified for clinical stronglyloidiasis among immunocompromised or immunosuppressed patients (Purtilo *et al.*, 1974). *Toxoplasma gondii, Entamoeba histolytica,* and *Giardia lamblia* are among the protozoa that have been associated with natural or induced immunoincompetence. Space does not permit review of the mushrooming subdiscipline of the genetics of susceptibility and resistance to infection, one which will undoubtedly change the nature of infectious disease thinking in the 1980s (Skamene *et al.*, 1980).

Recently, wormy persons were further characterized by examination of the intestinal helminths (Croll and Ghadirian, 1981) of the people of Jazin, an agricultural village near Esfahan, Iran. Human excreta is systematically collected

TABLE V

The Prevalence of *Ascaris lumbricoides* Infection at Various Times
after Chemotherapeutic Treatment[a]

Age class (years)	Number in age group of subsample (111 people)	Prevalence (%) at posttreatment sampling times[b]				
		7	30	60	90	365
0–4	10	0.0	50.0	60.0	80.0	90.0
5–9	24	4.2	41.7	66.7	87.5	91.7
10–14	22	4.5	54.5	68.2	90.9	81.8
15–19	10	10.0	30.0	60.0	70.0	90.0
20–24	12	8.3	33.3	58.3	83.3	83.3
25–29	4	0.0	25.0	50.0	75.0	100.0
30–34	9	0.0	22.2	55.5	88.9	100.0
35–39	8	12.5	50.0	62.5	87.5	87.5
40–44	2	0.0	50.0	100.0	50.0	50.0
45+	10	0.0	40.0	80.0	70.0	70.0

[a]From Croll *et al.*, 1981.
[b]The times are given in days posttreatment.

and marketed as fertilizer, and the region supports one of the highest rates of *Ascaris lumbricoides* in the world (Croll *et al.*, 1981). One hundred and twenty volunteers were treated with broad spectrum anthelmintics and all of the parasites passed in the subsequent 2 days were collected, identified, and counted. This provided a cross-sectional survey of the frequency distribution of *A. lumbricoides, Trichuris trichiura, Necator americanus,* and *Ancylostoma duodenale* (Fig. 1). The recruitment of fresh worm burdens was monitored through the following year (Table V).

All helminths were overdispersed and subsequent analysis enabled the following conclusions to be drawn about these species in Jazin:

1. Wormy persons could be described only for single species because there was no indication that carrying a heavy burden of one species either predisposed or excluded an individual from being in the highly infected cohort for another species. This was true even for biologically similar species such as *Ascaris lumbricoides* and *T. trichiura* or *N. americanus* and *Ancylostoma duodenale.*
2. Wormy persons for any single species at the beginning of the program were neither significantly included nor excluded from being wormy persons for that species after recruitment of fresh burdens.

In parallel studies in Gargaria, a village of West Bengal, India, stool and blood were examined for ova and cysts or microfilariae of *Wuchereria bancrofti* respectively. The parasites were similarly overdispersed (Fig. 2) and wormy per-

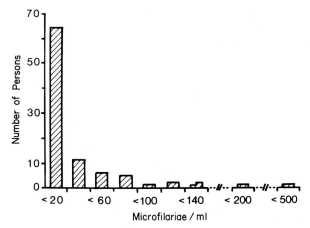

FIG. 2. The frequency distribution of microfilariae of *Wuchereria bancrofti* in Gargaria, West Bengal.

sons for microfilariae were not necessarily the same as those for intestinal parasites.

Many additional field studies are needed to unravel the complex interactions of exposure, susceptibility, and overdispersion in helminth populations. Part of the approach will require a much more detailed and refined methodology for the definition of *exposure* in the context of human behavioural actions.

IV. The Distribution of Helminths in Communities and Its Association with Socioagricultural Practices

Babol is the main town of the central-eastern region of the Caspian littoral zone of Iran. Surrounding it are several villages, each of about 500 inhabitants, with the villages tending to specialize in one or two different major agricultural practices. Between 1975 and 1977, nine villages were sampled by single stool examinations for intestinal parasites, with a total of 2181 villagers yielding a total prevalence for parasites (excluding pathogenic and nonpathogenic amoebae) of 74.6% (Ghadirian *et al.*, 1979).

Vegetables were cultivated in coastal villages (e.g., Hali Bagh) with a high water table, poor drainage, and salty subsoil. The inhabitants were heavily infected with *Ascaris lumbricoides* and *Trichuris trichiura* (Fig. 3). Rice, the dominant crop further inland, was the focus for hookworms. In Gol Afshan,

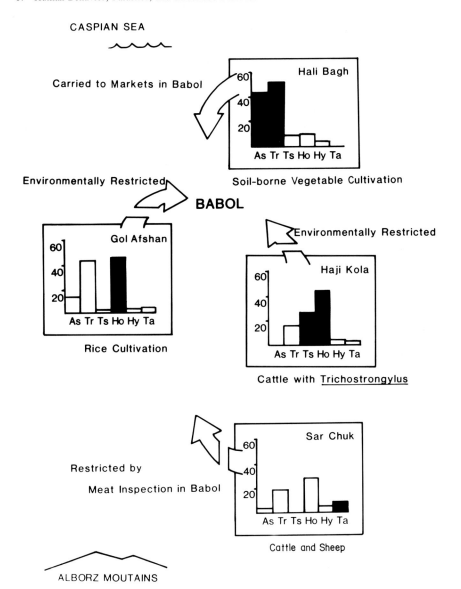

FIG. 3. Socioagricultural factors and parasitic infections at Babol in northern Iran. As = *Ascaris lumbricoides*, Tr = *Trichuris trichiura*, Ts = *Trichostrongylus sp.*, Ho = hookworm, Hy = *Hymenolepis nana*, Ta = *Taenia saginata*.

hookworm infected 46% of the population; furthermore, it was abundant in that age group of males who worked in the paddy fields. In nearby Haji Kola, in addition to rice, dairy cattle were farmed which carried high levels of *Trichostrongylus* spp. It was here that the highest levels of human trichostrongyliasis were reached (Fig. 3), with a hookworm prevalence of 46%. In the foothills of the Alborz Mountains, goat, cattle, and sheep herders suffer from nasal myiasis and *Taenia saginata*. Although *T. saginata* is only poorly detected in stool samples, it did reach 8% in Sar Chuck where the villagers favor beef heart as a delicacy. The prevalence of *Hymenolepis nana* was also higher in certain areas, but no explanation for this was found.

Babol has been sampled repeatedly for parasites, and the experience of those involved was sought. Infections of *Ascaris lumbricoides* and *Trichuris trichiura* were common from the vegetables that reached the markets from Hali Bagh. However, hookworms and *Trichostrongylus* spp. were infrequent because they resulted from work in rice paddies or cattle husbandry and were effectively excluded from Babol. Similarly, the rudimentary meat inspection exercised in the town had almost removed *Taenia saginata* from the townsfolk. The widespread nature of trichuriasis probably reflects both its refractoriness to chemotherapy and its longevity (Fig. 3).

Village latrines were introduced in this region in the 1970s but remained largely unused. Mass treatment with levamisole of 16,600 persons had been used repeatedly between 1972 and 1977, but reinfection was typical and reoccurred rapidly.

This study illustrates that geography and climate, even over the range of a few kilometres, determine the way of life in rural settings, and that the way of life determines the nature and intensity of parasites. Clearly, a more local, more directed, and more culturally sensitive use of the resources might have provided much better results. Transport of food between adjacent villages presents a health hazard and provides methods of intervention. This approach attempts to integrate the principles of human ecology and behavior with our understanding of infectious diseases. As Fabrega (1974) put it:

> Culture, in ordering behaviour (including diet, energy expenditure, subsistence patterns, marriage rules, child-rearing, exposure to diseases) . . . to some extent orders biology. . . . Culture orders the categories through which biological changes become manifest.

V. Culture, Attitudes, and Human Behavior

The direct quantification of human behavior, an essential first step, must be related to an examination of the attitudes, beliefs, and motivations that cause it

(Chen Paul, 1970; Heyneman, 1971; Dalton, 1976; Dunn, 1979). "Although bridges, latrines and laundry sites can be built (to combat schistosomiasis), without such studies, there is no assurance that they will be used (Dunn, 1979)." Indeed, in the West we have encountered behavioral problems and extensive noncompliance with the advice of epidemiologists with respect to cigarette smoking, the use of seat belts, and obesity. This integration of behavior with attitude has even been extended to include culture. Anthropologists have focused upon health and the social behaviors which are implicated. The specific social dimensions often studied include these relationships: mother–child, employer–laborer, male–female, intercaste, and interclass. Reviewing the field, Montgomery (1973) concluded that a more precise definition of the transmission of infection in anthropological terms had not been achieved.

Alland's important ideas (1969) require an act of faith for his anthropological approach. He rightly asserts that the morbidity profile of a population is dependent upon encounters with parasites. Even if they are not understood, certain cultural practices will have an objective effect on morbidity rates. The complexity of these will often go beyond the existing native medical theory. Thus, behaviors will have been selected that favor reduced morbidity and survival, even if the factual basis for them is not appreciated. Nonetheless it is important to remember that self-sufficient and stable populations may also have incorporated methods of numerical self-regulation. The Abrou of the Ivory Coast studied by Alland, although showing many cultural and environmental adaptations that seem medically adaptive, have others, such as the poor nutrition of children at times of drought and famine, that seem to be distinctly maladaptive. One of the greatest challenges confronting research into this subject is that human behavior has been molded by health status as perceived through symptom complexes. Furthermore, single parasite species infections are frequently less common than multiple species infections. Fevers, abdominal pains, headache, lymphadenopathy, and changes in bowel habits often confuse many clinicians. It is perhaps difficult to imagine an intuitive causal relationship between health-promoting behaviors and the specific avoidance of strongyloidiasis, giardiasis, malaria, brucellosis, and filariasis. At the more general level, coprophobia, avoidance of vectors, and cleanliness may have been deliberately favored in most cultures.

When interpreting man's behavior in the context of "health," there are eight categories of observation. There are those actions that are consciously related to health promotion or maintenance, and those that deliberately enhance ill-health or mortality. Similarly, there are both nondeliberate and deliberate actions or habits that are favorable to either health or ill-health. Finally, each of these four must be defined by the population at risk *and,* independently, by the outside observer (Dunn, 1979). In Chad, it was found that villagers adapted to disability and deformity, which undoubtedly reduced their working capacity, by finding new and simpler functions in their communities (Buck *et al.,* 1970). Only when new diseases or exacerbations disrupted their lives did they recognize their illness. Such social and psychological compensation reduces the objective perception of health and illness.

The acceptable approach, and the best, for changing human attitudes is through communication and information—in short, by education.

VI. Complexity, Diversity, and Sociocultural Integration

In assessing the morbidity and mortality resulting from infectious diseases in the tropics today, various students of the subject have wondered how long the current situation has existed. Bradley (1977) "looked back wistfully at the Utopian natural ecosystems of man" and concluded that, "if this was an idyllic primordial state it was a long way back."

In his discussion of the health of hunter–gatherers, Dunn (1968) compared the parasitic burdens of various populations (Table VI). He found that hunter–gatherers were "an element of their ecosystem" and that there was "little or no buffering between them and the other components of the system." Using measures of biological diversity and complexity to compare environments, he noted that the Semang of tropical Malaysia and the Pygmy of Equatorial Africa, each from complex environments, carried 22 and 20 intestinal parasite species, respectively. In contrast those aboriginal peoples of the dry deserts of Australia and the Kalahari, living in less biologically complex environments, carried far fewer. Citing Pampigliene, Nelson (1972) asserts that a prevalence of 50% of the monkey nematode *Strongyloides fülleborni* in the Pygmies of the Congo is the highest yet recorded in man.

In a more detailed parasitological study, the effects of population density, land availability, mobility, food gathering, dwelling construction, and animal contact on the transmission of parasites were described for seven aboriginal groups of Malaysia (Dunn, 1972).

The countries in which risks of parasitic diseases are the greatest are also those in rapid sociocultural transition. Social change will affect the prevalence of parasites altering the activities significant to the host–parasite interface, in communities now entering the protective but unstable yoke of sanitation, hygiene, and chemotherapy. Patrick and Tyroler (1972) have stressed the need for studying the consequences of rapid social change on the health status of the people. They developed a useful "modernization index" for the Papago Indians of Arizona, and a similar conceptual framework was generated for villagers in the highlands of New Guinea (Sinnett and Whyte, 1973).

The accompanying diagram attempts to conceptualize the current discon-

TABLE VI

Parasitic Helminths and Protozoa in Four Hunting and Gathering Peoples[a]

	Bushman (Africa)	Australian Aborigine		Semang (Malaya)	Pygmy (Africa)
		(Entire continent)	(Central Australia)		
Plant	Desert	Desert	Desert	Tropical rain forest	Tropical rain forest
Complexity index[b]	5.6	5.6	5.6	270–405	270–405
Number of helminth species	2	6	1	10	11
Number of species of intestinal protozoa	0	1	0	9	6
Number of species of blood protozoa	1	2	0	3	3
Total parasite species	3	9	1	22	20

[a]Adapted from Dunn, 1968.

[b]A function of vegetation complexity and secondarily of other biological complexity; not synonymous with diversity.

tinuities between the goals of medical practice and its sociocultural context (Fig. 4). Contrasted are the situations in a typical ''developing'' tropical nation and that of a typical ''developed'' temperate nation.

Public health and hygiene are little more than a directed attempt to minimize biological diversity. Disposal of human wastes, quarantine, vaccination, elimination of vermin and of vectors and microbes, food inspection, health examination of immigrants, and legislation regarding exotic pets are all specific attempts to reduce the exposure of man and his animals to potential pathogens. In developed countries, this has given a relatively ordered shape to the biological complexity and diversity of man's interactions with his pathogens. This order, of course, is supported by the social, cultural, and legislative systems that maintain it. In developing countries, before modern intervention, there was a greater biological diversity available for man's relationships. This, as Dunn (1968) shows us, varied with the local socioenvironmental conditions. Where endemic, malaria may cause a 10% case fatality rate in newborns, but it is regulated by the immunological status of the population and becomes one of many infectious diseases causing moderate morbidity. Most authors would now agree that the complexities of man's relationships with his living world a generation ago were directly equated to the complexities of his sociocultural system. In some cases, this was health promoting; in others it may have regulated the population with respect to food, territory, or climate.

Activities that are causing changes in parasitic diseases in the developed nations are mostly those that have increased biological complexity. Thus, immigration from tropical countries, including large numbers of refugees, has introduced unfamiliar diseases (Barrett-Connor, 1978). Enormous increases in inter-

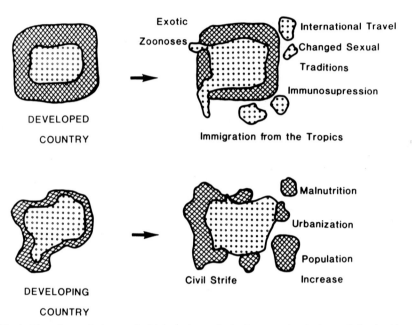

BIOLOGICAL COMPLEXITY AND SOCIOCULTURAL INTEGRATION

A GENERATION AGO   CURRENT SITUATION

DEVELOPED
COUNTRY

Exotic
Zoonoses

International Travel

Changed Sexual
Traditions

Immunosupression

Immigration from the Tropics

DEVELOPING
COUNTRY

Malnutrition

Urbanization

Population
Increase

Civil Strife

FIG. 4. The effects of changes in biological complexity between developing and developed regions.

national travel to tropical areas, introduction of exotic pets, consumption of more exotic foods, and adventurism in uninformed outdoor pursuits have all led to the exposure of man to a greater diversity of pathogens. The liberalization of sexual customs and the wide use of immunosuppressive drugs have served to increase exposure and susceptibility to infection. The sociocultural discontinuity is now moving to reflect this increased biological complexity (Fig. 4).

In the tropical developing nations, the opposite could be said to be happening. From a complex but relatively stable balance between biology and sociology, the introduction of latrines, public water systems, mass anthelmintic programs, mosquito eradication, and the erection of clinics and public health laboratories have begun to reduce and standardize biological complexity. At the same time (not necessarily resulting directly from these attempts), there has been a chaotic change in many sociocultural systems because of such conditions as malnutrition, urbanization, civil strife, and population increases of unprecedented proportions. Although of exaggerated proportions and minor significance in the developed world, this model helps to emphasize the reciprocal problems in both kinds of nations now threatened by changing patterns of parasitic disease.

In his Malaysian studies, Dunn (1972) found that with a movement from the tropical rain forest to more simplified habitats, certain flukes and *Hymenolepis nana* disappeared. A similar case could be made for the decline of *Taenia saginata* and *Diphyllobothrium* sp. in Canada, both requiring intermediate hosts (Croll and Gyorkos, 1979). However, although this occurs, there is an increase in both prevalence and intensity of certain parasites sharing the biological properties of weeds: *Ascaris lumbricoides, Trichuris trichiura, Giardia lamblia,* and *Entamoeba histolytica.* It is noteworthy that these were not only the most abundant in the more settled Temuan group of Malaya, but also the dominant intestinal parasitic pathogens of North America and Western Europe. Cohen (1976), making a theoretical examination of factors influencing stability in host–parasite population interactions, makes a similar point about the strategic merits of intervention into the equilibrium of complex life cycles and of "weed" parasites with their simple, direct transmission and prodigious fecundity.

> Over the coming years a shift is required from the previous global eradication approach to a revised strategy for a malaria action programme based on local and regional situations. The programme is being based on tactical variants to cover all types of epidemiological situations and offers possibilities for control commensurate with the financial and manpower resources available to the Member States concerned with the state of development of their health services. An intensified programme of research is being promoted as part of the UNDP/World Bank/WHO Special Programme for Research and Training in Tropical Diseases (W.H.O., 1980).

Acknowledgments

I know that Neil would have wanted to thank his many colleagues, throughout the world, for the stimulus of their discussions that led to the conception of this chapter and book. Special thanks are due to Ms. Theresa Gyorkos for her kindness and dedication in helping to prepare Neil's chapter for publication. Thanks are also due to Mrs. Diane King and Mrs. Carol Berezowsky for typing the manuscript and preparing the figures, respectively. Finally I would like to thank Mr. Patrick Kelly of Academic Press and Dr. John Cross for their vision and efforts in completing Neil's final contribution to medical parasitology.

Doreen A. Croll

References

Abou Daoud, K., and Schwabe, C. W. (1964). Epidemiology of echinococcosis in The Middle East III. A study of hydatid disease patients from the city of Beirut. *Amer. J. Trop. Med. Hyg.* **13,** 681–685.
Alland, A., Jr. (1969). Ecology and Adaptation to Parasitic Disease. *In* "Environment Cultural

Behaviour Ecological Studies in Cultural Anthropology'' (A. P. Vayda, ed.), pp. 80–89. Natural History Press, New York.

Anderson, R. M. (1976). Dynamic aspects of parasite population ecology. *In* "Ecological Aspects of Parasitology", pp. 431–462. North-Holland Publ., Amsterdam.

Audy, J. R. (1958). The localization of disease with special reference to the zoonoses. *Trans. R. Soc. Trop. Med. Hyg.* **52,** 308–328.

Audy, J. R. (1972). Aspects of human behaviour interfering with vector control. *In* "Vector Control and the Recrudescence of Vector-Borne Diseases," pp. 67–82. *Pan Am. Health Organ. Sci. Publ.* #238.

Bang, F. B., Bang, M. G., and Bang, B. G. (1975). Ecology of respiratory virus transmission: a comparison of three communities in West Bengal. *Amer. J. Trop. Med. Hyg.* **24,** 326–346.

Barrett-Connor, E. (1978). Latent and chronic infections imported from South-East Asia. *JAMA* **239,** 1901–1906.

Bennett, F. J., Kagan, I. G., Barnicot, N. A., and Woodburn, J. C. (1970). Helminth and protozoal parasites of the Hazda of Tanzania. *Trans. R. Soc. Trop. Med. Hyg.* **64,** 857–880.

Bhajan, M. B., Martinez, J., Ruiz-Tiben, E., and Jobin, W. R. (1978). Socioeconomic changes and reduction in prevalence of schistosomiasis in Puerto Rico. *Bol. Assoc. Med. P. R.* **70,** 106–112.

Bradley, D. J. (1977). Human pest and disease problems: contrasts between developing and developed countries. *In* "Origins of Pest, Parasite, Disease and Weed Problems" (J. M. Cherrett, and G. R. Sagar, eds.), pp. 329–345. Blackwell, Oxford.

Buck, A. A., Anderson, R. I., Sasaki, T. T., and Kawata, K. (1970). "Health and Disease in Chad." Johns Hopkins Press, Baltimore, Maryland.

Burridge, M. J., and Schwabe, C. W. (1977). Hydatid disease in New Zealand: an epidemiological study of transmission among Maoris. *Amer. J. Trop. Med. Hyg.* **26,** 258–265.

Chen Paul, C. Y. (1970). Indigenous concepts of causation and methods of prevention of childhood disease in a rural Malay community. *J. Trop. Pediatr.* **16,** 33–42.

Cohen, J. E. (1976). Schistosomiasis: A human host parasite system. *In* "Theoretical Ecology: Principles and Applications" (R. M. May, ed.), pp. 237–256. Blackwell, Oxford.

Crofton, H. D. (1971). A quantitative approach to parasitism. *Parasitology* **62,** 179–195.

Croll, N. A., and Ghadirian, E. (1981). Wormy persons: contributions to the nature and patterns of overdispersion in persons with hyperinfection of *Ascaris lumbricoides, Ancylostoma duodenale* and *Trichuris trichiura. Trop. Geogr. Med.* **33,** 241–248.

Croll, N. A., and Gyorkos, T. W. (1979). Parasitic disease in humans: the extent in Canada. *Can. Med. Assoc. J.* **120,** 310–312.

Croll, N. A., Ghadirian, E., and Sukul, N. C. (1982). Exposure and susceptibility in human helminthiasis. *Tropical Doctor* **12,** 136–138.

Croll, N. A., Anderson, R. M., Gyorkos, T. W., and Ghadirian, E. (1981). The population biology and control of *Ascaris lumbricoides* in a rural community in Iran. *Trans. R. Soc. Trop. Med. Hyg.* **76,** 187–197.

Dalton, P. P. (1976). A sociological approach to the control of *Schistosoma mansoni* in St. Lucia. *Bull. W.H.O.* **54,** 587–595.

Dunn, F. L. (1968). Epidemiological Factors: health and disease in hunter–gatherers. *In* "Man the Hunter" (R. B. Lee, and I. DeVere, eds.), pp. 221–228. Aldine, Chicago.

Dunn, F. L. (1972). Intestinal parasitism in Malayan aborigines. *Bull. W.H.O.* **46,** 99–113.

Dunn, F. L. (1979). Behavioural aspects of the control of parasitic diseases. *Bull. W.H.O.* **57,** 499–512.

Fabrega, H., Jr. (1974). "Disease and Social Behaviour: An Interdisciplinary Perspective." MIT Press, Cambridge, Massachusetts.

Farooq, M., and Mallah, M. B. (1966). The behavioural patterns of social and religious water-contact activities in the Egypt-49 bilharziasis project area. *Bull. W.H.O.* **35,** 377–387.

Fleck, A. C., Jr., and Ianni, F. A. J. (1958). Epidemiology and anthropology: some suggested affinities in theory and method. *Hum. Organ.* **16,** 38–40.

Forrester, A. T. T., Nelson, G. S., and Sander, G. (1961). The first record of an outbreak of trichinosis in Africa south of the Sahara. *Trans. R. Soc. Trop. Med. Hyg.* **55,** 503–513.

Ghadirian, E., Croll, N. A., and Gyorkos, T. W. (1979). Socioagricultural factors and parasitic infections in the Caspian littoral region of Iran. *Trop. Geogr. Med.* **31,** 485–491.

Gillett, J. D. (1975). Mosquito-borne disease: a strategy for the future. *Sci. Prog. (Oxford)* **62,** 395–414.

Gillett, J. D. (1979). The universities and health in the tropics: the problem and an answer. *In* "Pressures and Priorities." Report, Congress of Universities of the Commonwealth, 12th, Vancouver, 1978.

Hausfeld, R. G. (1970). An anthropological method for measuring exposure to leprosy in a leprosy-endemic population at Karimui, New Guinea. *Bull. W.H.O.* **43,** 863–877.

Heyneman, D. (1971). Mis-aid to the Third World: Disease repercussions caused by ecological ignorance. *Can. J. Public Health* **62,** 303–313.

Holmes, O. W. (1892). "The works of Oliver Wendell Holmes." 13 vols. Houghton, Boston, Massachusetts.

Jenner, E. (1798). "An inquiry into the causes and effects of the variolae vaccinae, a disease discovered in some of the western counties of England, particularly Gloucestershire and known by the name of cowpox." Sampson Low, London.

Jordan, P., Christie, J. D., and Unrau, G. O. (1980). Schistosomiasis transmission with particular reference to possible ecological and biological methods of control. A review. *Acta Trop.* **37,** 95–135.

Maxcy, K. F. (1956). "Rosenau Preventive Medicine and Public Health." Appleton, London.

May, J. M. (1950). Medical geography: its methods and objectives. *Geogr. Rev.* **40,** 9–41.

Montgomery, E. (1973). Ecological aspects of health and disease in local populations. *Annu. Rev. Anthropol.* **2,** 27–61.

Nelson, G. S. (1972). Human behaviour in the transmission of parasitic diseases. *In* "Behavioural Aspects of Parasite Transmission" (E. U. Canning, and C. A. Wright, eds.), pp. 109–122. Academic Press, New York.

Nnochiri, E. (1968). Parasitism and the socio-economic environment of urban citizens. *In* "Parasitic Disease and Urbanization in a Developing Community," pp. 18–35 and 105–112. Oxford Univ. Press, London and New York.

Panum, P. L. (1940). "Observations made during the epidemic of measles on the Faroe Islands in the year 1846." Delta Omega Society, New York.

Patrick, R., and Tyroler, H. A. (1972). Papago Indians modernization: a community scale for health research. *Hum. Organ.* **31,** 127–136.

Pavlovsky, E. N. (1963). "Natural Foci of Human Infections." Israel Program for Scientific Translations, Jerusalem.

Petersdorff, R. G., and Feinstein, A. R. (1981). An informal appraisal of the current status of medical sociology. *JAMA* **245,** 943–950.

Pugh, R. N. H., and Gilles, H. M. (1978). Malumfashi Endemic Diseases Research Project, III. Urinary schistosomiasis: a longitudinal study. *Ann. Trop. Med. Parasitol.* **72,** 471–482.

Purtilo, D. T., Meyers, W. M., and Connor, D. H. (1974). Fatal strongyloidiasis in immunosuppressed patients. *Am. J. Med.* **56,** 488–493.

Roundy, R. W. (1978). A model for combining human behaviour and disease ecology to assess disease hazard in a community; rural Ethiopia as a model. *Soc. Sci. Med.* **12,** 121–130.

Skamene, E. (1980). "Genetic Control of Natural Resistance to Infection and Malignancy" (E. Skamene, P. A. L. Kongshavn, and M. Landy, eds.), pp. 209–214. Academic Press, New York.

Schwabe, C. W. (1969). "Veterinary Medicine and Human Health," 2nd ed. Williams & Wilkins, Baltimore, Maryland.

Sinnett, R. F., and Whyte, H. M. (1973). Epidemiological studies in a highland population of New Guinea: environment, culture and health status. *Hum. Ecol.* **1,** 245–277.

Woodruff, A. W., Bisseru, B., and Bowe, J. C. (1966). Infection with animal helminths as a factor in causing poliomyelitis and epilepsy. *Br. Med. J.* **1,** 1576–1579.

World Health Organization (1979). "Parasitic Zoonoses." *W.H.O. Tech. Rep. Ser.* 637.

World Health Organization (1980). Communicable disease prevention and control. Global medium-term programme. Sixth General Programme of Work covering a specific period (1978–1983), CDS/MTP/80.1. Geneva, Switzerland.

Zahra, A. (1980). "A global overview of communicable disease and their control." Second World Congress on Antisepsis, New York City, June 12–14, 1980.

2

Human Behavior and Parasitic Zoonoses in North America

PETER M. SCHANTZ

Helminthic Diseases Branch
Parasitic Diseases Division
Center for Infectious Diseases
Centers for Disease Control
Public Health Service
Department of Health and Human Services
Atlanta, Georgia

Introduction

The rate and pattern of parasitic infection transmission in a given locality are products of a complex and dynamic interaction of hosts, parasites, and environment. The relative significance of each variable will vary with the situation. Among the most important host factors influencing the transmission of parasitic infections is culturally determined human behavior. On no group of parasitic diseases is the influence of human behavior more evident than on the zoonoses, which are defined as "those diseases and infections which are naturally transmitted between vertebrate animals and man (W.H.O., 1959)."

The interactions of human beings with animals are many and varied. Through hunting, animal husbandry, keeping pets, and numerous other recreational and avocational activities human beings engage in contact with a large variety of lower animal species in ways that expose them to those species' pathogens. Another important dimension of man's interactions with animals is his fondness for foods of animal origin. The nonrandom distribution of many zoonotic diseases in heterogeneous human populations often results from culturally determined differences in behavior relating to animals, and certain variants of behavior are more likely to result in the transmission of disease.

Before the domestication of lower animals, human beings subsisted as hunters and gatherers with more limited animal contact. Human exposure to zoonotic infectious agents occurred when hunters invaded the habitats of sylvatic hosts and ate their meat. The domestication of ever-increasing numbers of lower animal species provided commensurate opportunities for sharing their pathogens by creating synanthropic links that facilitated exposure to zoonotic infectious agents. Certain animal husbandry practices (e.g., crowding of animals, feeding garbage to pigs, feeding sheep viscera to dogs) further enhanced opportunities for disease transmission among animals, thereby multipling the probability of human exposure. The movement of domesticated animals and their pathogens throughout the world with migrating human populations (a continuing process) led to the widespread dispersion of many zoonotic diseases and their present cosmopolitan distribution.

The student of zoonotic diseases recognizes the rural areas of many developing countries as ideal settings for investigations. In such rural villages persons commonly share their homes with various animal species under conditions of poor sanitation and hygiene that inevitably lead to frequent exposure to each other's pathogens. Because veterinary services are often lacking and human medical care usually inadequate, zoonoses are often among the diseases of major economic importance and public health concern in developing countries. In contrast, the situation in most industrialized countries is markedly different. The process of urbanization and suburbanization has led to another extreme as in the United States where less than 2% of the population is engaged in farming, a proportion that continues to decline. Consequently, contact exposure to zoonotic diseases of farm animals is limited to farmers, veterinarians, abattoir workers, and others with occupational exposure to livestock species. On the other hand, the numbers of dogs, cats and other pet animals have increased tremendously since World War II, reflecting increased prosperity and suburbanization. Today, nearly 41 million dogs are distributed among one-third to one-half of American households (Franti and Kraus, 1974; Franti *et al.*, 1980; Griffith and Brenner, 1977; Schneider and Vaida, 1975; Wilbur, 1976); estimates that include unowned dogs are 60 to 80 million. The total number of cats is estimated at 30 million (Flick, 1973; Franti *et al.*, 1980; Griffith and Brenner, 1977). Because at least 55% of all households have either a cat or dog, opportunities for exposure to infectious agents of pet dogs and cats have reached an all-time high.

In this chapter, trichinosis, cystic and alveolar hydatid disease, and toxocariasis are used to illustrate the influence of human behavioral factors on the distribution and transmission of zoonotic diseases. The natural modes of transmission, the type of disease produced in humans, and the use of human behavior in developing strategies for prevention and control are described.

II. Trichinosis

Trichinosis is caused by nearly microscopic nematode worms of the genus *Trichinella,* the larval stages of which localize in the muscles of pigs and other carnivorous animals, including humans. Because *Trichinella* spp. are highly adaptive parasites, trichinosis is one of the most ubiquitous parasitic infections. Virtually all mammals and some birds are susceptible; more than 100 species of wild animals have been identified as natural hosts for this parasite (Zimmerman, 1970). As would be expected, human *Trichinella* spp. infections are recognized worldwide although incidence varies greatly. Although some textbooks continue to refer to a single species, *Trichinella spiralis,* recent studies suggest that the parasite is not a homogeneous species. A number of variant populations are known with differing degrees of infectivity to host species and unique biological characteristics of epidemiologic significance. It has not been determined whether those differences are sufficient to confer separate species or subspecies status to the variants or strains of *T. spiralis* (Boev *et al.,* 1969).

People become parasitized from eating undercooked meat of infected animals. Animal husbandry practices provide conditions favoring establishment of synanthropic cycles and persistence of the parasite in domestic food animal species. Cultural influences on meat preferences and methods of preparation are important factors in determining the likelihood of human exposure to trichinosis.

A. Parasite Development and Pathogenesis of Disease

Trichinella spp. are transmitted from one host to another by ingestion of infected meat. Development of the parasite is similar in all host species. After ingestion, infected meat is digested, releasing larval trichinae into the new host's intestine where they rapidly mature into adults, mate, and produce large numbers of offspring. The larval offspring pass from the intestine into the circulatory system, invading the muscles in which they migrate extensively before becoming encapsulated within a microscopic cyst. The cycle can only be continued when the raw or improperly processed flesh of an infected animal is consumed by a susceptible host.

Most animals appear relatively resistant to the effects of the infection, and clinical disease is rarely recognized in species other than humans. Infections in humans vary from negligible symptoms to a severe, sometimes fatal, disease. When only a few larvae are ingested, believed to be the most common occurrence, the light infection is usually unnoticed. Heavier trichnosis infections characteristically produce diarrhea followed by fever, generalized swelling, muscle pain, and fatigue lasting for several weeks or more and resulting from the adult parasites in the intestines, and the larvae migrating through the muscles. The heaviest infections can be fatal, usually because of severe damage to heart or brain.

B.   Parasite Maintenance Cycles

Although most persons who are aware of trichinosis associate the disease with ingestion of infected pork, the parasite's occurrence in swine is only a spin-off from maintenance cycles in wild animals. In North America, in-depth studies of wildlife reservoirs of trichinosis have been performed in Alaska (Rausch *et al.*, 1956), British Columbia (Schmitt *et al.*, 1978), Iowa (Zimmerman and Hubbard, 1969), and the Rocky Mountain Region (Worley *et al.*, 1974). Limited findings in other regions indicate that infection also occurs in wild animals throughout most of the continent. In the temperate zones of North America, *Trichinella spiralis* is maintained in sylvatic cycles involving bears, wolves, foxes, coyotes, and wild cats. Scavenging, and to a lesser extent, predation, appear to be the primary modes of transmission (Zimmerman, 1970). A synanthropic cycle probably became established in domestic swine when pigs ingested infected wild animals. The perpetuation of *T. spiralis* in the swine reservoir is almost entirely a result of husbandry practices that facilitate transmission (Fig. 1). The primary sources of infection (commercial and household garbage, wildlife carcasses) usually must be made available to swine by man. It is unlikely that significant levels of infection would be maintained in swine without the practice of garbage feeding, which forces pigs to cannibalize by ingesting raw pork scraps.

In the United States, the infection rate in garbage-fed pigs is five times higher than in those not so fed (Zimmerman and Zinter, 1971). Although the number of pigs that have been fed garbage are a distinct minority (less than 2%) of the total

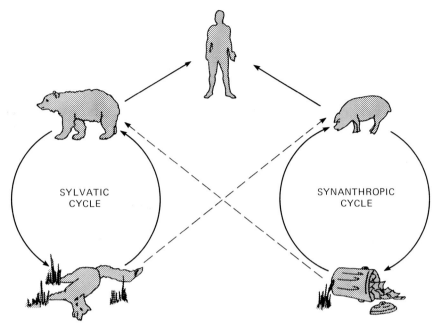

FIG. 1. Schematic representation of maintenance cycles of *Trichinella spiralis* showing interrelationships between sylvatic and synanthropic cycles.

butchered hogs, nearly 300,000 inspected in March 1981 included approximately 15,000 that had been fed uncooked garbage (U.S.D.A., 1981). Although most states have regulations that prohibit garbage feeding entirely, or require that garbage fed to swine be cooked, these are difficult to enforce and illegal garbage feeding is believed to be common. One investigation of six infected herds in states that prohibit garbage feeding indicated that the most probable sources of infection were table scraps (three herds), restaurant garbage (one herd), and wildlife carcasses (two herds) (Zimmerman and Zinter, 1971).

The host species involved in sylvatic maintenance cycles in Arctic regions are somewhat different from those in temperate zones. They include polar, grizzly, and black bears, wolves, foxes, wolverines, lynx, and numerous mustelids and rodents (Rausch *et al.*, 1956; Nelson, 1968). Marine mammals found infected include the walrus, the ringed seal, the bearded seal, and the white whale. The infection of marine mammals has not been completely explained although Fay (1960) suggested that some species, such as walrus, are occasionally carnivorous, and that other species may pick up infections from transport hosts such as necrophagous crustaceans, amphipods, or fish that have eaten infected carrion. *Trichinella* spp. which occur in arctic animals have a number of biological characteristics distinguishing them from other populations of the nematode, and it has been suggested that these deserve separate species status (e.g., *T. nativa* Britov and Boev, 1972). Some of these characteristics, such as relative resistance to freezing temperatures (Schantz *et al.*, 1979b), appear to confer advantages for survival in the arctic environment. Arctic isolates of *Trichinella* spp. are not highly infective for swine, and naturally infected swine have never been recorded in Alaska.

Sources of infection for human beings include pork and meat of numerous sylvatic animals. Although infection in pigs plays no important role in maintenance of the parasite in nature, it has always been responsible for most human infections.

C.   Human Behavior and Trichinosis

Trichinosis was first recognized in North America in 1842, and scattered reports indicate that numerous outbreaks totaling hundreds of cases occurred during the first half of this century. The disease was made reportable in some states in the late nineteenth century, and in 1947 the U.S. Public Health Service began collecting statistics on trichinosis at the national level. In the late 1940s approximately 400 cases with 10 or 15 deaths were reported each year. The number of reported cases then declined progressively until about 1966. Subsequently, the annual number of reported cases appears to have stabilized at between 100 and 150 cases, with an average of one death per year (CDC, 1981a).

Data on human trichinosis in the United States are derived from the Centers for Disease Control (CDC) Trichinosis National Surveillance Activity, which collects detailed epidemiologic information on reported cases. Between 1967 and 1980 a pork product was incriminated as the source of infection in three out of every four cases in which a likely source was identified. The remaining cases were divided about equally between those caused by ground beef, apparently adulterated with pork, and those caused by ingestion of the meat of wild animals (CDC, 1981a). Typically, the incriminated pork product was a federally inspected product purchased at a local supermarket or butcher shop (67%). Less frequently, the meat was purchased at a restaurant or obtained directly from the farm where the pig was raised.

Americans through long custom generally tend to cook pork products until well done, rendering them safe. Outbreaks of trichinosis have occurred most frequently among citizens of ethnic backgrounds whose culinary preferences include raw pork. For example, in a 1940 autopsy survey deceased persons of German or Italian descent were infected at a rate of approximately 29%, compared with a 2% rate in Jews, whose religious laws proscribe pork (Wright *et al.*, 1944). This higher risk of infection in certain ethnic groups continues today. Examination of the surnames of persons involved in outbreaks due to consumption of pork products reveals that the proportion of affected persons of German,

Italian, Polish, or Portuguese ancestry is disproportionately higher than is their overall representation in the population of the United States (Schantz *et al.*, 1977). A typical sequence of events leading to an outbreak includes the purchase from commercial sources of fresh pork which is then prepared at home according to traditional ethnic recipes as fresh, spiced sausage. This is distributed to family and friends and consumed raw.

Recent immigrants are often not aware that pork in the United States is not inspected for trichinosis. Two outbreaks of trichinosis were recognized in New York between 1971 and 1973 involving 23 Thai immigrants who had consumed traditional Thai dishes made of fermented American pork (Imperato *et al.*, 1974). Although most of the present population of the United States is two, three, or four generations removed from immigrant forebears and Americanized in their food habits, a minority retain certain food habits of their ancestral countries.

Every year, some cases of trichinosis result from the ingestion of "rare" hamburger or ground beef. Although cattle, because they are strict herbivores, are not naturally infected with *T. spiralis,* ground beef products are often adulterated by the intentional or inadvertent mixing of beef and pork. In a multistate survey performed in 1975, pork was found in 6% of ground beef samples purchased at supermarkets (Schantz *et al.*, 1977). Investigation of ground beef associated outbreaks has demonstrated that the ground beef was mixed with pork either intentionally for profit motives or through ignorance of the dangers of using the same meat grinder for beef and pork.

Acquisition of trichinosis directly from sylvatic cycles is not uncommon; such cases have always been a minority. Between 1967 and 1980, 88 cases of trichinosis following consumption of bear meat represented 5.3% of the total number of 1671 cases reported in the United States for that period. Bear meat-associated cases of trichinosis occur throughout North America, mostly in the Arctic. Since 1949, of 119 trichinosis cases reported in Alaska 58 (48%) followed ingestion of bear meat (Ellana and Lum, 1980). Bears are a major meat source for Eskimos and other native arctic Americans, and cases would probably be much more common were it not for the general practice, passed down through generations, of cooking bear meat thoroughly to avoid illness. That outbreaks do occasionally result from human error is illustrated by a recent example involving eight Alaskan residents who attended a dinner of raw frozen meat thought to be caribou, but which was later discovered to be bear meat (CDC, 1981b). The meat was eaten after being dipped in seal oil which may have disguised its usually distinctive taste.

Although walrus (*Odobenus rosmarus*) has been an important meat item in the diet of generations of Arctic populations, only since 1975 have cases of trichinosis associated with this meat source been reported in Alaska. Investigations of five outbreaks of walrus-associated trichinosis revealed an interesting example of the interaction of culture and disease (Ellana and Lum, 1980). All 61 trichinosis cases occurred among residents of four coastal villages that have not traditionally used walrus meat as a primary subsistence food. Increased numbers of walrus have made this game species available in areas outside its usual range (including the four villages), and the inhabitants eat walrus meat as *kwak,* which is raw frozen meat. In contrast, among Siberian Yuit and Iniut populations who regularly hunt and consume walrus, the meat is thoroughly boiled or prepared in other ways that destroy trichinae. Furthermore, traditional walrus hunters selectively avoid old male walrus (in which trichina infections may be more frequent). Experience with trichinosis in generations past may have engendered these practices that protect against the disease. In contrast, villagers who hunt walrus occasionally have no such tradition and may be at higher trichinosis risk (Ellana and Lum, 1980).

D.   Human Behavior and Trichinosis Control

Knowledge of the human factors involved in *Trichinella* spp. transmission and infection risk has important implications for control and prevention. Although man can do little to disrupt transmission of *Trichinella* spp. in sylvatic cycles, interruption of synanthropic transmission would greatly reduce the public health problem; infected pork is currently responsible for at least three-fourths of human cases in North America. Thus, if all swine producers could be effectively educated about the hazards of raw garbage, table scraps, wild animal carcasses, or other infected animal feeds, further control measures would be unnecessary.

Over the years Americans have become aware of the dangers of eating uncooked pork, and most pork consumed in the United States is thoroughly cooked. The identification of citizens of European ancestry and recent immigrants of ethnic groups that traditionally consume raw pork as "high-risk" groups suggests these are target groups for special health education.

Since the knowledge and technology to greatly reduce or eliminate trichinosis exist in the United States, it is not clear why it remains one of the few developed countries in which trichinosis continues to be a public health problem. Many European governments with greater trichinosis problems, which implemented eradication programs long ago, have observed the decline and near disappearance of human cases (Pawlowski, 1981). Because pork consumers are directly at risk, public apathy is surprising. Year after year, the disease accounts for hundreds of preventable cases of serious, painful illness and occasional death. The lack of attention by pork producers and agricultural authorities to the problem is also surprising, because negative publicity about trichinosis depresses consumer demand for pork. It is not obvious what will cause American consumers and public health officials to expect and demand trichina-free pork, available in many countries with far fewer resources.

III. Cystic Hydatid Disease (Echinococcosis)

Echinococcosis is an infection caused by cestodes of the genus *Echinococcus*, whose life cycles involve two mammalian hosts. Definitive hosts are carnivores, in which adult worms are present in the intestines. Intermediate hosts are various species of herbivorous and omnivorous animals, in which larval or metacestode forms develop. Humans and other intermediate hosts become infected by ingesting eggs passed in the feces of infected definitive hosts. The metacestode forms are referred to as hydatid cysts, and the disease they cause is commonly referred to as hydatid disease.

Classic cystic hydatid disease is caused by *Echinococcus granulosus*. This species is adapted to dogs and to various domestic and sylvatic animal intermediate hosts. It exists throughout the world; in many regions it is a major public health and economic problem.

A. Parasite Development and Pathogenesis of Disease

Humans become infected when they ingest tapeworm eggs passed in feces of infected dogs. After ingestion, the eggs hatch, releasing into the small intestine embryos that penetrate the intestinal mucosa and pass into the host's circulatory system, which then carries them to liver, lungs, and other sites where cyst development begins. In humans, the slowly growing hydatid cysts can attain a volume of many liters and contain many thousands of protoscolices. Variable clinical manifestations are determined by cyst site, size, and condition. The slowly growing hydatid cyst is often tolerated until its size causes dysfunction. If the cyst ruptures, the sudden fluid release can precipitate allergic reactions ranging from mild to fatal (anaphylaxis). Dissemination of protoscolices can result in multiple secondary hydatid cysts. Most mortality is associated with surgery for hydatid cyst removal; mortality varies from 1 to 4% in such cases (Schantz, 1982).

B. Parasite Maintenance Cycles

The occurrence of *Echinococcus granulosus* in a particular host assemblage (e.g., wolf–moose; dog–sheep; dog–horse) usually implies a well-established host–parasite relationship, with adaptations reflected in the "strain" characteristics. According to Rausch (1967), *E. granulosus* evolved in and was maintained in cycles involving wolves and wild ungulates. In early Neolithic times in Europe

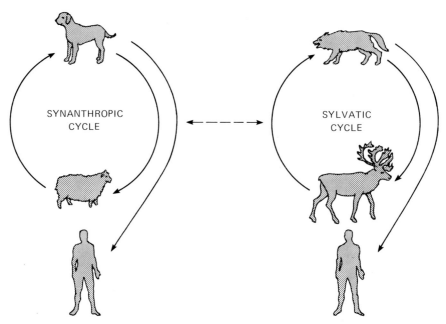

FIG. 2. Schematic representation of maintenance cycles of *Echinococcus granulosus* showing interrelationships between sylvatic and synanthropic cycles.

(and perhaps elsewhere) as the wolf and several ungulates became domesticated, a synanthropic cycle became possible in which the dog replaced the wolf as the definitive host and domestic ungulates became the intermediate hosts (Fig. 2). The cestode, widely dispersed with its hosts, adapted itself to a variety of domestic and sylvatic host species. Sheep may be the most important intermediate hosts, but swine, cattle, goats, horses, and camels are susceptible and can be more important in certain regions. Dogs and other definitive hosts become infected after ingesting organs of infected intermediate hosts containing hydatid cysts. Under natural conditions, such transmission is the result of a predator–prey relationship existing between hosts. In a synanthropic cycle, however, transmission is considerably modified by human behavior. The widespread rural practice of feeding dogs the viscera of home-butchered sheep, for example, facilitates transmission of the pastoral strain, consequently increasing the risk of infecting humans.

C.   Human Behavior and Cystic Hydatid Disease

Local differences in prevalence and patterns of transmission are determined by factor complexes involving host, agent, environment, and human behavior.

[Recent reviews on the epidemiology of cystic hydatid disease include those by Schwabe (1968), Rausch (1967), Gemmel and Johnstone (1977), Williams *et al.* (1971), and Schantz (1982).] Some human influences on *Echinococcus granulosus* transmission are discussed in this section.

Before the domestication of animals, and in some high-latitude regions today, *E. granulosus* occurred in wolves and wild ungulates under conditions in which humans only rarely became infected. By domestication of these hosts, humans created nearly optimal conditions for the continued transmission of this cestode, for its dispersal throughout the world, and for their own entry into its life cycle. In rural endemic areas of both advanced and developing countries, the widespread use of dogs for working livestock and the concomitant habit of feeding them on viscera of home-butchered sheep or other livestock are common. Thus, an artificial system more efficient than the natural systems in perpetuating the life cycle has been developed. Under such conditions, canine infection occurs commonly and repeatedly, contaminating the environment extensively with cestode eggs. Human populations living under such conditions are frequently exposed, and the probability that any given individual will become infected depends, in part, upon factors such as personal hygiene and cleanliness. These in turn are often functions of educational, socioeconomic, and cultural characteristics.

Direct contact with infected dogs, particularly the characteristic playful and intimate contact between children and their pets, seems to be the most important source of human infection. Cestode eggs adhere to hairs around the anus of the infected dog and can also be found on muzzle and paws. Indirect means of contact via water and contaminated vegetables or through the intermediary of flies and other arthropods may also result in human infections.

In North America both sylvatic and pastoral forms of *E. granulosus* occur. In the western provinces of Canada and in Alaska the sylvatic strain occurs in cycles involving wolves, moose, and caribou (Cameron, 1960; Rausch, 1960; Wilson *et al.*, 1968). Wilson *et al.* (1968) estimated that about 75% of the total population of 50,000 Eskimos, Aleuts, and Indians who live in Alaska are in *E. granulosus*-endemic areas. Most human infections are limited to Indian tribes that trap and hunt, then feed their dogs on the lungs and other offal of caribou and moose (Fig. 3). The infected dogs return to the villages and are kept tethered close to or within the homes. Fecal contamination around the dwellings is probably the most important source of infection (Cameron, 1960; Rausch, 1960).

In the lower 48 United States, the pastoral form of *E. granulosus* occurs in various localities. Analytic review of the United States echinococcosis literature by Pappaioanou *et al.* (1977) revealed that the pattern of risk has changed markedly with time, indicating a variety of cultural and economic practices that have facilitated the perpetuation of the life cycles.

Evidence suggests that *E. granulosus* was introduced (probably from Europe) into the swine population of the southeastern United States before 1900. Trans-

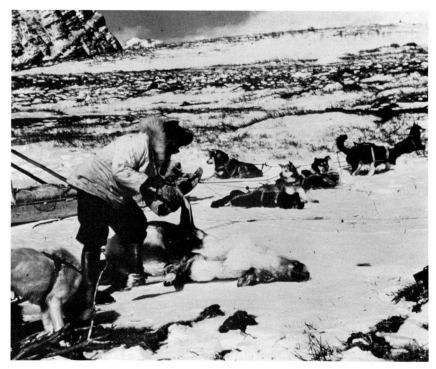

FIG. 3. Eskimo of the Nunamiut tribe skinning a caribou taken in the Brooks Mountain range, Alaska. Lungs and other viscera of caribou are usually fed to the dogs (photograph courtesy of Dr. Robert L. Rausch).

mission was probably perpetuated among backyard swine, maintained as scavengers or fed on household garbage by sharecroppers and small landholders. The infection spread from this original focus via movements of swine or dogs (there may have been subsequent introductions from abroad) into similar small swine holdings in the lower Mississippi valley. Home slaughter of pigs was characteristically practiced on such farms before World War II, and the relationship between man and dog was often very close (Pappaioanou *et al.*, 1977). Most human cases reported associated with these transmission foci were in black persons.

Since the 1950s, improved living standards combined with decreased home slaughter and application of more rigid swine-raising controls apparently reduced transmission in the swine–dog cycle resulting in a decline in cases. In contrast, transmission in cycles involving dogs and sheep has increased. *E. granulosus* infection was absent or very rare in the U.S. sheep population until recently; in the 1940s, human infections associated with the sheep–dog cycle appeared in

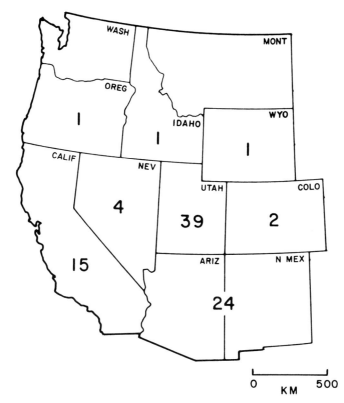

FIG. 4. Distribution in western United States of 87 reported autochthonous cases of *Echinococcus granulosus* infections in humans, 1940–1980. Number = cases in state (after Crellin *et al.*, 1982).

California, and from there it has been dispersed to other western states. In large areas of the West (Fig. 4) where transhumant sheep ranching uses dogs that are fed home-butchered sheep viscera or dead sheep (including about 17,500 square miles containing 38% of California's approximately one million stock sheep population, central Utah containing over one million sheep in six or more counties, and some of the major Indian reservations of the Southwest), conditions for hydatid disease transmission, intensification, and spread are highly favorable.

In California, where three different systems of sheep husbandry are practiced, *E. granulosus* transmission is almost exclusively associated with a transhumant system of sheep raising in which sheepmen leasing cropped-over land, or using government-owned forest and other lands, move their sheep throughout the year (Schwabe, 1979). This system of husbandry, practiced in California mainly by persons of Basque extraction, utilizes many dogs that have traditionally been fed sheep carcasses and offal (Araujo *et al.*, 1975). In contrast, sheep raising on the

Pacific coast north and south of San Francisco depends on permanently fenced pasture—very few dogs are involved and virtually no hydatid transmission occurs. From California, *E. granulosus* was apparently transported by dogs or sheep to Utah where 39 human cases have been diagnosed since 1946 (Crellin *et al.*, 1982). Although transhumant sheep raising is practiced throughout the state, *E. granulosus* transmission is largely confined to centrally located Sanpete County, where the use of local people as herders, dog management practices, and the existence of community herds have contributed to the perpetuation of the *E. granulosus* life cycle (Crellin *et al.*, 1982).

The introduction of *E. granulosus* into Arizona and New Mexico before 1965 appears to be the most recently identified extension of the cestode's range, which may be increasing (Schantz, 1977). Since 1965, infections acquired locally have been diagnosed in 24 American Indians of the Navajo (16), Zuni (4), and Santo Domingo (2) tribes, and 2 in non-Indians. Epidemiologic investigations revealed that the dogs responsible for the human infections became infected from two possible sources. One source was sheep raised locally in rural areas of the Navajo reservation where the infection is enzootic in the dog–sheep cycle. A second source of human infection was dogs, infected by eating viscera of off-reservation sheep purchased from trading posts or peddlers, and butchered by individual families in urban areas of the Navajo reservation or the Zuni and Santo Domingo pueblos. Examination of available records at several reservation trading posts indicated that sheep were commonly purchased in Utah and Colorado, where abattoir inspection data had demonstrated the presence of hydatid cysts. Transport of sheep from these areas may have been the mechanism introducing infection onto the reservations; available evidence linked six of the seven cases diagnosed in 1974 to this source of infection (Schantz, 1977).

Various cultural and animal husbandry practices of the Navajo are highly conducive to the continued transmission of cestodes in the dog–sheep cycle. When the Spanish introduced sheep and goats to the Navajo about 250 years ago, sheep raising became (and remains) the major form of subsistence. There are few families who do not derive some of their income from the sale of sheep or wool, or who do not occasionally butcher animals for food (Fig. 5). The Navajo's relationship with his livestock animals is more than economic; it has been argued that the adoption of sheep raising as a major subsistence activity has provided the foundation for the Navajo maintenance of social separateness from the Anglo-American culture (Downs, 1974). The presence of numerous dogs in rural homes, and the prevailing poor hygienic conditions, increase opportunities for exposure of family members to cestode eggs. It is not clear why echinococcosis prevalence remains low; there is a high potential for continued or increased transmission (Schantz, 1977). The movement of infected sheep or dogs from California, Utah, Arizona, and New Mexico may introduce echinococcosis into adjacent states (Crellin, 1982).

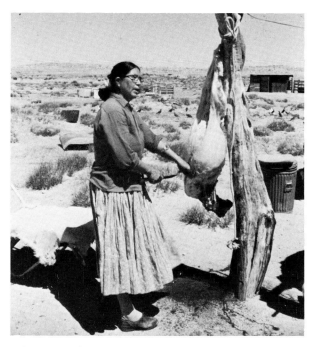

FIG. 5. Navajo woman of Arizona butchering sheep. Although the entire edible carcass is generally used for human consumption, portions considered unfit for human consumption are given to the dogs.

D. Human Behavior and Control of Cystic Hydatid Disease

Hydatid disease control has been described as being fundamentally a problem of health education (Beard, 1969) which attempts to persuade the population to change practices that perpetuate cestode transmission. The apparent association of human risk of infection with *Echinococcus granulosus* in the United States with particular population groups (hunting Indian tribes in Alaska; blacks in the Southeast; Basques, Indians, and Mormon sheepranchers in parts of the West) and occupations (backyard swine raising, transhumant sheep ranching) suggests that the immediate educational efforts required to contain and combat hydatid disease in the United States should concentrate on identified high-risk groups.

Rausch (1967) predicted that changing social conditions in the Arctic would affect the pattern of occurrence of zoonotic diseases. Among these changes, the decline of the hunting lifestyle among the younger generations and the replacement of sled dogs by motor-driven vehicles have reduced opportunities for transmission of *E. granulosus*. A downward trend in numbers of new cases in humans has been noticed in recent years.

IV. Alveolar Hydatid Disease

Alveolar hydatid disease (AHD) is caused by *Echinococcus multilocularis,* whose final and intermediate hosts are, respectively, foxes and their rodent prey. In humans, this species causes one of the most lethal parasitic infections known. The greater host specificity of *E. multilocularis* and its restriction to a relatively small number of sylvatic animal hosts limit the geographic distribution of this agent, reducing potential human exposure.

A. Parasite Development and Pathogenesis of Disease

As with *Echinococcus granulosus,* infection with larval *E. multilocularis* follows ingestion of eggs. The primary localization of the larval mass, in natural intermediate hosts as well as in humans, is the liver. In humans, the larval mass proliferates indefinitely by exogenous budding, progressively invading the surrounding tissues and resembling a malignancy in behavior and appearance. Local extension of the lesion and metastases to the lungs and the brain can follow. Because alveolar hydatid disease is often not diagnosed until well advanced, the lesion may often be inoperable. With or without surgery, mortality range is about 50–75% (Wilson and Rausch, 1980).

B. Parasite Maintenance Cycles

In comparison to *E. granulosus, E. multilocularis* is characterized by a greater degree of host specificity, particularly in the larval stages. The natural definitive and intermediate hosts of this cestode are foxes and small rodents. In the comparatively simple biotic conditions of the arctic tundra zone, the cestode is maintained in cycles involving the arctic fox, *Alopex alopex,* and several kinds of voles; in more complex biomes, a greater variety of host species is involved. The red fox, *Vulpes vulpes,* is the most important definitive host throughout most of the range of distribution outside of the Arctic Circle. Other carnivores that are naturally infected, including domestic dogs and cats, coyotes, and wolves, may occasionally have important epidemiological roles. *E. multilocularis* infection is limited geographically to the northern hemisphere; it is endemic in Alaska, some regions of Canada, central Europe, Asia, and northern Japan (Rausch, 1967).

C. Human Behavior and Alveolar Hydatid Disease

Confined to sylvatic hosts over much of its range, *Echinococcus multiocularis* is ecologically separated from man. Nevertheless, in some areas alveolar hydatid disease is a major health problem. Lukashenko (1975) reported that 1000 cases of infection had been diagnosed in the Iakut Republic in northeastern Siberia between 1950 and 1965, and that a prevalence of 8.9 cases per 1000 inhabitants had been noted in some regions. Human exposure is often determined by occupational and avocational factors; hunters, trappers, and other persons who work with fox fur are most frequently exposed (Lukashenko, 1971). Dogs that become infected by capturing and eating infected voles are even more important as a source of human infection. When infected voles occur in villages as commensal rodents, as they do in some Eskimo villages of the tundra zone in North America, the cycle of the cestode is readily completed, resulting in a hyperendemic focus (Fay, 1973; Rausch, 1967). The poor sanitary conditions usually prevail in such villages permit extensive accumulation of dog feces and enhance the risk of human infection. Thirty-four cases of AHD were diagnosed in Alaskan Eskimos from 1947 through 1980 (Wilson and Rausch, 1980).

Recent studies have demonstrated a large and increasing area of infection in south central Canada (Manitoba, Saskatchewan, and Alberta) and in the north central United States (North Dakota, South Dakota, Minnesota, Iowa, Nebraska, Montana, and Wyoming). The important sylvatic hosts in this region are red foxes, coyotes, deer mice, and field voles (Leiby et al., 1970). The cestode may have been recently introduced to this region by transport of infected dogs from Alaska (Rausch, 1967) or by southward migration of infected arctic foxes. The first human case definitely associated with the central North American focus was diagnosed in 1977 in Minnesota (Gamble et al., 1979). Infection rates in foxes in Minnesota increased fivefold, from 5 to 26%, between 1967 and 1979 (Ballard and Vande Vusse, 1981). The availability of suitable hosts and the lack of ecological barriers in adjacent areas offer the potential for further spread in the United States. This evolving phenomenon presents a dilemma for owners of dogs and cats in rural areas, where they may become infected by preying on infected rodents and then in turn infect their human owners. A greater human health hazard will develop if an independent cycle of transmission evolves in domestic cats and house mice (Fig. 6). Naturally infected domestic cats have been found in Japan, Canada, the United States, and Germany, and infected house mice have been found in the United States at least once (Leiby and Kritsky, 1972). If such a synanthropic cycle becomes established, the cestode will be introduced into new geographical areas, including urban and suburban localities, greatly increasing the potential for human exposure.

D. Human Behavior and Control of Alveolar Hydatid Disease

Eliminating *Echinococcus multilocularis* from sylvatic animal hosts would be impractical under most circumstances. Personal preventive measures, in areas

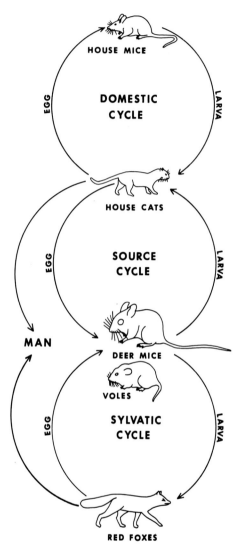

FIG. 6. Life cycles (known and hypothetical) of *Echinococcus multilocularis* in central North America (with the permission of P. D. Leiby and D. C. Kritsky, 1972, *J. Parasitol.* **56,** 1141).

where the infection is endemic, include avoidance of contact with foxes or other potentially infected definitive hosts. Intense public education to improve hygienic practices and a concurrent reduction in the number of dogs (through replacement by motorized vehicles) has been partially effective in lowering parasite prevalence in dogs in one Eskimo village where the infection was hyper-endemic (Wilson and Rausch, 1980).

Restricting movement of dogs from endemic areas may retard the geographic spread of this cestode. Such legislation was enacted in 1951 to prevent the spread from St. Lawrence Island to mainland Alaska (Rausch and Schiller, 1956) before it was realized that this movement had already taken place. The unrestricted translocation of foxes from North Dakota and other *E. multilocularis*-endemic areas by hunting clubs will accelerate the dispersion of the zoonosis in the United States.

V. Toxocariasis

The common roundworm (*Toxocara canis*) of dogs is capable of infecting human beings and occasionally causes serious disease. But unlike *Echinococcus granulosus*, which is strictly limited in occurrence to dogs in certain western sheep raising areas, roundworm infections occur almost universally in pet dogs. *Toxocara* spp. are transmitted transplacentally from bitch to pups, and infection rates are very high in young dogs. Because dogs are popular pets in the United States and Canada, the parasite eggs are widely disseminated in the environment. Although education and sanitary improvements have reduced promiscuous defecation by human beings, thus decreasing soil contamination with eggs of human-adapted helminths, dogs enjoy relative immunity from such restrictions, continuing to deposit their excreta in private and public places. Ten to 30% of soil samples taken from public playgrounds and parks have been found contaminated with *Toxocara* eggs. Interest in this parasitic zoonosis reflects a growing awareness of potential human health problems associated with large numbers of pet animals in urban and suburban areas (Glickman and Schantz, 1981). The roundworm (*T. cati*) of cats is widespread, common, and may also infect humans; current evidence suggests that it does so much less frequently than does *T. canis* (Schantz and Glickman, 1981).

A. Parasite Development and Pathogenesis of Disease

People become infected by ingesting the infective eggs of *Toxocara* spp. present in soil or other materials. Direct contact with infected dogs and cats plays a secondary part in transmission because of the prolonged external incubation period that is required before the eggs become infective. The eggs hatch in the small intestine, and the larvae (350–450 × 16–20 μm) penetrate the mucosa, migrate to the liver via the portal circulation, follow vascular channels to the lungs, and then enter the systemic circulation and somatic tissues. Larvae migrate extensively through the body and have been found in virtually every tissue and organ system including liver, lungs, heart, and brain. The clinical and pathological manifestations result from the mechanical damage caused by the migrating larvae and the inflammatory response, often severe, that they stimulate.

Infection by only a few larvae, a common occurrence, is usually asymptomatic. The two distinct forms of the disease are classical visceral larva migrans (VLM) and ocular larva migrans (OLM). Typically, the VLM syndrome is diagnosed in children 1 to 4 years of age. Most cases in the literature have been characterized, almost uniformly, by fever, leukocytosis, persistent eosinophilia, hypergammaglobulinemia, and hepatomegaly. The few fatalities apparently attributable to toxocariasis have resulted either from extensive involvement of the myocardium or central nervous system, or from exaggerated immunologic response.

Invasion of the eye by *Toxocara* sp. larvae (OLM) is not uncommon. Because the differential diagnosis can include retinoblastoma and specific clinical findings are frequently lacking, some eyes infected by the larvae become needlessly enucleated. OLM differs in several important respects from VLM: many ocular cases are reported in adults, and the mean age at diagnosis is 7 to 8 years as compared to 1 to 4 years for VLM; ocular disease is usually seen in the absence of other signs or symptoms of VLM; and a history of pica is less common. An interpretation of the current understanding of the different pathogeneses of these two forms of toxocariasis has been reported by Glickman and Schantz (1981).

B. Parasite Maintenance Cycles

Toxocara canis is a nematode roundworm of the family Ascaridae whose adult forms live in the proximal small intestines of their canid definitive hosts. The life cycle of *T. canis* illustrates fascinating adaptations that ensure survival and transmission to successive generations of hosts. Dogs and other canids can become infected with *T. canis* by (1) ingestion of infective eggs, (2) ingestion of larvae in tissues of paratenic hosts, (3) transplacental migration of larvae from a pregnant bitch to her developing pups, (4) transmammary passage in milk of larvae from a lactating bitch to nursing pups, or (5) ingestion of late stage larvae or immature adults in the vomitus or feces of infected pups. *T. canis* probably infects canids in all tropical and temperate regions of the world. Published reports indicate that toxocariasis is prevalent throughout North America at latitudes below 60°N (Schantz and Glickman, 1981). The prevalence of infection in puppies 2–6 months of age has been reported to be greater than 80%, whereas in adult dogs 1 year of age or older infection rates decline to less than 20%. The high prevalence in pups is caused by the effectiveness of transplacental and transmammary transmission. There is little evidence to contradict the generalization that virtually all pups are infected with larvae of *T. canis* (Scothorn *et al.*, 1965).

C. Human Behavior and Toxocariasis

High prevalence of *Toxocara* infection in dogs and cats, frequency of pet ownership in American households, and promiscuous defecation by dogs in public places combine to produce widespread environmental contamination with *Toxocara* eggs, providing ample opportunities for zoonotic transmission. It is potentially important to zoonotic transmission of toxocariasis that households with young children (<12 years of age) are more likely to have pet dogs or cats than are households with older children (Selby *et al.*, 1980). In families with dogs, the potential for household contamination with *T. canis* eggs is high.

For people without household pets, the local park or playground may pose a similar risk. Studies in parts of North America have found that 10–32% of soil samples collected from parks, playgrounds (including children's sandboxes), schoolyards, and other public places are contaminated with *Toxocara* eggs (Dada and Lindquist, 1979; Dubin *et al.*, 1975; Ghadirian *et al.*, 1976; Headlee, 1936).

Serologic surveys indicate that infection, if not disease, is widespread. Glickman and Schantz (1982) recently reported on the testing of 8457 serum specimens drawn from a representative sample of the U.S. population. Positive antibody titers were found in 2.8% of the sample; subjects from the southern and northeastern states had the highest seroprevalence. Rates varied significantly with age, race, and socioeconomic level. Seroprevalence, highest in children less than 12 years old, declined markedly with advancing age. Seroprevalence was higher for blacks than whites of all ages, and it was highest among persons of the lowest socioeconomic classes.

We do not know the frequency of clinical disease in humans, because toxocariasis is not a reportable disease in the United States and because the diagnosis is difficult to confirm by laboratory methods. Neither worms nor eggs are passed in human feces, and biopsy techniques are often unrewarding despite widespread tissue invasion. Furthermore, the nonspecific nature of the clinical signs and symptoms often results in substantial underdiagnosis. Despite problems in ascertainment, we know that toxocariasis occurs whenever humans live in close association with dogs. More than 1900 diagnoses of this disease have been reported from 48 countries and every region of the United States (Ehrhard and Kernbaum, 1979). Interestingly, most cases of toxocaral disease are reported from industrialized countries. This may reflect the availability of diagnostic technology adequate for demonstration of the type of retinal lesion resulting from larval invasion and the more firmly ensconced tradition of reporting diseases in industrialized countries. Nevertheless, the prevalence of dogs in rural areas of developing countries, combined with their generally lower levels of hygiene, tends to produce even greater opportunities for zoonotic transmission.

Exposure to contaminated environments is not in itself sufficient to produce infection or disease. In recent studies of commonly exposed groups, kennel workers, veterinarians, and veterinary assistants did not have greater serologic evidence of toxocariasis than did matched nonexposed control groups (Jacobs *et al.*, 1977; Glickman and Cypess, 1977). In contrast, Woodruff *et al.* (1978) demonstrated positive ELISA titers in 15.7% of 102 British dog breeders and exhibiters and their employees. This was significantly higher than the rate of positive titers among 922 healthy adults from Britain (2.6%). The authors believed that dog breeders might be exposed to particular risk because of the high rate of congenital infections in pups, but the lack of higher seroprevalence in other occupationally exposed groups suggests that observance of routine hygiene by trained persons is adequate to avoid infection.

Epidemiological studies of toxocariasis in the United States indicate that children with pica and dogs in the same household present the greatest risk factors. In two studies, significant associations were found between infected persons and the presence of pups less than 3 months of age in the housebold within 1 year of onset of ocular illness (Schantz *et al.*, 1979; 1980). In another study of 100 young children seen at a Pittsburgh lead screening clinic, dog ownership was significantly associated with the presence of antibodies for *Toxocara* (Glickman *et al.*, 1981).

The strong association in the United States between household dogs and human cases contrasts with findings in Britain, where about 50% of patients with clinical toxocariasis have never owned a dog or cat, and have had only slight and transient contact with them (Woodruff *et al.*, 1978). Woodruff *et al.* suspected that most of these cases had been exposed to *Toxocara* eggs in the soil in parks and public places.

Pica, which occurs in 10 to 30% of children between 1 and 6 years of age (Bicknell, 1975), is an important risk factor for toxocariasis. The word "pica" comes from the Latin name for the magpie bird (*Pica pica*), which is notorious for its habit of gathering a variety of objects to satisfy its hunger and curiosity. Pica in humans can be defined as the habitual ingestion of nonfood substances, and it is considered a form of deviant behavior if it continues "beyond the normal developmental stage of occasional indiscriminate and experimental mouthing and swallowing (Bicknell, 1975)." The materials ingested as a result of pica depend on their availability in the environment as well as on conscious selection factors. Pica may be limited to the ingestion of specific substances such as soil, clay, starch, feces, plaster or paint, crayons, matches, and hair, or it may encompass a wide variety of objects.

Pica is more than just a socially unacceptable habit in children. Children with bizarre appetites are at high risk of several important diseases, including poisoning from the ingestion of paints containing lead or accidental poisoning by a variety of household products and drugs. Dirt-eating or geophagia is the type of pica that confers greatest risk of toxocariasis; most patients with clinical disease have had this habit. Glickman *et al.* (1981), screening 100 children of ages 1–6 years from a lead clinic in Pittsburgh for *Toxocara* spp. antibody, observed a significant association between feces, soil, or grass pica and elevated *Toxocara* spp. antibody levels, but not between those forms of pica and elevated blood lead level. Children with feces, soil, or grass pica were 20 times more likely to have elevated *Toxocara* spp. antibody levels than children with other or no forms of pica. A positive association was found between paint or plaster pica and elevated blood lead levels, but not for this type of pica and elevated *Toxocara* spp. antibody levels.

Estimates of the prevalence of pica vary widely because of difficulties in ascertaining accurate information from the parents and the lack of uniformity in defining the term. It is apparent, however, that the prevalence of pica is greatest in children aged 1–6 years, significantly higher in blacks than whites, and slightly greater in boys than girls. Pica is quite frequently associated with mental retardation, hyperactivity, and epilepsy. It has been hypothesized that pica accounts for the higher toxocaral seroprevalence in epileptics and mentally retarded individuals (Glickman *et al.,* 1979; Brook *et al.,* 1981). Interestingly, culturally determined pica behavior persists in adulthood among black women (Vermeer and Frate, 1979). Because the preferred clays are often obtained from surface soils that may occasionally be contaminated with dog or cat feces, such persons may possibly be exposed to *Toxocara* spp. infection. We have hypothesized that this may account for the higher toxocaral seroprevalence among black women as compared with black men or persons of both sexes of other races (Glickman and Schantz, 1981).

D.   Human Behavior and Toxocariasis Control

Control and prevention of toxocariasis in pets and humans requires comprehensive measures to prevent transmission among animals and between animals and humans, and to reduce environmental contamination with *Toxocara* spp. eggs. Measures generally recommended include:

1. Reducing the numbers of uncontrolled, ownerless dogs and cats as well as unwanted or poorly supervised pets.
2. Preventing the fouling of pavements and public places with dog feces; excluding dogs from children's playgrounds and areas of parks where children play.
3. Enforcing leash laws and promoting the social concept of responsible pet ownership.

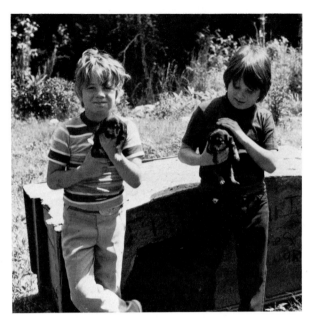

FIG. 7. Young boys handling pups. Children, due to intimate and casual handling of dogs, are most at risk when exposed to infectious agents harbored by pet animals.

4. Educating the public, particularly pet owners, about the zoonotic potential of roundworms in dogs and cats.
5. Eliminating roundworms from infected dogs and cats by appropriate preventive treatments.

Because the number of dogs in the United States is increasing, there appears to be little immediate prospect for decreasing potential exposure to dogs and their excreta, although appeals to enforce leash laws and proposed legislation prohibiting dogs from public parks and playgrounds are reaching increasingly responsive ears in many urban communities. "Scoop" laws requiring pet owners to clean up after their pets have recently been enacted in a number of cities and reportedly have aided perceptibly in decreasing fecal contamination in public places. Because of the importance of pica as a risk factor for toxocariasis and other diseases, children with pica should be excluded from environments thought to be contaminated with eggs of *T. canis,* and every effort should be made to eliminate the habit.

Surveys of dog owners in the United States indicate that families with young children are the primary dog-owning group because the major reason for acquiring a dog is as a pet for children (Anon, 1979; Selby *et al.,* 1980). Children, due to their intimate and casual handlings of dogs and frequent disregard for good hygienic practices, are most vulnerable when exposed to infectious agents harbored by their pets (Fig. 7). It is a cause for some concern, then, that most pet owners are unaware that any diseases other than rabies can be acquired from pets (Schantz and Glickman, 1981).

An interesting observation reported in follow-up studies of toxocariasis cases is that approximately 80% of dog-owning families had regularly utilized veterinary services for their pet (Schantz et al., 1979a; 1980). Despite this potential source of preventive medical education, less than one-third of the families knew about the public health hazards posed by dog parasites. Without such knowledge, pet owners will be unaware of the need for measures to minimize the risk of infection for family members. To reduce the likelihood of zoonotic transmission, practicing veterinarians should advise pet owners of potential zoonotic risks and encourage prophylactic care for pets (Schantz and Glickman, 1981).

References

Anon. (1979). Profile of the dog owner. *Bull. Inst. Study Anim. Probl.* **1**, 4.

Araujo, F. P., Schwabe, C. W., Sawyer, J. C., and David, W. G. (1975). Hydatid disease transmission in California. A study of the Basque connection. *Am. J. Epidemiol.* **102**, 291–299.

Ballard, N. B., and Vande Vusse, F. J. (1981). Distribution and prevalence of *Echinococcus multilocularis* in Minnesota foxes. *Annu. Meet. Am. Soc. Parasitol.*, Toronto. *Abstr.* #85, p. 46.

Beard, T. C. (1969). Hydatid control, a problem in health education. *Med. J. Aust.* **2**, 456.

Bicknell, J. (1975). "Pica: A Childhood Symptom", pp. 4–25. Butterworth, London.

Boev, S. N., Shaikenov, B., and Sokolova, L. A. (1979). (A disputed question of the taxonomy of trichinellae) (*In Russian*). *Parasitologija* **13**, 144–149.

Brook, I., Fish, C. H., Schantz, P. M., and Cotton, D. D. (1981). Toxocariasis in an institution for the mentally retarded. *Infect. Cont.* **2**, 317–320.

Cameron, T. W. M. (1960). The incidence and diagnosis of hydatid cysts in Canada: *Echinococcus granulosus* var. *canadensis*. *Parassitologia (Rome)* **2**, 281.

Centers for Disease Control (1981a). Trichinosis Surveillance Annual Summary 1980.

Centers for Disease Control. (1981b). Trichinosis associated with meat from a grizzly bear. *Morb. Mort. Week. Rep.* **30**, 115–121.

Crellin, J. R., Andersen, F. L., Schantz, P. M., and Condie, S. J. (1982). Factors influencing distribution and prevalence of *E. granulosus* in Utah. *Am. J. Epidemiol.* **116**, 463–474.

Dada, B. J. O., and Lindquist, W. D. (1979). Studies on flotation techniques for the recovery of helminth eggs from soil and the prevalence of eggs of *Toxocara* spp. in some Kansas public places. *J. Am. Vet. Med. Assoc.* **174**, 1208–1210.

Downs, J. F. (1974). "Animal Husbandry in Navajo Society and Culture". Univ. of California Press, Berkeley.

Dubin, S., Segall, S., and Martindale, J. (1975). Contamination of soil in two city parks with canine nematode ova including *Toxocara canis:* A preliminary study. *Am. J. Public Health* **65**, 1242–1245.

Ehrhard, T., and Kernbaum, S. (1979). *Toxocara canis* et toxocarose humaine. *Bull. Inst. Pasteur (Paris)*, **77**, 225–287.

Ellana, L., and Lum, M. K. W. (1980). Changing pattern of Arctic trichinosis: Relationship of culture and disease. *Proc. Alaskan Sci. Conf., 31st,* Am. Assoc. Adv. Sci., Sept. 17–19, Anchorage, Alaska, p. 80.

Fay, F. H. (1973). The ecology of *Echinococcus multilocularis* Leuckart, 1863 (Cestoda: Taeniidae) on St. Lawrence Island, Alaska. *Ann. Parasitol. Hum. Comp.* **48**, 523.

Fay, H. (1960). Carnivorous walrus and some Arctic zoonoses. *Arctic* **13**, 111–122.

Flick, S. C. (1973). Endoparasites in cats: current practice and opinions. *Feline Pract.* July-August, 21–34.

Franti, C. E., and Kraus, J. F. (1974). Aspects of pet ownership in Yolo County, California. *J. Am. Vet. Med. Assoc.* **164**, 166–171.

Franti, C. E., Kraus, J. F., Borhani, N. E., Johnson, S. L., and Tucker, S. D. (1980). Pet ownership in rural northern California (El Dorado County). *J. Am. Vet. Med. Assoc.* **176**, 143–149.

Gamble, W. G., Segal, M., Schantz, P. M., and Rausch, R. L. (1979). Alveolar hydatid disease in Minnesota: First human case acquired in the contiguous United States. *JAMA* **241**, 904.

Gemmell, M. A., and Johnstone, P. D. (1977). Experimental epidemiology of hydatidosis and cysticercosis. *Adv. Parasitol.* **15**, 311.

Ghadirian, E., Viens, P., Strykowski, H., and Dubreul, F. (1976). Prevalence of *Toxocara* and other helminth ova in dogs and soil in the Montreal metropolitan area. *Can. J. Public Health* **67**, 495–496.

Glickman, L. T., and Cypess, R. H. (1977). *Toxocara* infection in animal hospital employees. *Am. J. Public Health* **67**, 1193–1195.

Glickman, L. T., Cypess, R. H., Crumrine, P. K., and Gitlin, D. A. (1979). *Toxocara* infection and epilepsy in children. *J. Pediatr.* **94**(1), 75–78.

Glickman, L. T., Chaudry, I. U., Costantino, J., Clack, F. B., Cypess, R. H., and Winslow, L. (1981). Pica patterns, toxocariasis and elevated blood lead in children. *Am. J. Trop. Med. Hyg.* **30**, 77–80.

Glickman, L. T., and Schantz, P. M. (1981). Epidemiology and pathogenesis of zoonotic toxocariasis. *Epidemiol. Rev.* **3**, 230–250.

Griffiths, A. O., and Brenner, A. (1977). Survey of cat and dog ownership in Champaign County, Illinois. *J. Am. Vet. Med. Assoc.* **170**, 1333–1340.

Headlee, W. H. (1936). The epidemiology of human ascariasis in the metropolitan area of New Orleans, Louisiana. *Am. J. Hyg.,* **24**, 479–521.

Imperato, P. J., Harvey, R. P., Shookhoff, H. B., and Chaves, A. D. (1974). Trichinosis among Thais living in New York City. *JAMA* **227**, 526–529.

Jacobs, D. E., Woodruff, A. W., Shah, A. I., and Prole, J. H. B. (1977). *Toxocara* infections and kennel workers. *Br. Med. J.* **7**, 51.

Leiby, P. D., Carney, W. P., and Woods, C. E. (1970). Studies on sylvatic echinococcosis. II. Host occurrence and geographic distribution of *Echinococcus multilocularis* in the north central United States. *J. Parasitol.* **56**, 1141.

Leiby, P. D., and Kirtsky, D. C. (1972). *Echinococcus multilocularis:* a possible domestic life cycle in central North America and its public health implications. *J. Parasitol.* **58**, 1213.

Lukashenko, N. P. (1971). Problems of epidemiology and prophylaxis of alveococcosis (multilocular echinococcosis): a general review—with particular reference to the U.S.S.R. *Int. J. Parasitol.* **1**, 125.

Lukashenko, N. P. (1975). ''Alveokokkoz (al'veolyarnyi ekhinokokkoz).'' Meditsina, Moscow. 328 pp.

Nelson, G. S. (1968). The transmission of *Trichinella spiralis* from wild animals to man and domestic animals. *In* ''Some Diseases of Animals Communicable to Man in Britain'' (O. Graham-Jones, ed.), pp. 77–89. Pergamon, Oxford.

Pappaioanou, M., Schwabe, C. W., and Sard, D. M. (1977). An evolving pattern of human hydatid disease transmission in the United States. *Am. J. Trop. Med. Hyg.* **26,** 732–742.

Pawlowski, Z. S. (1981). Control of trichinellosis. *Proc. Int. Conf. on Trichinellosis, 5th* (C. W. Kim, and E. J. Ruitenberg, eds.), pp. 7–20. Reedbooks, London.

Rausch, R., and Schiller, E. L. (1956). Studies on the helminth fauna of Alaska. *Parasitology* **46,** 395–419.

Rausch, R., Babero, B. B., Rausch, R. V., and Schiller, E. L. (1956). Studies on the helminth fauna of Alaska. XXVII. The occurrence of larvae of *Trichinella spiralis* in Alaskan mammals. *J. Parasitol.* **42,** 259–271.

Rausch, R. L. (1960). Recent studies on hydatid disease in Alaska. *Parassitologia (Rome)* **2,** 391.

Rausch, R. L. (1967). On the ecology and distribution of *Echinococcus* spp. (Cestoda: Taeniidae), and characteristics of their development in the intermediate host. *Ann. Parasitol. Hum. Comp.* **42,** 19.

Schantz, P. M. (1977). Echinococcosis in American Indians living in Arizona and New Mexico. Review of recent studies. *Am. J. Epidemiol.* **106,** 370–379.

Schantz, P. M., and Glickman. L. T. (1979). Canine and human toxocariasis: the public health problem and the veterinarian's role in prevention. *J. Am. Vet. Med. Assoc.* **175,** 1270–1273.

Schantz, P. M., Juranek, D. D., and Schultz, M. G. (1977). Trichinosis in the United States 1975. Increase in cases attributed to numerous common-source outbreaks. *J. Infect. Dis.* **136,** 712–715.

Schantz, P. M., Meyer, D., and Glickman, L. T. (1979a). Clinical, serologic, and epidemiologic characteristics of ocular toxocariasis. *Am. J. Trop. Med. Hyg.* **28,** 24–28.

Schantz, P. M., Woodard, T. L., Sinclair, S., and Isenstein, R. S. (1979b). Resistance to freezing of the arctic strain of *Trichinella spiralis*. Ann. Meet. Am. Assoc. Vet. Parasitol., Seattle, July 1979, p. 15.

Schantz, P. M., Weis, P. E., Pollard, Z. F., and White, M. C. (1980). Risk factors for toxocaral ocular larva migrans: a case-control study. *Am. J. Public Health* **70,** 1269–1272.

Schantz, P. M., and Glickman, L. T. (1981). Roundworms in dogs and cats: Veterinary and public health considerations. *Compend. Contin. Educ. Pract. Vet.* **3,** 773–784.

Schantz, P. M. (1982). Echinococcosis. *In* "Handbook of Zoonoses" (J. Steele, and P. Arambulo, eds.), Vol. III, pp. 231–277. CRC Press, Boca Raton, Florida.

Schmitt, N., Saville, J. M., Greenway, J. A., Sotvell, P. L., Friis, L., and Hole, L. (1978). Sylvatic trichinosis in British Columbia. *Public Health Rep.* **93,** 189–193.

Schneider, R., and Vaida, M. L. (1975). Survey of canine and feline populations: Alameda and Contra Costa Counties, California, 1970. *J. Am. Vet. Med. Assoc.* **166,** 481–486.

Schwabe, C. W. (1968). Epidemiology of echinococcosis. *Bull. W.H.O.* **39,** 131.

Schwabe, C. W. (1979). Epidemiological aspects of the planning and evaluation of hydatid disease control. *Austr. Vet. J.* **55,** 109–117.

Scothorn, M. W., Koutz, F. R., and Groves, H. F. (1965). Prenatal *Toxocara canis* infection in pups. *J. Am. Vet. Med. Assoc.* **146,** 45–48.

Selby, L. A., Rhoades, J. D., Irvin, J. A., Carey, G. E., and Wade, R. G. (1980). Values and limitations of pet ownership. *J. Am. Vet. Med. Assoc.,* **176,** 1274–1276.

U.S. Department of Agriculture (1981). "National Status on Control of Garbage-Feeding." *APHIS,* Vet. Serv., March.

Vermeer, D. E., and Frate, D. A. (1979). Geophagia in rural Mississippi: Environmental and cultural contexts and nutritional implications. *Am. J. Clin. Nutr.* **32,** 2129–2135.

WHO Technical Report Series, No. 169 (1959). "Zoonoses: Second Report of the Joint WHO/FAO Expert Committee," p. 125.

Wilbur, R. H. (1976). Pets, pet ownership, and animal control: social and psychological attitudes, 1975. In *Proc. Nat. Conf. Dog and Cat Control,* pp. 21–34. American Humane Association.

Williams, J. F., Adaros, H. L., and Trejos, A. (1971). Current prevalence and distribution of hydatidosis, with special reference to the Americas. *Am. J. Trop. Med. Hyg.* **20,** 224.

Wilson, J. F., Diddams, A. C., and Rausch, R. L. (1968). Cystic hydatid disease in Alaska. A review of 101 autochthonous cases of *Echinococcus granulosus* infection. *Am. Rev. Respir. Dis.* **98,** 1.

Wilson, J. F., and Rausch, R. L. (1980). Alveolar hydatid disease: A review of clinical features of 33 indigenous cases of *Echinococcus multilocularis* infection in Alaskan Eskimos. *Am. J. Trop. Med. Hyg.* **29,** 1340–1355.

Woodruff, A. W., DeSavigny, D., and Jacobs, D. E. (1978). Study of toxocaral infection in dog breeders. *Br. Med. J.* **2,** 1747–1748.

Worley, D. E., Fox, J. C., and Winter, J. B. (1974). Prevalence and distribution of *Trichinella spiralis* in carnivorous mammals in the Northern Rocky Mountain Region (USA). *Proc. Int. Conf. Trichinellosis, 3rd* (C. W. Kim, ed.), pp. 597–602. Intext, New York.

Wright, W. H., Jacobs, L., Walton, A. C. (1944). Studies on trichinosis. XVI. Epidemiological considerations based on the examination for trichinae of 5,313 diaphragms from 189 hospitals in 37 states and District of Columbia. *Public Health Rep.* **59,** 669–681.

Zimmerman, W. J., and Hubbard, E. D. (1969). Trichiniasis in wildlife of Iowa. *Am. J. Epidemiol.* **90,** 84–92.

Zimmerman, W. J. (1970). Trichinosis in the United States. *In* ''Trichinosis in Man and Animals'' (S. E. Gould, ed.), pp. 378–400. Thomas, Springfield, Illinois.

Zimmerman, W. J., and Zinter, D. E. (1971). The prevalence of trichinosis in swine in the United States 1966–70. *Health Serv. Ment. Health Adm. U.S., Health Rep.* **86,** 937–945.

3

Human Behavior and Zoonotic Diseases in Malaysia

B. L. LIM and J. W. MAK
Institute for Medical Research
Kuala Lumpur
Malaysia

I. Introduction

Although the majority of parasitic and other microbial zoonoses in Malaysia afflict rural communities, others such as salmonellosis may cause explosive, institutional outbreaks in urban centers. In many of these situations man becomes infected by coming into either direct or indirect contact with animal reservoirs of the pathogens when he encroaches on their habitats during occupational, social, or recreational activities. Zoonotic Brugian filariasis affects large numbers of people in rural areas; although not fatal, the disease may cause considerable morbidity and the loss of many man-hours of work during acute attacks, and result in social stigmata because of such chronic manifestations as elephantiasis of the limbs. Leptospirosis can end fatally, and were it not for effective chemotherapy, diseases such as this and scrub typhus would have a much greater impact on the health and economy of the nation. Parasitic zoonoses such as angiostrongyliasis and pentastomiasis, although infrequently reported, are probably underdiagnosed; because large numbers of infected reservoir hosts are present, such zoonoses may represent only the "tip of the iceberg" of the actual number of human infections.

Diseases caused by subperiodic *Brugia malayi* infection will be present as long as man lives and works in an ecological setting that includes animal reservoirs of the disease. Indeed, existing control strategies have failed to interrupt the chain of transmission of zoonotic subperiodic *B. malayi* in areas where a high prevalence of the infection exists in host leaf monkeys (*Presbytis* spp.). Although effective preventive measures are available for some of the other diseases, ignorance, lack of vigilance, or careless behavior by those likely to be exposed to the pathogens involved may result in infection.

As it will not be possible to include all the zoonoses seen in Malaysia, the choice of diseases for discussion is based on their relative prevalence, their medical importance, available research, and problems that have been encountered in their control.

II. Some Important Zoonotic Diseases

A. Angiostrongyliasis

Angiostrongyliasis is a disease, caused by the nematode *Angiostrongylus* sp., of the central nervous system. In Malaysia, the causative agent is *Angiostrongylus malaysiensis*, the adults of which are found in commensal and forest rats. The intermediate hosts are terrestrial and aquatic molluscs. The first-stage larvae pass from the infected rats in the feces, and molluscs ingest the first-stage larvae whereupon they develop to the infective or third-stage larvae. Rats feed on these infected molluscs, and the parasite develops to the adult stage in their lungs.

In Malaysia, the parasite was first described as *Angiostrongylus cantonensis*. Evidence of strain specificity among three geographical taxa of *A. cantonensis*, the Thai, Hawaiian, and Malaysian strains, was found by Heyneman and Lim (1967) and Lim and Heyneman (1968). Based on these differences in pathogenicity and morphology, the Malaysian parasite was restudied and described as *A. malaysiensis* by Bhaibulaya and Cross (1971). *A. malaysiensis* is found throughout the country in commensal and feral rats and in the molluscan hosts (Lim *et al.*, 1965; 1976; Lim, 1967). The prevalence of infection in these hosts is associated with different biological habitats. The degree of susceptibility of the

TABLE I

Prevalence of *Angiostrongylus malaysiensis* Third-Stage Larvae in Land Molluscs
from Various Habitats in Malaysia

Habitats	Number examined	Terrestrial snails				
		M.r.[a]	*A.f.*	*Q.s.*	*S.o.*	*B.s.*
Town	500	2.8 (145)[b]	32.4 (112)	0	0.4 (6)	0
Scrub	500	31.0 (183)	19.6 (87)	9.6 (12)	1.6 (4)	0.8 (3)
Lalang	500	0	2.8 (29)	0	0	0
Ricefield	500	0	1.7 (10)	0	0	0
Oil palm	500	70.4 (285)	3.6 (434)	1.8 (42)	2.0 (11)	0.4 (2)
Rubber plantation	500	5.8 (61)	0.8 (12)	0	0	0

		Aquatic snails			
		P.s.	*B.i.*	*I.e.*	*L.r.*
Ricefield	500	24.8 (18)[b]	16.8 (16)	21.0 (5)	10.4 (3)
Pond	500	15.6 (12)	2.4 (4)	1.6 (2)	0
Stream	500	3.4 (16)	1.0 (3)	0.6 (2)	0

[a]*M.r.* = *Macrochlamys resplendens*, *A.f.* = *Achatina fulica*, *Q.s.* = *Quantula striata*, *S.o.* = *Subulina octona*, *B.s.* = *Bradybaena similaris*, *P.s.* = *Pila scutata*, *B.i.* = *Bellamya ingallsiana*, *I.e.* = *Indoplanorbis exutus*, *L.r.* = *Lymnaea rubiginosa*.

[b]Figures in parentheses denote mean number of larvae per positive snail.

molluscan host to the parasite varies with the host species. Of five species of terrestrial snails examined, the infection rates were found to be higher in *Macrochlamys resplendens* and *Achatina fulica* than in other snail species (Table I). Higher infection rates of these snail species were found in scrub and oil palm habitats. The prevalence of infections in the four species of aquatic snails examined from different habitats showed no marked difference, but *Pila scutata* showed a higher rate than the other species. Infection rates of all snail species examined were higher in rice fields than in the other habitats examined. Slugs are very susceptible hosts for the parasite; of the four species examined, *Micropармarion malayanus* and *Girasia peguensis* had the highest prevalence rates. Similarly, more infections were seen in scrub and oil palm habitats (Table II).

The principal definitive hosts of this parasite are the commensal rats (Table III); forest rats do not seem to play an important part in the propagation of the parasite (Table IV). Infection rates in these commensal rats were found to be related to those of molluscan intermediate hosts in the various habitats, as in scrub and oil palm. Among the field rats, *Rattus tiomanicus* was found to be a more susceptible host; in the towns, *R. norvegicus* was more susceptible (Table III).

Among the intermediate molluscan hosts, one species of land snail (*Achatina*

TABLE II

Prevalence of *Angiostrongylus malaysiensis* Third-Stage Larvae in Land Slugs
from Various Habitats in Malaysia

Habitat	Number examined	*Microparmarion malayanus*	*Lavicaulis alte*	*Girasia peguenia*	*Lemperula* sp.
Town	500	5.8 (142)[a]	1.6 (12)	2.4 (82)	3.1 (57)
Scrub	500	49.6 (245)	5.0 (84)	22.0 (272)	9.4 (14)
Lalang	500	31.0 (101)	6.8 (22)	1.6 (14)	3.4 (18)
Ricefield	500	29.7 (75)	5.6 (7)	5.2 (9)	3.8 (7)
Oil palm	500	73.0 (298)	24.4 (252)	25.4 (268)	22.0 (168)
Rubber plantation	500	61.9 (121)	4.8 (6)	18.5 (168)	2.9 (8)

[a]Figures in parentheses denote mean number of larvae per positive slug.

fulica) and one aquatic snail (*Pila scutata*) are of potential importance in the transmission of the disease to man. In Thailand, Punyadasni and Punyagupta (1961) and Punyagupta (1965) discovered that patients with eosinophilic meningoencephalitis had ingested pickled aquatic snails (*P. ampullacca*). The land snail, *A. fulica,* which is commonly eaten in certain parts of Taiwan (Republic of China), has been implicated in several cases of cerebroangiostrongyliasis (Hsieh, 1967). *A. fulica* is not eaten by man in Malaysia, but is sometimes fed to ducks.

Lim *et al.* (1978) studied the consumption of *P. scutata* by local human populations in Malaysia and found that among the three ethnic groups (Malays, Indians, and Chinese), the Chinese are the principal consumers of this snail. Resurveys of *Pila scutata* consumed as food in various villages and sold in the markets throughout the country were made. Five hundred grams of *P. scutata*, 25–40 mm, consisted of 26 individuals. The net weight of these 26 snails (without the shells) was about 87 g; 51 g remained after removal of the visceral portions. Based on these data, an estimate was made of the numbers of individual snails and net weights with and without the viscera (Table V).

The survey (Lim *et al.*, 1978) revealed that relatively few *P. scutata* were consumed by Malaysians. More were consumed by rural than by urban folks; urban Chinese and Indians eat these snails for medicinal purposes. Boils, eye infections, alcoholic intoxication, heat and toxicity, dysentery and diarrhea, and bodily and muscular aches and pains are so treated. In rural populations, the snails were eaten as food as well as for medicine (Lim *et al.*, 1978). Survival of the infective larvae embedded in the muscular tissues of snails after the snail has been seasoned with spices and cooked is unlikely. The Chinese, on the other hand, eat the snail whole (including viscera) and usually half cooked. The wormload of larvae of the infected snail ranges from 2–150 (with a mean of 18) infective larvae (Table I), which is probably too low for subsequent infection of

TABLE III

Prevalence of *Angiostrongylus malaysiensis* in Commensal Rats from Various Habitats in Malaysia

Habitat	R.d.[a]		R.e.		R.t.		R.a.		R.n.	
	a[b]	b	a	b	a	b	a	b	a	b
Town	2712	9.3 (4)[c]	172	4.7 (2)	—	—	—	—	1287	23.0 (11)
Scrub	388	31.9 (8)	140	24.3 (4)	576	34.7 (8)	136	50.0 (8)	—	—
Lalang	140	12.5 (2)	192	1.6 (2)	552	10.9 (4)	352	11.4 (7)	—	—
Ricefield	304	14.8 (3)	344	25.0 (2)	460	25.0 (5)	841	14.7 (8)	—	—
Oil palm	124	48.4 (6)	44	45.5 (4)	2945	35.0 (10)	180	30.0 (16)	—	—
Rubber plantation	240	4.2 (2)	366	6.5 (2)	272	9.9 (4)	24	8.3 (4)	—	—

[a] *R.d.* = *Rattus rattus diardii*, *R.e.* = *Rattus exulans*, *R.t.* = *Rattus tiomanicus*, *R.a.* = *Rattus argentiventer*, *R.n.* = *Rattus norvegicus*.

[b] The a columns give the number of animals examined whereas the b columns give the % positive.

[c] The figures in parentheses denote the mean number of worms per infected animal.

TABLE IV

Prevalence of *Angiostrongylus malaysiensis* in Forest Rats and Shrews from Various Habitats in Malaysia

Habitat	R.m.[a]		R.b.		R.s.		R.a.		R.c.		R.w.		R.sa.	
	a[b]	b	a	b	a	b	a	b	a	b	a	b	a	b
Fringe	454	1.5 (4)[c]	48	6.3 (5)	185	1.1 (3)	295	0.7 (4)	112	4.5 (7)	285	0.4 (3)	212	0.9 (4)
Forest	648	0	424	0	328	0	48	0	215	0	348	0	785	0

[a]R.m. = *Rattus muelleri*, R.b. = *Rattus bowersi*, R.s. = *Rattus surifer*, R.a. = *Rattus annandalei*, R.c. = *Rattus cremoriventer*, R.w. = *Rattus whiteheadi*, R.sa. = *Rattus sabanus*.

[b]The a columns give the number of animals examined whereas the b columns give the % positive.

[c]The figures in parentheses denote the mean number of worms per infected animal.

TABLE V

Pila scutata Consumed as Food by Rural and Urban Populations in Peninsular Malaysia

State	Villages		Urban market		Weight of wet flesh with viscera (kg)		Weight of flesh without viscera (kg)	
	Yearly estimated intake (kg)	Estimated number of snails consumed	Yearly estimated intake (kg)	Estimated number of snails consumed	Village	Town	Village	Town
Perlis	600	31,200	600	31,200	104.4	104.4	61.2	61.2
Kedah	600	31,200	600	31,200	104.4	104.4	61.2	61.2
Perak	750	39,000	150	7,800	130.5	26.1	76.5	15.3
Selangor	70	3,640	250	13,000	12.2	43.5	7.1	25.5
Malacca	160	8,320	300	15,600	27.8	52.2	16.3	30.6
Johore	50	2,600	50	2,600	8.7	8.7	5.1	5.1
Kelantan	500	26,000	300	15,600	87.0	52.2	51.0	30.6
Trengganu	500	26,000	300	15,600	87.0	52.2	51.0	30.6
Pahang	500	26,000	200	10,400	87.0	34.8	51.0	20.4
Totals	3,730	193,960	2,750	143,000	649.0	478.5	380.4	280.5

man especially when snails are half cooked. Significantly, when this snail is consumed for medicinal value it is not normally eaten in large quantities; this minimizes the risk of human infection.

Angiostrongylus malaysiensis is found in areas where two main intermediate hosts (*Macrochlamys resplendens* and *M. malayanus*) and the final hosts occur in high densities, especially in oil palm and scrub vegetation. The transmission cycle of the parasite in town is minimal because the activities of urban rodents are more confined to houses, restricting the chances of contact with intermediate hosts outside houses. In field habitats, freshwater molluscs, also involved in the lifecycle, apparently are important additional intermediate hosts. The freshwater snail, *Pila scutata,* which is consumed as food and medicine, is the only molluscan intermediate host that can be considered as a potential source of human infection in Malaysia. Heyneman and Lim (1967) demonstrated that fresh vegetables, particularly lettuce, may also be involved in the transmission of the parasite to man.

A. malaysiensis has been reported as pathogenic to man. The first five human cases of eosinophilic meningoencephalitis in Malaysia in which this parasite was implicated were reported from Kuching [Sarawak (Watts, 1969)] and the sixth case was found in Kuala Lumpur in Peninsular Malaysia (Bisseru *et al.,* 1972).

Although there has been no further report of human cases, accidental infection by the parasite because of consumption of freshwater snails and contaminated fresh vegetables is always possible.

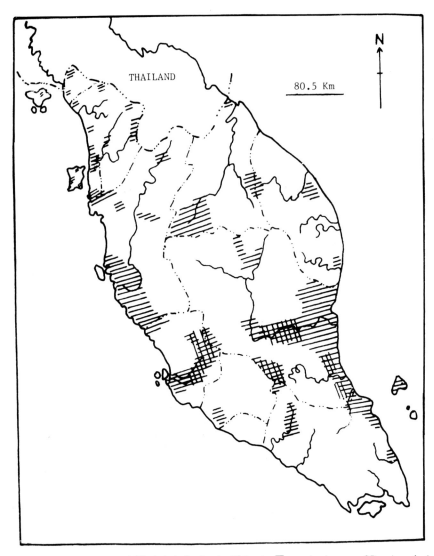

FIG. 1. Endemic areas of filiariasis in Peninsular Malaysia. ▨ = endemic areas of *Brugia malayi;*
▧ = *foci of Wuchereria bancrofti.*

B. Zoonotic Brugian Filariasis

Brugia malayi, Brugia timori, and *Wuchereria bancrofti* are responsible for
human filariasis in Southeast Asia. Of these, *B. malayi* is the dominant species.
B. timori is known to be endemic only in the islands of Timor, Flores, Rote, and

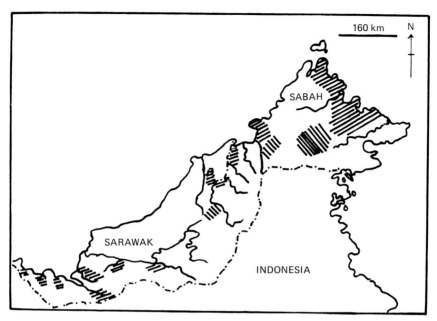

FIG. 2. Endemic areas of filiariasis in Sabah and Sarawak, Malaysia. ▨ = endemic areas of *Brugia malayi;* ▧ = endemic areas of *Wuchereria bancrofti.*

Alor in Indonesia (Oemijati and Lim, 1966; Kurihara and Oemijati, 1975). Both *B. malayi* and *W. bancrofti* are endemic in Malaysia (Figs. 1 and 2). Two major strains of *B. malayi* are present, periodic and subperiodic, with biological and epidemiological differences. Since Poynton and Hodgkin (1939) first suggested the potential transmission of subperiodic *B. malayi* from *Macaca fascicularis* to man, further studies on the prevalence of the infection in wild and domestic animals (Edeson *et al.,* 1955), and on the successful experimental transmission of the parasite between animals and man (Edeson and Wharton, 1958; Dondero *et al.,* 1972), have strengthened the belief that the disease can be a zoonosis.

In many endemic areas of Brugian filariasis, the control strategy has relied mainly on mass chemotherapy with diethylcarbamazine citrate (DEC-C) against both periodic and subperiodic *Brugia malayi*. Differences in the efficiency of mass chemotherapy with DEC-C in different localities have been experienced, depending on which form (or even both forms) of the parasite was present. Although the Malaria Control Programme has been found to have a complementary beneficial effect on the control of periodic *B. malayi* in areas where endophilic and endophagic *Anopheles* spp. mosquitoes are the principal vectors (Mak *et al.,* 1977), problems of zoonotic transmission and the exophilic and exophagic characteristics of *Mansonia* spp. vectors (Wharton, 1962) have undermined control efforts with DEC-C against subperiodic *B. malayi*. This is evident in a study area near swamp forests in Pondok Tanjong, Taiping, where leaf monkeys (*Presbytis* spp.) abound; mass control with DEC-C applied for five or six cycles did not stop the transmission of subperiodic *B. malayi*, and microfilarial rates remained rather high compared with pretreatment levels (Fig. 3). Similarly, in another subperiodic *B. malayi* endemic area (Johore), three cycles of mass treatment did not substantially decrease the microfilarial rate (Fig. 4) compared to periodic *B. malayi* in Penang (Fig. 5).

Although 31 of 447 (6.9%) domestic cats were found to be infected with subperiodic *B. malayi*, they appeared to have been infected from man (Mak *et al.*, 1980), unlike the situation in wild animal reservoirs. A number of wild carnivores and nonhuman primates are infected with subperiodic *B. malayi*, but in Malaysia only leaf monkeys (*Presbytis obscura, P. cristata,* and *P. melalophos*) are highly infected (Lim and Mak, 1978). Indeed, in certain areas 76.3% of these leaf monkeys were parasitized. Because *Mansonia* spp. vector mosquitoes bite both man and animals (Wharton, 1962), it is likely that humans are constantly exposed to subperiodic *B. malayi* infective third-stage larvae (L_3) suggesting that zoonotic transmission is responsible for the inefficiency of mass chemotherapy with DEC-C in these areas.

Where Brugian filariasis is endemic, a number of factors must be considered in evaluating filariasis control schemes. Essential baseline data in addition to demographic characteristics and prevalence rates of infection in the population should be obtained to aid in the planning and choice of the control program. These include

1. The *Brugia* species and strain involved, morphological studies of the microfilariae, and periodicity studies of microfilarial carriers are essential. Subperiodic *B. malayi* when present suggests the need for a closer look at wild and domestic animals as potential reservoirs of the infection.

2. The prevalence and species of filarial parasites in wild and domestic animals must be studied by animal trapping. The presence of subperiodic *B. malayi* and other filarial parasites that use mosquitoes as vectors will contribute not only to the variety of L_3 but to the antigenic stimulation of the human population with filariids of nonhuman origin. If seroepidemiological studies for the evaluation of endemicity are contemplated, this problem would have to be considered.

3. Entomological surveys to identify vectors and to determine their relationships with human and animal reservoirs should be conducted. Positive identification of the species of L_3 will mean a more rational interpretation of entomological survey data.

The problems raised by animal reservoir hosts in the evaluation of filariasis control schemes can be summarized as follows:

A sufficiently large number of animal reservoirs of subperiodic *B. malayi*

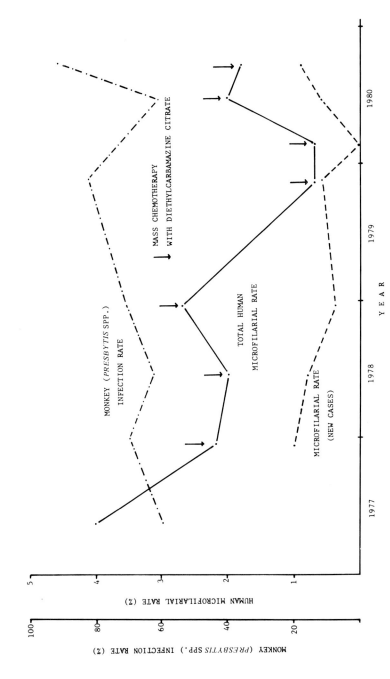

FIG 3. Effect of mass chemotherapy with diethylcarbamazine citrate at 6 mg/kg daily for 6 days on rate of human microfilarial infection from subperiodic *Brugia malayi*; Pondok Tanjong, Taiping.

MONKEY (*PRESBYTIS* SPP.) INFECTION RATE

MASS CHEMOTHERAPY WITH DIETHYLCARBAMAZINE CITRATE

TOTAL HUMAN MICROFILARIAL RATE

MICROFILARIAL RATE (NEW CASES)

HUMAN MICROFILARIAL RATE (%)

MONKEY (*PRESBYTIS* SPP.) INFECTION RATE (%)

Y E A R

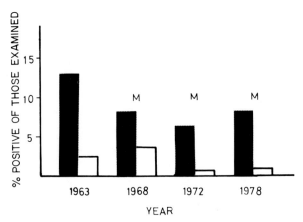

FIG. 4. Effect of mass treatment (M) with diethylcarbamazine DEC at 6 mg/kg weekly for 6 weeks in Kampong Bandar, Muar, Johore. ■ = microfilarial rate; □ = elephantiasis rate.

could, in the presence of *Mansonia* spp. vectors, negate mass chemotherapeutic control efforts. Animal reservoir hosts of *Brugia* spp. will contribute to the diversity of L_3 in vectors. In most Southeast Asian countries, *Brugia* spp. present in animal reservoirs include *B. malayi, B. pahangi, B. tupaiae,* and other *Brugia* spp. Others such as *B. timori* can be experimentally transmitted to cats and gerbils (Partono *et al.*, 1977), suggesting that natural animal infections may be possible. It is extremely difficult to differentiate *Brugia* L_3 with light micros-copy, and the diversity of *Brugia* spp. L_3 will probably complicate evaluation of the control program if the infective mosquito is used as an index of the risk of the population to infection. Not all the *Brugia* spp. listed have been tested to evalu-ate their infectivity to man. Immunological experience with L_3 of nonhuman filarial parasites will also complicate interpretation of seroepidemiological sur-vey results if used in estimating the effectiveness of control programs.

C. Malaysian Schistosomiasis

Since the first case of *Schistosoma japonicum*-type infection was discovered incidentally during an autopsy of an Orang Asli female from Fort Betau, Pahang, Peninsular Malaysia (Murugesu and Por, 1973), a further eight cases have been found, mostly from reviews of autopsy materials (Leong *et al.*, 1975). A tenth case was seen in another Orang Asli who presented with nephrotic syndrome and a liver biopsy showing evidence of *S. japonicum*-type infection (Murugesu *et al.*, 1978). The ages of these ten patients (five males and five females) ranged from 11 to 68 years, and, based on autopsy studies, an infection rate of 5.5% (230 autopsies) was seen in Orang Asli one year of age and older. Seven of the cases were from Pahang State, and three from Perak State.

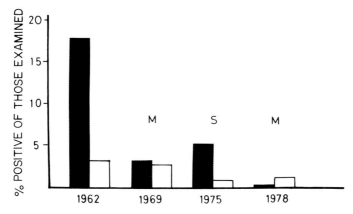

FIG. 5. Effect of DEC at 6 mg/kg weekly for 6 weeks on periodic *Brugia malayi* in *kampongs* Sungei Kedak, Permatang Bendahari, and Permatang Tok Labu, Province Wellesly North, Penang. M = mass treatment; S = selective treatment; ■ = microfilarial rate; □ = elephantiasis rate.

This infection caused mild to moderate fibrosis of the portal tracts of the liver. Granulomatous lesions were also seen around eggs measuring 53.7 μm (range 48–62 μm) × 36 μm (range 30–44 μm). The infection is probably zoonotically transmitted from wild animal reservoirs, a belief strengthened by the finding of *S. japonicum*-type eggs in the feces of one of nine *Rattus muelleri* caught in the endemic locality. Further, one of two new species of freshwater hydrobiid snails of subfamily Triculinae and new genus *Robertsiella* (*R. kaporensis* and *R. gismanni*) was found shedding cercariae of the parasite. These snails were found in heavily shaded, small, shallow streams with sandy gravel bottoms, among the roots of the *Saraca thaipingensis* trees which send thick roots into the river water (Greer *et al.*, 1980; Greer *et al.*, 1980a; Davis and Greer, 1980). Adult worms recovered from experimental transmission of cercariae from naturally infected snails into mice and hamsters were found to be morphologically similar to *S. japonicum* and *S. mekongi*. However, the exact taxonomic status of the Malaysian schistosome needs to be defined. Although human infections have been reported only in Orang Asli who live in close proximity to wild animal reservoirs, further studies are needed to map the distribution and epidemiology of the disease in other population groups.

D. Pentastomiasis

Pentastomiasis is caused by larval and nymphal stages of class Pentastomida. Adult pentastomids are usually parasitic in the respiratory tract and lungs of vertebrates. Man is an accidental host infected by ingestion of inadequately processed or cooked animal meat, or by other food contaminated with eggs of pentastomids.

Nymphal pentastomiasis was found in 22 Orang Asli aborigines of Peninsular Malaysia autopsied at the University of Malaysia Medical Center in Kuala Lumpur (Prathap *et al.*, 1969). Orang Asli who were initially hospitalized at the Gombak Aborigine Hospital were transported there by helicopter from jungle villages within a radius of 75 miles from Gombak. The Orang Asli people live a primitive life utilizing the villages as semipermanent bases from which they forage food from the jungle. Their food consists of a great variety of fruits, tubers, insects (especially grubs), and small vertebrates such as snakes, lizards, rodents, insectivores, carnivores, subhuman primates, and birds. The snakes consumed are often definitive hosts, infected with the nymphal pentastomes. Small animals are usually eaten raw, but large animals such as snakes, monkeys, and birds are skinned and cooked, although poorly.

Although the infection mechanism has not been documented, the food habits of these people suggest probable methods. None of the human infections reported were heavy; in individual infections, only a few nymphs were involved. These nymphs were of the genera *Porocephalus* and *Armillifer*, which infect the lungs of snakes as adults and the flesh of mammals as larvae and nymphs. A gravid female of these pentastomes will contain several thousand viable eggs, thus massive infections occur when an entire worm is consumed (Self, 1972). These latter observations supply evidence that the Orang Asli infections probably were not from consuming entire worms recovered from snakes but from food or drink contaminated by eggs distributed naturally via the mouth or anus of snakes. Another possible source is from butchered snakes, via contaminated hands, or from egg-contaminated flesh not cooked sufficiently to kill the eggs. Furthermore, there is reason to believe that soil- or wood-dwelling insect grubs that consume snake excreta can transmit the eggs to man mechanically when he eats these grubs uncooked. There is also the possibility of transmission by drinking water contaminated by snake excreta that contains eggs.

A study of the prevalence of the infestation in wild mammals has been valuable in understanding the endemic transmission of pentastomiasis in Malaysia (Table VI). All species of animals studied had nymphal pentastomes, although infection percentages among them are much lower than in man in the same area (Prathap *et al.*, 1969).

The knowledge that Insectivora and Chiroptera are infected certainly implicates insects as transmitting agents. From our knowledge of pentastome life cycles, we can be certain that this is a paratenic function; that is, the insects, especially grubs, swallow the eggs in snake excreta or in food contaminated by them. The eggs or larvae survive metamorphosis in bats to be transmitted to other bats through the adult insects.

Rodents, insectivores, and primates are generally omnivorous; their feeding habits are quite similar to those of the Orang Asli occupying the same jungle habitats. It is also well known that porocephalid pentastomes can infect a great

TABLE VI

Prevalence of Pentastomiasis in Wild Animals Examined from Malaysia

Orders	Number of species	Number of individuals examined	Number of species infected	Number of individuals infected	% individuals infected
Insectivora	2	128	2	2	1.56
Chiroptera	1	115	1	1	0.86
Rodentia (rats)	8	2758	8	27	0.09
Rodentia (squirrels)	3	582	3	4	0.68
Carnivora	8	48	8	10	20.08
Primata (primitive)	4	272	4	4	1.47
Reptilia (pythons)	2	184	2	69	37.50
Totals	28	4087	28	117	2.86

variety of animals (Self, 1969). Therefore, any group of mammal species with food habits similar to those of the aborigines will harbor pentastome nymphs in environments where infected snakes abound, and where mammal food habits are conducive to the transmission of eggs from the snakes. Consequently, the food habits of the Orang Asli, similar to those of coexisting wild mammals which serve as natural intermediate hosts for the pentastomes, may expose them to infection. The wild mammals are totally responsible for maintaining the endemic focus of the pentastomes; occurrence in the aborigines is incidental.

Although the carnivores in question are classified as flesh eaters, they (as do many other species of the same order) eat most items of food consumed by man and undoubtedly are infected from the same sources. Thus, the epidemiology of the disease is associated with the socioeconomic and food habits of the rural populations, particularly with the Orang Asli in Malaysia. Although this disease has not yet been reported among the other racial groups in rural areas, cases may be found during further investigations.

E. Leptospirosis

Leptospirosis, a common zoonotic infection in Malaysia, affects rural populations much more than urban, especially those persons engaged in agricultural pursuits. Antibody surveys among "normal" populations, using the sensitized erythrocyte lysis (SEL) test, have shown that rural children are exposed to infection as young as 4–6 years old and are constantly reinfected throughout life. Significant antibody levels are seen in 13% of the population (Tan, 1979), and it is indeed fortunate that the majority of the infecting serovars in Peninsular Malaysia are of low virulence although able to stimulate protective antibodies

(Tan and Lopes, 1972). Approximately 25% of all oil palm and rubber estate laborers, padi planters, and farmers have significant antibody levels, a reflection of the close contact that agricultural workers have with animal reservoirs. Fishermen, who spend most of their time at sea, did not show significant titers. Indeed, even among the same occupational groups the prevalence of significant antibody titers varies with the intensiveness of the contact between man and rats. Laborers on smaller rubber estates near forests are constantly exposed to foraging jungle rats (e.g., *Rattus bowersi, R. muelleri,* and *R. sabanus*) in which an overall infection rate of 17% has been found (Tan, 1970a). The prevalence of significant antibody titers in these laborers is 43–46%. In contrast, laborers of large, well managed estates, with houses away from the jungle fringe, have antibody prevalence rates of 0–3%. On oil palm estates, *R. jalorensis* occurs in great numbers, feeding on the fruits. Although the infection rate among these rats is 3%, their large numbers contribute to the high prevalence rates of leptospiral antibody titers in the laborers, an occupational group with prevalence rate of 32.6%.

Although a wide range of wild and domestic animals have been found with leptospiral infections, the most important natural reservoirs, which maintain the wild parasite populations, are ground rats. However, not all rats are efficient reservoirs in terms of susceptibility and duration of excretion of leptospires; *Rattus norvegicus, R. argentiventer, R. exulans,* and *R. muelleri* are extremely efficient (Smith *et al.,* 1961a). Although the distribution of these rats overlaps, species abundance varies with habitat type; the dominant species will be the important reservoir host in that locality. In towns sampled, rat species varied widely. In the seaport (Klang), *R. norvegicus* predominated; the infection rate was 32% with the serovar *javanica* predominating (Smith *et al.,* 1961b). *R. argentiventer* predominates in rice fields, also with the serovar *javanica* most common. In scrub and secondary forest (at least in the early stages), *R. jalorensis* and *R. exulans* are most common; the predominant serovar was *autumnalis.* In primary forests the giant rats *R. bowersi, R. muelleri,* and *R. sabanus,* the spiny rats *R. rajah* and *R. whiteheadi,* and the tree rats *R. canus* and *R. cremoriventer* are found. *R. muelleri* is found primarily in valley bottoms, and *R. sabanus* on the drier hill slopes.

Even when animal reservoir hosts are present, favorable environmental conditions are essential for efficient transmission. Requisite factors include water, soil, and surface waters with a pH $\geq$ 6.0, and soil condition is critical (Smith *et al.,* 1961a). The number of clinical cases presenting to hospitals tends to increase during the last quarter of the year, corresponding to the peak annual rainfall (Tan, 1970a); this is explained by the greater risk, during floods, of contamination of surface waters with leptospires from jungle animal reservoirs. A study among normal rice planters showed 24.2% seropositives during the wet season in August, compared to 7.2% during the dry season in April (Tan, 1970b). There was a corresponding change in the pH of the water and soil in the rice fields during these periods, from a range of 5.9–5.2 in the wet season to a mean of 4.8 in the dry season. The low pH during the dry season is unfavorable for leptospiral survival and multiplication.

Although rats have been incriminated as the most important animal disease reservoirs in Malaysia, infected domestic animals also disseminate the disease. Fifty-five percent of dogs, 35% of cattle, 23% of pigs, 15% of horses, and 8% of goats were found seropositive by the microscopic agglutination test (Joseph, 1979).

Clinically, nearly six times as many Malaysian males as females are infected, a reflection of the difference in exposure of the two sexes as a result of occupational and cultural factors. Another indication of the relationship between occupation and leptospiral infection is seen in the prevalence rates of the disease in racial groups. Indians–Pakistanis have a prevalence rate of 17.3 per 100,000 as compared to 6.8 per 100,000 in the general population (Tan, 1970c). A large population of Indians who work in rubber and oil palm estates is more exposed to leptospirosis than is the general population.

In recent years, there has been a change in predominant serovars isolated from clinical cases. For 1958–1968, the most frequent serovars were *autumnalis* and *hebdomadis;* in 1978 they were *javanica* and *pomona* (Tan, 1979); it remains to be seen whether there has been a corresponding change in the serovars isolated from animal reservoirs. Mortality rate in Malaysia from confirmed leptospirosis has been about 16% (Tan, 1970c), and this zoonotic disease still has considerable importance for the health of the rural population.

F. Scrub Typhus

Scrub typhus, a chigger-borne rickettsiosis which is an important disease in much of Southeast Asia, is prevalent in Malaysia (Traub and Wisseman, 1974). The disease is transmitted by the bite of an infected chigger, the larval stage of a trombiculid mite. Vectors of scrub typhus are limited to the single genus *Leptotrombidium,* and tend to be habitat-specific rather than host-specific (Harrison and Audy, 1951a; 1951b; Nadchatram, 1970). In Malaysia, several *Leptotrombidium* vector species, restricted to specific habitats, are known. The vector *L.(L.) fletcheri* is found in *lalang* grass (*Imperata cylindrica*) throughout Malaysia; *L. (L.) deliense* is abundant in almost all forest types and scrub (Hubert and Baker, 1963) and in oil palm estates (Dohany *et al.,* 1979). *L. (L.) arenicola* is found in sandy beaches near coastal regions (Traub, 1960; Upham *et al.,* 1971), but not on rocky shores.

The trombiculid mite vectors, particularly the genus *Leptotrombidium,* are associated with rats of genus *Rattus* and subgenus *Rattus* (*Rattus*) which are essentially grounddwellers (Traub and Wisseman, 1974). The disease is associated with rural ecology (Audy, 1948), and the risk populations are mostly rural people such as plantation and field workers and military personnel on field exercises.

A total of 1593 blood samples for isolation and 771 for serology were analyzed from four indicator species (*R. exulans, R. argentiventer, R. tiomanicus,* and *R. sabanus*) from the various habitats (Table VII). The selected species were not always confined to a single habitat, nor are the host species responses to infections with *Rickettsia tsutsugamushi* yet known. Comparisons cannot therefore be made without bias until responses to infection can be quantified in the laboratory. Nevertheless, some of the species were captured in more than one habitat which allowed some comparison of habitat among species. For example, *R. argentiventer* was caught in significant numbers in both the village and *lalang.* In the village, which contained fruit and coconut trees, brush, herbaceous vegetation and grass, this rat was less common, suggesting that it used such habitat less frequently; the *R. argentiventer* rickettsial isolation rates and seropositives were lower in the village than in the *lalang.* In *R. tiomanicus,* the rickettsial isolation rates in these two habitats were nearly equal, but the seropositives in the village were lower than in the *lalang* or in the scrub. No marked difference was found between seropositives of *R. exulans* in village and *lalang,* but the rickettsial isolation and seropositive rates in the forest rat, *R. sabanus,* were very high (Table VII).

These data suggest that transmission of rickettsiae to rats was occurring at a high rate in the *lalang.* Perhaps the close proximity of the *lalang* to the scrub habitat, and the apparent free movement of the rats between these habitats (the typical scrub rat, *R. tiomanicus,* was actually caught more frequently in the *lalang* than in the scrub) with regard to the habitat differences, could obscure the results in scrub typhus transmission to rats. Although very few scrub or *lalang* rats were caught in the forest, a high rate of rickettsial isolation was obtained in forest animals. The results support the original thesis that enzootic transmission of rickettsiae to rats is very active in the forest. Audy (1961) pointed out that the prevalence of scrub typhus in man varies according to the habitats he frequents and, in some geographic areas, with the season of the year. He also claimed that in most parts of Southeast Asia abandoned agricultural land grown over with scrub vegetation was of greatest risk to man. This was also true in many other transitional or preclimax habitats, such as river banks subjected to periodic inundations. Although stating that man seldom contracts infections in primary forests, he alluded to a "jungle tsutsugamushi" transmission cycle. He postulated that in the Malaysian forest endemic foci or "typhus islands," if present, were sparse, and that the endemic areas were confined to the deforested areas. Traub and Wisseman (1968) reported successional changes in host and vector populations in Malaysia as their habitats changed through time. Cadigan *et al.* (1972), in studies of Orang Asli, found that people in deep jungle villages had a

TABLE VII

Scrub Typhus (*Rickettsia tsutsugamushi*) Isolations and Serological Data in Four Selected *Rattus* Species in Five Types of Habitat in Peninsular Malaysia[a]

Habitat	R. exultans		R. argentiventer		R. tiomanicus		R. sabanus		Total	
	I[b](N)[c]	S[d](N)	I(N)	S(N)	I(N)	S(N)	I(N)	S(N)	I(N)	S(N)
Village	15 (83)	17 (106)	24 (33)	37 (38)	24 (140)	26 (151)	—	—	21 (256)	26.7 (295)
Lalang	31 (13)	14 (14)	46 (56)	60 (73)	27 (158)	45 (175)	—	—	34.7 (227)	39.7 (262)
Scrub/Edge	0 (3)	0 (3)	50 (12)	19 (16)	26 (47)	45 (49)	60 (5)	53 (34)	50.8 (67)	54.8 (102)
Forest	—	—	—	—	—	—	31 (106)	38 (112)	31 (106)	38 (112)
Oil palm	—	—	—	—	0.5 (937)	—	—	—	0.5 (937)	—
Totals	15.3 (99)	10.3 (123)	40 (101)	38.7 (127)	19.4 (1282)	38.7 (375)	45.5 (111)	45.5 (146)	24 (1593)	49 (771)

[a]After Lim *et al.* (1977) and Shirai *et al.* (1978).

[b]I: % rickettsial isolations.

[c]N: number of samples.

[d]S: % serological positives.

higher prevalence of antibodies against *R. tsutsugamushi* than did those in fringe habitats (scrub) or in typical rural villages (*kampongs*). It is clear that the transmission is active in *lalang* and less so in the villages, but the results for the scrub habitats (although an unusually high isolation rate was not obtained) tend to be obscured by both the close proximity of the study area to the *lalang* and the apparently free movement of rats between the two areas. The present study of rickettsiae in these rats provides a measure of rickettsial activity in trombiculids, but not necessarily in those mites that bite man. The isolation rates of rickettsiae from mammals and their antibody prevalence rates can be used as indications of the level of endemicity of this zoonosis, if not of its hyperendemicity or risk to man.

It is apparent that scrub typhus is a "manmade" disease. The tolerance of waste land is obviously an important factor in the creation of hyperendemic foci, and the subsequent utilization of waste land is to a great extent responsible for some of the infections. The individuals who become infected are those such as farmers, woodcutters, and military personnel whose habits bring them into contact with infected mite islands, indicating this is an occupational disease.

G. Other Zoonotic Diseases

A number of other zoonotic diseases occurring frequently in Malaysia have not been studied in detail. Salmonellosis, caused by the host of many *Salmonella* serotypes other than *Salmonella typhi* (*S. paratyphi* A and B), is considered a zoonosis. In Malaysia, the most common clinical manifestations of salmonellosis are gastroenteritis (71%), enteric fever (6.8%), meningitis (3%), localized abscesses (2.4%), urinary tract infections (0.9%), and others including the carrier state (16%) (Bhagwan Singh, 1967). Singh also showed that the commonest serotypes involved were *Salmonella typhimurium, S. derby, S. stanley, S. infantis, S. weltevreden, S. lexington, S. virchow, S. anatum, S. boris-morbiticans,* and *S. enteritidis.* Since 1965, *S. derby* and *S. weltevreden* have overtaken *S. typhimurium* as the cause of gastroenteritis outbreaks. Anandan *et al.* (1969) studied bacterial diseases in Orang Asli, and found 16 serotypes involved: *Salmonella newport, S. oslo, S. lexington, S. hvittingfoss, S. weltevreden, S. enteritidis* var. *chaco, S. infantis, S. javanica, S. typhosa, S. bovismorbificans, S. senftenberg* var. *newcastle, S. litchfiela, S. chingola, S. brunei,* and *Salmonella* 4, 5, 12:6. In 'healthy' Orang Asli communities from the fringe and deep jungles, 2.1% of the sample population were found to have *Salmonella* spp. in their stools. *Salmonella* spp. were isolated from 4.5% of all Orang Asli patients with diarrhea (Haug *et al.* 1969).

Ninety-six rectal swabs examined from chickens, dogs, goats, and cats were found negative for *Salmonella* spp. However, Bhagwan Singh (1967), in a study of 200 fecal specimens and 51 mesenteric lymph node samples from 251 pigs, isolated *S. anatum*, *S. bovis-morbificans*, and *S. weltevreden* once each from the feces, and *S. anatum* and *S. paratyphi* once each from the lymph nodes. Of 86 *Rattus rattus diardii* fecal samples examined, *Salmonella oslo* and *S. weltevreden* were isolated once each; 14 *R. rattus jalorensis*, 7 *R. rattus argentiventer*, and 7 *R. rattus exulans* examined were all negative. *S. derby* and *S. typhimurium* were isolated once each from feces of 90 sheep. Cattle (57), buffalo (51), goats (10), and a flying lemur (*Galopteras varigatus*) were all negative. Jegathesan *et al.* (1976) isolated *S. typhimurium* and *S. schwazengrund* once each from 38 shellfish, which are usually eaten by Malaysians in a partially cooked state.

The *Salmonella* spp. isolated from wild and domestic animals and shellfish, specifically *S. derby*, *S. weltevreden*, and *S. typhimurium*, have also been isolated from patients with salmonellosis. Cercarial dermatitis is also occasionally seen, especially among rice planters. Farmers who work in their flooded rice fields are infected by cercariae of *Schistosoma spindale* (Buckley, 1938), *Trichobilharzia* sp., and other species of avian and mammalian schistosomes (Basch, 1964). The snail intermediate hosts of these schistosomes are commonly found in the rice fields of Negri Sembilan. The legs, ankles, and arms are affected because they are in contact with the water during rice planting.

III. Summary

Zoonotic parasitic and other microbial diseases most often afflict rural communities in Malaysia, as they are intimately associated with occupational and social activities which bring man into direct or indirect contact with animal reservoir hosts and their respective pathogens. Control efforts directed at some of these diseases, such as subperiodic *Brugia malayi*, have been rather unsuccessful; in light of the problems identified, more effective strategies are needed. Considerable numbers of infected reservoir animals of the respective pathogens exist in the various ecosystems, maintaining the enzootic cycle; human infection occurs when man encroaches on animal habitats. In many instances, once infected man can maintain the transmission cycle within his own community (as in Brugian filariasis). In others (such as leptospirosis), the chances of transmission to the human community are remote. When man becomes a host to the infection, as in angiostrongyliasis and pentastomiasis, the infection then dead ends, and the medical significance is more individual than communal. Although some of the zoonoses are serious and potentially fatal, others such as cercarial dermatitis are mild, causing only transient pathological conditions.

References

Anandan, J., Lim, T. W., and Haug, N. L. (1969). Studies of bacterial disease in West Malaysian Orang Asli (Aborigines): previously unrecorded *Salmonella* serotypes. *Med J. Malaya* **23**, 269–271.

Audy, J. R. (1948). Natural history and scrub typhus. *Malay. Nat. J.* **3**, 114–129.

Audy, J. R. (1961). The ecology of scrub typhus. *In* "Studies in Disease Ecology" (J. M. May, ed.). Hafner, New York.

Basch, P. F. (1964). Some Malayan schistosomes. *Med. J. Malaya* **19**, 45.

Bhagwan Singh, R. (1967). Human *Salmonella* infections in Malaysia Barat. *Med. J. Malaya* **22**, 118–129.

Bhaibulaya, M., and Cross, J. H. (1971). *Angiostrongylus malaysiensis* (Nematoda: Metastrongylidae), a new species of rat lung-worm from Malaysia. *Southeast Asian J. Trop. Med. Public Health* **2**, 527–533.

Bisseru, B., Gill, S. S., and Lucas, J. K. (1972). Human infection with rat lungworm, *Angiostrongylus cantonensis* (Chen, 1935) in West Malaysia. *Med. J. Malaya* **26**, 164–166.

Buckley, J. J. C. (1938). On a dermatitis in Malaysia caused by the cercariae of *Schistosoma spindale* Montgomery, 1906. *J. Helminthol.* **16**, 117.

Cadigan, F. C., Andre, R. G., Bolton, M., Gan, E., and Walker, J. S. (1972). The effect of habitat on the prevalence of human scrub typhus in Malaysia. *Trans. R. Soc. Trop. Med. Hyg.* **66**, 582–587.

Davis, G. M., and Greer, G. J. (1980). A new genus and two new species of Triculinae (Gastropoda: Prosobranchia) and the transmission of a Malaysian mammalian *Schistosoma* sp. *Proc. Acad. Nat. Sci. Philadelphia* **132**, 245–276.

Dohany, A. L., Lim, B. L., and Huxsoll, D. L. (1979). Vectors of scrub typhus and their hosts on a mature oil palm estate. *Southeast Asian J. Trop. Med. Public Health* **10**, 510–513.

Dondero, T. J., Mullin, S. W., and Balasingam, S. (1972). Early clinical manifestations in filariasis due to *Brugia malayi*: observations on experimental infections in man. *Southeast Asian J. Trop. Med. Public Health* **3**, 569–575.

Edeson, J. F. B., and Wharton, R. H. (1958). The experimental transmission of *Wuchereria* infection from man to animals. *Proc. Int. Congr. Trop. Med. Malaria, 6th* **2**, 466–471.

Edeson, J. F. B., Wharton, R. H., and Buckley, J. J. C. (1955). Filarial parasites resembling *Wuchereria malayi* in domestic and forest animals in Malaya. *Trans. R. Soc. Trop. Med. Hyg.* **46**, 604–605.

Greer, G. J., Ow-Yang, C. K., Inder-Singh, K., and Lim, H. K. (1980). Discovery of a site of transmission of a *Schistosoma japonicum*-like schistosome in Peninsular Malaysia. *Trans. R. Soc. Trop. Med. Hyg.* **74**, 425.

Greer, G. J., Lim, H. K., and Ow-Yang, C. K. (1980a). Report of a freshwater hydrobiid snail from Pahang, Malaysia: a possible host of schistomes infecting man. *Southeast Asian J. Trop. Med. Public Health* **11**, 146–147.

Harrison, J. L., and Audy, J. R. (1951a). Host of the mite vectors of scrub typhus. I: A checklist of recorded hosts. *Ann. Trop. Med. Parasitol.* **45**, 171–185.

Harrison, J. L., and Audy, J. R. (1951b). Host of the mite vectors of scrub typhus. II: An analysis of the list of recorded hosts. *Ann. Trop. Med. Parasitol.* **45**, 186–194.

Haug, N. L., Davis, C. E., Anandan, J., and Lim, T. W. (1969). Studies of bacterial disease in West Malaysian Orang Asli. Distribution of enteropathogens. *Med. J. Malaya* **24**, 24–31.

Heyneman, D., and Lim, B. L. (1967a). Lack of cross-infection immunity as evidence for biological specificity among three geographical strains of *Angiostrongylus cantonensis* (Nematode: Metastrongylidae). *Med. J. Malaya* **21**, 375–377.

Heyneman, D., and Lim, B. L. (1967b). *Angiostrongylus cantonensis:* proof of direct transmission with its epidemiological implications. *Science* **158,** 1057–58.

Hsieh, H. C. (1967). *Angiostrongylus cantonensis* and eosinophilic meningitis or meningoencephalitus due to its infections. *Taiwan Clin. Med.* **3,** 1–5.

Hubert, A. A., and Baker, H. J. (1963). Studies on the habitats and populations of *Leptotrombidium* (*Leptotrombidium*) *akamushi* and *L. (L.) deliense* in Malaya. (Acarina: Trombiculidae). *Am. J. Hyg.* **78,** 131–142.

Jegathesan, M., Lim, T. W., Lim, E. S., Ding, S. H., and Lim, B. L. (1976). Bacterial enteropathogens in Malaysian shellfish. *Trop. Geogr. Med.* **28,** 91–95.

Joseph, P. G. (1979). Leptospirosis in animals in West Malaysia. *Malays. J. Pathol.* **2,** 15–21.

Kurihara, T., and Oemijati, S. (1975). Timor type microfilaria found in Flores island, Indonesia. *Jpn. J. Parasitol.* **2,** 78–80.

Leong, S. H., Murugesu, R., and Chong, K. C. (1975). Schistosomiasis in the Orang Asli (a report of 9 cases). *Proc. Malaysian–Singapore Congr. Med.,* 10th, **10,** 184–186.

Lim, B. L. (1967). Occurrence of *Angiostrongylus cantonensis* in rats around Kuching, Sarawak. *Ann. Trop. Med. Parasitol.* **61,** 429–431.

Lim, B. L., and Heyneman, D. (1968). Further cross-infection immunity studies of three strains of *Angiostrongylus cantonensis. Proc. Semin. Filariasis Immunol. Parasit. ʼnfect.,* pp. 68–72.

Lim, B. L., Lim, T. W., and Yap, L. F. (1976). *Angiostrongylus malaysiensis* from Tauran, Sabah with reference to the distribution of the parasite in Malaysia. *Southeast Asian J. Trop. Med. Public Health* **7,** 384–389.

Lim, B. L., and Mak, J. W. (1978). Non-human primates as reservoirs of zoonotic diseases with special references to Brugian filariasis in Peninsular Malaysia. *In* "Recent Advances in Primatology; Vol. 4, *Medicine*" (D. J. Chivers, and E. H. R. Ford, eds.), pp. 55–65. Academic Press, London.

Lim, B. L., Muul, I., and Chai, K. S. (1977). Zoonotic studies of small animals in the canopy transect at Bukit Lanjan Forest Reserve, Selangor, Malaysia. *Malay. Nat. J.* **31,** 127–139.

Lim, B. L., Ow-Yang, C. K., and Lie, K. J. (1965). Natural infection of *Angiostrongylus cantonensis* in Malaysian rodents and intermediate hosts and preliminary observations on acquired resistance. *Am. J. Trop. Med. Hyg.* **14,** 610–617.

Lim, B. L., Yap, L. F., Krishnasamy, M., Ramachandran, P., and Mansor, S. (1978). Freshwater snail consumption and angiostrongyliasis in Malaya. *Trop. Geogr. Med.* **30,** 241–246.

Mak, J. W., Cheong, W. H., Hassan, A. O., Sivanandam, S., and Mahadevan, S. (1977). Filariasis in Perlis, Peninsular Malaysia. *Med. J. Malays.* **31,** 198–203.

Mak, J. W., Yen, P. K. F., Lim, K. C., and Ramiah, N. (1980). Zoonotic implications of cats and dogs in filarial transmission in Peninsular Malaysia. *Trop. Geogr. Med.* **32,** 259–264.

Murugesu, R., and Por, P. (1973). The first case of schistosomiasis in Malaysia. *Southeast Asian J. Trop. Med. Public Health* **4,** 519–523.

Murugesu, R., Wang, F., and Dissanaike, A. S. (1978). *Schistosoma japonicum*-type infection in Malaysia—report of the first living case. *Trans. R. Soc. Trop. Med. Hyg.* **72,** 389–391.

Nadchatram, N. (1970). Correlation of habitat, environment and colour of chiggers, and their potential significance in the epidemiology of scrub typhus in Malaysia (Prostigmata: Trombiculidae). *J. Med. Entomol.* **7,** 131–144.

Oemijati, S., and Lim, K. T. (1966). Filariasis in Timor. Pacific Science Congress, 11th. *Maj. Kedokt. Indones.* **21,** 67–73.

Partono, F., Dennis, D. T., Purnomo, and Atmosoedjono, S. (1977). *Brugia timori:* experimental infection in some laboratory animals. *Southeast Asian J. Trop. Med. Public Health* **8,** 155–157.

Poynton, J. O., and Hodgkin, E. P. (1939). Two microfilariae of the Kra monkey (*Macaca irus*). *Trans. R. Soc. Trop. Med. Hyg.* **32,** 555–556.

Prathap, K., Lau, K. S., and Bolten, J. M. (1969). Pantastomiasis: a common finding at autopsy among Malaysian Aborigines. *Am. J. Trop. Med. Hyg.* **18**, 20–27.

Punyadasni, V., and Punyagupta, S. (1961). Two cases of eosinophilic meningitis following ingested raw snails possibly due to *Angiostrongylus cantonensis*. *Med. Assoc. Thailand* No. 26.

Punyagupta, S. (1965). Eosinophilic meningoencephalitis in Thailand: Summary of nine cases and observations on *Angiostrongylus cantonensis* as a causative agent and *Pila ampullacea* as a new intermediate host. *J. Trop. Med. Hyg.* **14**, 370–374.

Self, J. T. (1969). Biological relations of the Pentastomida: A bibliography of the Pentastomida. *Exp. Parasitol.* **24**, 63–119.

Self, J. T. (1972). Pentastomiasis: host responses to larval and nymphal infections. *Trans. Am. Micros. Soc.* **91**, 2–8.

Shirai, A., Robinson, D. M., Lim, B. L., Dohany, A. L., and Huxsoll, D. L. (1978). *Rickettsia tsutsugamushi* infections in chiggers and small mammals on a mature oil palm estate. *Southeast Asian J. Trop. Med. Public Health* **9**, 356–359.

Smith, C. E. G., Turner, L. H., Harrison, J. L., and Broom, J. C. (1961a). Animal leptospirosis in Malaya. 1. Methods, zoogeographical background, and broad analysis of results. *Bull. W.H.O.* **24**, 5–21.

Smith, C. E. G., Turner, L. H., Harrison, J. L., and Broom, J. C. (1961b). Animal leptospirosis in Malaya. 2. Localities sampled. *Bull. W.H.O.* **24**, 23–34.

Tan, D. S. K. (1970a). Leptospirosis in rural West Malaysia. *Med. J. Malays.* **24**, 261–266.

Tan, D. S. K. (1970b). Leptospirosis in the ricefields of West Malaysia. *Southeast Asian J. Trop. Med. Public Health* **1**, 483–491.

Tan, D. S. K. (1970c). Clinical leptospirosis in West Malaysia. *Southeast Asian J. Trop. Med. Public Health* **1**, 102–111.

Tan, D. S. K. (1979). Leptospirosis in West Malaysia—epidemiology and laboratory diagnosis. *Malays. J. Pathol.* **2**, 1–6.

Tan, D. S. K., and Lopes, D. A. (1972). A preliminary survey of the status of leptospirosis in the Malaysian armed forces. *Southeast Asian J. Trop. Med. Public Health* **3**, 208–211.

Traub, R. (1960). Malaysian Parasites. XLV. Two new species of chiggers of the genus *Leptotrombidium*. *Stud. Inst. Med. Res. F.M.S.* **29**, 198–204.

Traub, R., and Wisseman, C. L., Jr. (1968). Ecological considerations in scrub typhus. *Bull. W.H.O.* **29**, 219–230.

Traub, R., and Wisseman, C. L., Jr. (1974). The ecology of chigger-borne rickettsiosis (scrub typhus). *J. Med. Entomol.* **11**, 237–303.

Upham, R. W., Hubert, A. A., Phang, O. W., Yusof bin Mat, and Rapmurd, G. (1971). Distribution of *Leptotrombidium (Leptotrombidium) arenicola* (Acarina: Trombiculidae) on the ground in West Malaysia. *J. Med. Entomol.* **8**, 401.

Watts, M. B. (1969). Five cases of eosinophilic meningitis in Sarawak. *Med. J. Malaya* **24**, 89–93.

Wharton, R. H. (1962). The biology of *Mansonia* mosquitoes in relation to the transmission of filariasis in Malaya. *Inst. Med. Res.* (Kuala Lumpur, Malaysia) Bull. No. 11, pp. 45–48.

4

Filariasis in Southeast Asia

V. ZAMAN

Department of Microbiology
Faculty of Medicine
National University of Singapore
Singapore

I. Introduction

This chapter is concerned mainly with the prevalence of human filarial infection in Southeast Asia. As an introduction, the history, morphology, life cycle, epidemiology, and laboratory diagnosis of the parasite are briefly covered. Experimental studies and chemotherapy are not discussed here because excellent reviews have appeared recently (Edeson, 1972; Deham and McGreevy, 1977; Hawking, 1979).

Filariasis in Southeast Asia is caused mainly by lymphatic-dwelling filarials belonging to the genera *Wuchereria* and *Brugia*. In the case of *Wuchereria* only one species (*W. bancrofti*) is involved; in *Brugia*, there are two species (*B. malayi* and *B. timori*). An animal filaria (*B. pahangi*) is capable of infecting humans (Edeson *et al.*, 1960), but the extent of the disease in human populations is not known.

II. History

The ancient Asian literature has many descriptions of elephantiasis, an important manifestation of filariasis. The Indian medical men attributed the enlargement of legs (*Sli pada,* Sanskrit) to derangement of three *doshas;* these were wind (*ratha*), phleghm (*kapha*), and bile (*pitha*). *Sli pada* of more than one year's duration was regarded as incurable. Indian writings also state that the condition occurred more commonly where stagnant water was present and mosquito breeding occurred. For treatment, the Indian physicians used blood letting (Hoeppli, 1959). In the islands of the Pacific, elephantiasis was attributed to many causes including heredity, the consumption of certain foods, and frequent contact with water. The patients rarely received treatment because they were regarded as incurable (Hoeppli, 1959). The ancient Malay literature did not discuss etiology, but gives the treatment of orchitis (and presumably elephantiasis) as the application of herbal ointments and plasters (Gimlette and Burkill, 1930). According to traditional Chinese medicine, the treatment for elephantiasis and lymphangitis (called *liu-huo* or "flowing fire" by native populations) consisted of acupuncture and administration of herbs that faciliated the removal of "heat" and "moisture." Among the herbs still used is an infusion of fresh eucalyptus leaves ("A Barefoot Doctor's Manual," 1977).

III. Morphology (Faust *et al.*, 1976; Anderson *et al.*, 1976)

A. *Wuchereria bancrofti*

Male worms are elongated and thread-like, measuring about 40 μm in length by 0.1 μm in cross section. The cuticle is smooth with five transverse striations. The cephalic extremity is dilated and has two rows of 10 papillae. The caudal extremity in males is curved; the ventral surface has 24 papillae. There are two unequal spicules measuring 0.2 and 0.6 mm, respectively. The female is between 80 and 100 μm in length and 0.2 to 0.3 μm in cross section. It has two ovaries lying posteriorly and leading to two uteri; the uteri open into a short vagina via two oviducts. The vulva lies from 0.8 to 0.9 mm from the anterior end. The proximal part of the uterus is filled with immature embryos. As the eggs pass to the distal end, the microfilariae are formed; these distend the egg shells and transform them into "sheaths." The sheaths, larger than the microfilariae, generally project beyond the anterior and posterior ends.

The microfilariae (Fig. 1C) measure 210–320 μm long and about 8 μm wide. The anterior end is rounded and the posterior end attenuated. When alive they move gracefully, and in stained preparations the outline is regular and smoothly curved. The column of cells inside are known as "nuclei;" these are large, discrete, and well separated from each other. There are no terminal nuclei at the tip of the tail. The sheath stains lightly.

The distinctive caudal morphology is the main morphological feature used for differentiation of infecting larvae (L$_3$) from other species (Fig. 2). There are three caudal papillae, two ventral and one dorsal. As the papillae do not lie in the same plane, all three papillae are not usually visible simultaneously. In profile only one or two papillae may be seen clearly, which causes confusion in diagnosis. The papillae are large and appear to be slightly constricted near the base giving them a pedunculated appearance.

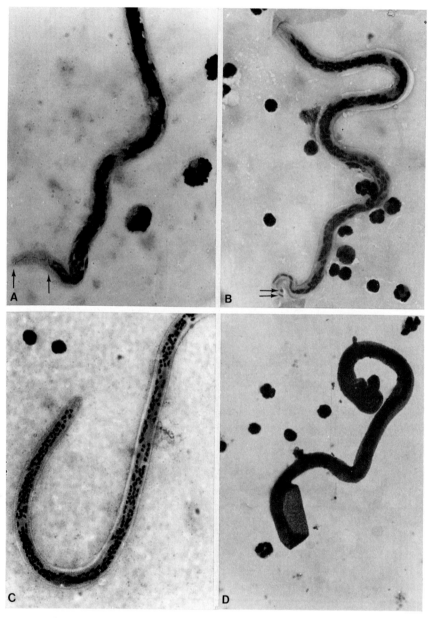

FIG. 1. (A) Microfilaria of *Brugia timori* showing the elongated cephalic space (marked by arrows) (× 870). Haematoxylin. (B) Microfilaria of *Brugia malayi* showing the terminal nuclei (marked by arrows) (× 870). Haematoxylin. (C) Microfilaria of *Wuchereria bancrofti* showing discrete nuclei (× 870). Haematoxylin. (D) Microfilaria of *Brugia malayi* showing intensely stained sheath (× 870). Giemsa.

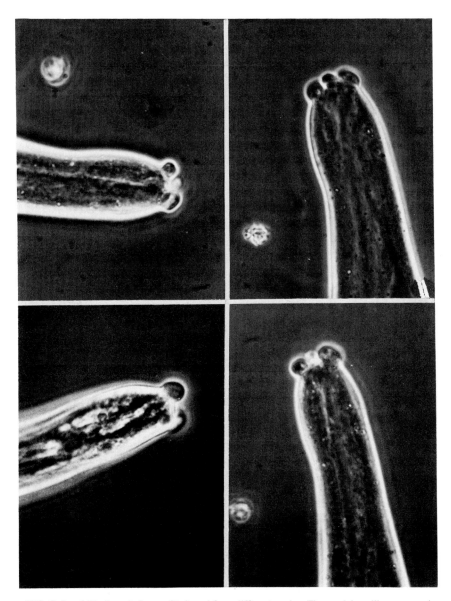

FIG. 2. L$_3$ of *Wuchereria bancrofti* viewed from different angles. The caudal papillae are prominent and slightly pedunculated. Phase contrast ($\times$ 780).

B. *Brugia malayi*

The adults resemble *W. bancrofti*. The cephalic extremity is dilated; caudal papillae are approximately 11 in number; the vulva is preoesophageal; the left spicule appears to be morphologically complex.

The microfilariae (Fig. 1B,C) measure 220–250 μm in length and about 6 μm in breadth. The outline is generally irregular and often appears twisted. The cephalic space is larger than in *W. bancrofti*. The body nuclei are coarse and tend to overlap. The tail has two terminal nuclei, the major characteristic of the species. The sheath is clearly visible in phase contrast preparation and stains darkly with Giemsa (Fig. 1C).

The infective Larvae (Fig. 3) are 1.3–1.7 μm long; unlike *W. bancrofti,* the caudal papillae are small and dome-shaped.

C. *Brugia timori*

Adult worms obtained from experimentally infected jirds (*Meriones unguiculatus*) were studied by Partono *et al.* (1977). These are filariform and creamy white with a distinct bulb-like head. The tail is long, tapered, and smoothly rounded. Circumoval papillae are arranged in circles with four on each side. Male body length is 13.4–22.8 (16.9) μm; body width at the anus is 53–62 (57) μm. Left and right spicules are unequal in length and dissimilar in appearance.

Female body length is 21.1–39.2 (26.7) μm; maximum width is 80–140 (99) μm. Numerous minute cuticular bones extend 127–184 (163) μm from tip of tail anteriorly.

The microfilariae (Fig. 1C) of *B. timori* differ from *B. malayi* (Fig. 1B,C) in greater body length, a long cephalic space with a length-to-width ratio of about 3:1. The subterminal and terminal nuclei are usually smaller than those of *B. malayi,* distending the surrounding cuticle only slightly.

In infecting larvae (Purnomo *et al.*, 1976), the head is slightly rounded and bears two rows of small papillae. The caudal extremity bears one conspicuous dorsal papilla and two less noticeable ventral papillae. The terminal papillae are broadly based and gently rounded as in *B. malayi*.

IV. Vectors

The vectors given for *Wuchereria bancrofti, Brugia malayi,* and *B. timori* (Table I) are based on a review by Ramalingam (1975).

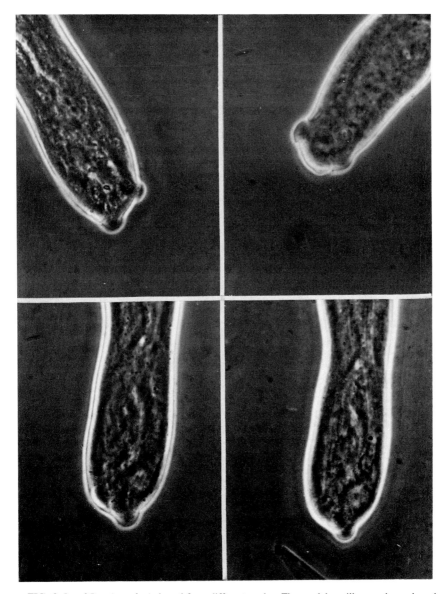

FIG. 3. L$_3$ of *Brugia malayi* viewed from different angles. The caudal papillae are dome shaped and not as large as *W. bancrofti*. Phase contrast ($\times$ 750).

TABLE I

Vectors of Filariasis in Southeast Asia

Country	Filarial species	Mosquito vectors
West Malaysia	*Wuchereria bancrofti*	*Culex quinquefasciatus*
		Anopheles letifer
		Anopheles maculatus
		Anopheles whartoni
East Malaysia	*Wuchereria bancrofti*	*Anopheles barbirostris*
		Anopheles leucosphyrus
Indonesia	*Wuchereria bancrofti*	*Culex quinquefasciatus*
		Culex bitaeniorhynchus
		Anopheles barbirostris
		Anopheles farauti
		Anopheles koliensis
		Anopheles punctulatus
		Anopheles bancroftii
		Aedes kochi
Indochinese peninsula	*Wuchereria bancrofti*	*Culex quinquefasciatus*
		Anopheles sinensis
Philippines	*Wuchereria bancrofti*	*Culex quinquefasciatus*
		Aedes poecilus
		Anopheles annularis
		Anopheles minimus
Singapore	*Wuchereria bancrofti*	*Culex quinquefasciatus*
Vietnam	*Wuchereria bancrofti*	*Culex quinquefasciatus*
Thailand	*Wuchereria bancrofti*	*Aedes niveus*
(nocturnal subperiodic forms)		
West Malaysia	*Brugia malayi*	*Anopheles campestris*
(periodic)		*Anopheles donaldi*
		Mansonia uniformis
		Mansonia annulifera
West Malaysia	*Brugia malayi*	*Mansonia dives*
(subperiodic)		*Mansonia bonneae*
		Mansonia annulata
		Mansonia uniformis
East Malaysia	*Brugia malayi*	*Mansonia dives*
(subperiodic)		*Mansonia bonneae*
Indonesia	*Brugia malayi*	*Mansonia annulata*
(periodicity undetermined)		*Mansonia indiana*
		Mansonia dives
		Mansonia bonneae
		Mansonia unformis
		Anopheles barbirostris
Indochinese peninsula	*Brugia malayi*	*Mansonia indiana*
Thailand	*Brugia malayi*	*Mansonia annulata*
		Mansonia uniformis

TABLE I (*Continued*)

Country	Filarial species	Mosquito vectors
		Mansonia indiana
		Mansonia dives
		Mansonia bonneae
		Anopheles barbirostris
Philippines	*Brugia malayi*	*Mansonia bonneae*
		Mansonia uniformis
Indonesia	*Brugia timori*	*Anopheles barbirostris*

V. Important Mosquito Vectors and Their Relationship to Human Ecology

A. *Culex quinquefasciatus* (Curtis and Feachem, 1981)

This species is generally regarded as urban, although it is occasionally re-corded in rural areas. It has benefited enormously from the industrialization and overcrowding of cities in all parts of Asia. Overcrowding has often led to the breakdown of the sewage disposal facilities and the contamination of drains with sewage and sullage. In addition to drains, the mosquitoes breed readily in pit latrines, bucket latrines, soakage pits used for washing water, water-filled recep-tacles, blocked streams that contain stagnant water, and sewage farms. In cities with proper sewage disposal systems, septic tanks act as excellent breeding grounds, especially when they have cracked or improper lids. Ponds that are contaminated with sewage and that also contain vegetation favor breeding more than those that are free of vegetation (Yao, 1975). Optimal breeding conditions occur when contamination rates reach a level of 1000 ppm of organic solids. However, not all *C. quinquefasciatus* breeding places are associated with sewage or sullage. In some rural areas in northern India, disused irrigation wells dug as part of the "grain revolution" in agriculture act as major sites of *Culex* breeding. Unfortunately, this species shows natural tolerance to D.D.T. and has also developed resistance to D.D.T., benzene hexachloride, dieldrin, and some organophosphorus compounds (Hamon and Mouchet, 1967). According to Ham-mon *et al.* (1964), resistance to insecticides has also played an important part in the wide prevalence of *C. quinquefasciatus* as insecticide-susceptible, competing species were eliminated.

B. *Mansonia* spp. (Burton, 1959–1960; Wharton *et al.*, 1962)

Many aquatic grasses and plants act as breeding sites for this mosquito (Fig. 4A). These include (i) floating plants such as *Pistia stratiotes, Sylvania auriculata,* and *Eichhornia crassipes;* (ii) floating and semifixed plants such as *Rattan* sp. (grass), *Gussieae repens, Isachne globosa, Hymenachne pseudointerrupta,* and *Panicum amplexicaules;* and (iii) fixed plants such as *Crinum thaianum* and *Thelypteris* sp..

The eggs are laid on the ventral surfaces of leaves floating in water and are cemented together to form typical clusters (Fig. 4A). The larvae hatch directly into water by breaking the apical portion of the cone-shaped egg (Fig. 4B). Larvae and pupae both obtain oxygen from the roots or other parts of aquatic plants (Fig. 5A,B). If deprived of the water plants, the larvae do not survive for more than a few days. *Mansonia dives, M. bonneae, M. annulata,* and *M. uniformis* are commonly found in swamp forests, and *M. annulata* in forest verges where open swamp and forest meet. In areas where *Mansonia* spp. act as the main vector, mechanical removal and destruction of aquatic vegetation is employed. However, aquatic plants often serve as a source of food for pigs, fishes, and crustaceans; their removal is, therefore, resented by rural people, and may have some adverse economic implications.

C. *Aedes poecilus*

This species prefers to breed in the axils of abaca and banana plants and is sometimes seen in tree holes. It is a night-biting mosquito and will enter houses for feeding, although it does not rest there during the day.

D. *Aedes niveus*

This species breeds in tree holes and bamboo stumps. Feeding occurs mostly during sunrise and sunset; in Malaya they are mostly canopy feeders.

E. *Anopheles barbirostris*

They breed in a variety of places including areas adjacent to rice fields, deep water containers, and wells. Because it does not rest indoors after taking a blood meal, the species is not readily susceptible to insecticide spraying.

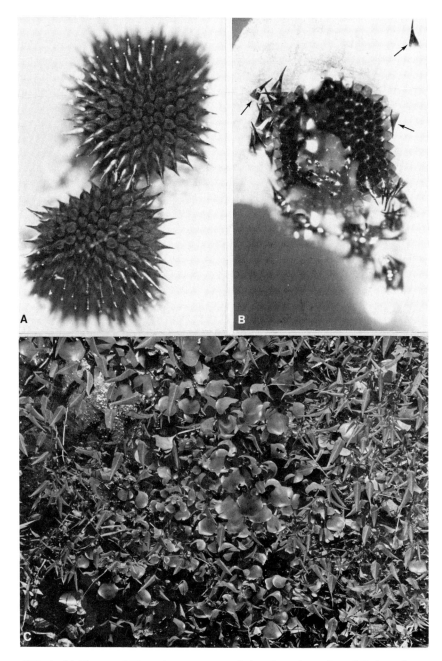

FIG. 4. (A) Clusters of *Mansonia* spp. eggs attached to the under surface of *Pistia* sp. leaves. (B) During the hatching of larva the apical portion of egg breaks off (marked by arrows). (C) Collection of water plants in a disused tin mine in Malaysia. Most of these plants are able to support *Mansonia* spp. mosquitoes.

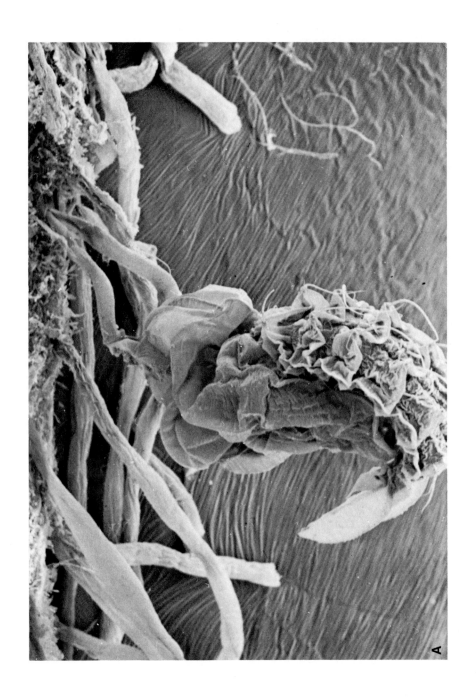

84

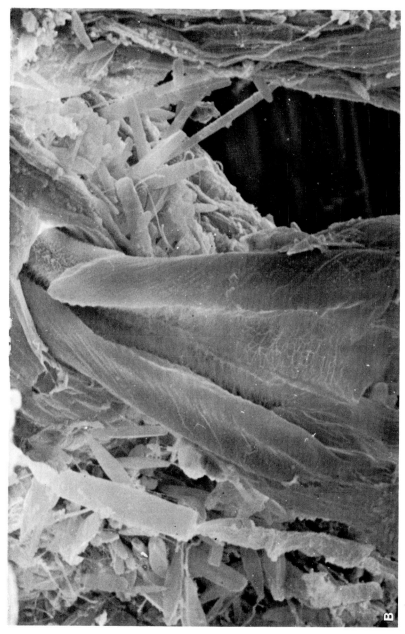

FIG. 5. (A) Scanning electron micrograph of a pupa of *Mansonia* spp. attached to water plants. (× 40). (B) Scanning electron micrograph of the breathing trumpet of the same pupa showing the part that has penetrated the plant tissues. (× 2400).

85

F. *Anopheles campestris*

This is a lowland species, most often found in alluvial plains and in broad river valleys and deltas. The breeding places are usually in deep water and frequently associated with vegetation. It may be found in burrow pits between coconut plantations, in ditches, in earth wells, and in corners of rice fields. It enters human habitation readily during the night, and significant numbers rest indoors.

G. *Anopheles leucosphyrus*

This is mainly a forest mosquito, often found in elevated areas in clear seepage pools. Adults do not rest in houses during the day but enter at night to bite, usually after 10 PM.

H. *Anopheles maculatus*

Found mainly in the foothills and rarely in the plains, it prefers to breed in clear seepage waters in clear sunlight. The female feeds both in outdoor locations and inside houses but does not rest indoors during daytime.

I. *Anopheles letifer*

A species found mainly in coastal plains, it prefers to breed in stagnant pools and drains. The female feeds in both outdoor and indoor locations but does not rest in houses during daytime.

J. *Anopheles whartoni*

This species resembles *A. letifer* in habits.

K. *Anopheles minimus*

Found mainly in the foothills, it prefers to breed in and along the edge of clear, slowly moving streams containing vegetation. The female feeds in both outdoor and indoor locations. It often rests in houses during the day, with preference for low resting places such as cots, along the lower part of walls, and floors.

L.   *Anopheles minimus flavirostris*

Usually found in foothills and hilly places, this species often breeds in clear sunlit streams. Adults rest indoors during the daytime.

M.   *Anopheles annulatus*

Found mainly in rice fields, stagnant pools, swamps and drains, it can rest in houses during the daytime.

N.   *Anopheles sinensis*

This is a zoophilous mosquito in Malaysia but in China prefers to bite man. It breeds in rice fields, clear water ponds, and ditches exposed to sun and containing vegetation.

VI.   Life Cycles

Filarial worms develop through five stages in their life cycle. The microfilariae, the diagnostic stage of the parasite, are found in the peripheral circulation. In this respect they often show nocturnal periodicity during which they circulate in the peripheral blood in the night and accumulate in the visceral blood, particularly the pulmonary blood vessels, during daytimes. On being ingested with the blood meal, the parasite undergoes further development if the vector is suitable. The suitability of the vector depends on various factors; the mechanisms that cause refractoriness in certain vectors have been reviewed by Denham and McGreevy (1977). The microfilariae lose their sheaths in the mosquito stomach and invade the stomach wall. Within 24 hr they migrate to the thoracic muscles where further development begins. Within the thoracic muscle, molting occurs, producing a stout first-stage larva. Another molt occurs in thoracic muscle before the parasite migrates to the head of the mosquito. The infective third-stage larva is fully developed in approximately 2 weeks time. The infective larvae migrate out from the proboscis when the mosquito takes a blood meal, entering the puncture wound made by the vector after the mouth parts have been withdrawn (Ewert, 1967). The larvae then reach the lymph glands and molt twice more before becoming adults, usually remaining in and around the lymph glands of the part of the body invaded. The adults develop primarily in the afferent vessels and subcapsular sinuses of the lymph nodes. Mating and subsequent discharge of microfilariae require several months. Sometimes the microfilariae do not appear in the peripheral blood until a year or more after the infection has been acquired.

VII. Periodicity

The number of microfilariae circulating in the blood corresponds to the biting activity of the vector. The nocturnal periodicity of *W. bancrofti* in many parts of Southeast Asia coincides with nightbiting by *C. quinquefasciatus*. Experiments (Katamine, 1970) have shown that the increase and decrease of microfilariae results from their periodic liberation from the lung capillaries. This in turn is connected to the physiological rhythms of man during work and sleep. A reversal in periodicity occurs if the sleep pattern is reversed.

VIII. Clinical Stages

The disease manifestation in filariasis passes through an acute to a chronic stage. The acute symptoms probably represent a hypersensitivity phenomenon from either the molting of the parasite in its development or a reaction to dead or dying worms. During the acute phase there may be fever, lymphadenitis, lymphangitis, orchitis, and epididymitis. Some patients develop urticarial (allergic) rash, generalized muscle pain, insomnia, anorexia, and headache. Microfilaemia often occurs during the acute phase of the disease and may be accompanied by eosinophilia.

The chronic stage of the disease, which may take many years to develop, is characterized by lymphoedema, hydrocele, and elephantiasis. If the lymphatics of the urinary bladder are involved, chyluria may develop, and if the peritoneal lymphatics are involved, ascites may occur. Enlargement of the lower limb is more common in *B. malayi* than in *W. bancrofti* infections, in which the genitalia are commonly involved.

The development of elephantiasis has been ascribed to repeated infections. These occur continually in endemic areas but only a small percentage of the population develops lesions. Host variability, therefore, appears to be an important factor. In a study done recently in Polynesia, 225 individuals were examined in an investigation of genetic influences on susceptibility to bancroftian filariasis.

Statistical analysis showed that there was a significant clustering of patients with filariasis within family groups. It was postulated, therefore, that genetic susceptibility to filarial disease occurs although no difference was found between susceptibles and nonsusceptibles using histocompatibility (HLA) antigens (Ottesen *et al.*, 1981).

A form of occult filariasis (Beaver, 1970) known as tropical pulmonary eosinophilia or eosinophilic lung is also seen in the region (Lie and Sandosham, 1968). Hypereosinophilia is an important feature of the condition. The patient generally has a chronic cough associated with asthma-like breathing difficulty that is more marked during the night. X rays of the lung often reveal mottling similar to miliary tuberculosis. The lung fields characteristically clear, and symptoms disappear, after a course of diethylcarbamazine (Fig. 6A,B). The pathology in this condition is produced by microfilariae, which have been observed in lung biopsy specimens. The microfilariae can be of various species, and the possibility that the reaction is caused by animal microfilariae has received some support in the past. However, it appears more likely that the hypersensitivity of the host, rather than the species of parasite, induces the reaction.

IX. Epidemiology

Wuchereria bancrofti has no animal reservoir although it has been developed experimentally in Taiwan monkeys (*Macaca cyclopis*) (Cross *et al.*, 1979).

Brugia malayi occurs in nocturnally periodic and subperiodic forms. The subperiodic form has also two types, the nocturnally subperiodic and diurnally subperiodic. Morphological differentiation of subperiodic and periodic *B. malayi* is difficult. The microfilariae of periodic strains ex-sheath more readily, and in Giemsa-stained preparations more ex-sheathed microfilariae are seen in the periodic strain. Differentiation is also possible using vector susceptibility as an index. In the case of the periodic strain, *Anopheles* spp. are more susceptible and *Mansonia* spp. more resistant; the situation is reversed with subperiodic strains. Although periodic infection can be transmitted experimentally to cats, rhesus monkeys, and gerbils, it appears that the main reservoir is human. The subperiodic form of *B. malayi* occurs as a natural infection in various domestic and wild animals and thus is a true zoonosis. Among the animals found to be naturally infected are dusky leaf monkey (*Presbytis* spp.), long-tailed macaque (*Macaca irus*), domestic cat (*Felis domestica*), civet cat (*Paradoxurus hermaphroditus*), and pangolin (*Manis javanica*) (Wilson, 1961).

The domestic cat has been used extensively to study the host–parasite relationships of *B. malayi* and *B. pahangi*. The response in cats appears to vary greatly,

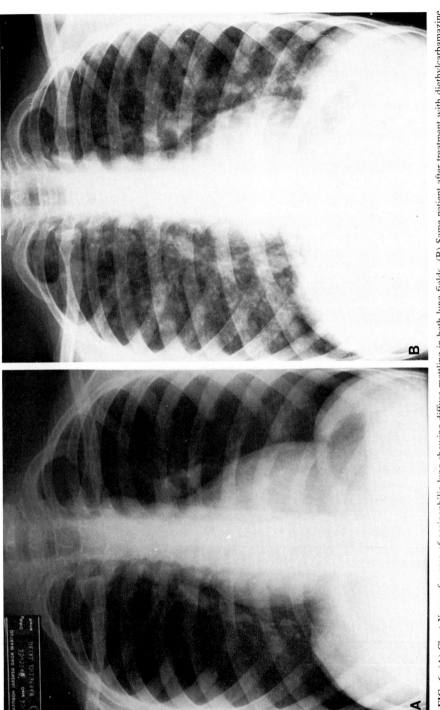

FIG. 6. (A) Chest X ray of a case of eosinophilic lung showing diffuse mottling in both lung fields. (B) Same patient after treatment with diethylcarbamazine. Mottling disappears after treatment.

and "English" cats have been found to be generally more resistant to infection than "Malaysian" cats (Denham and McGreevy, 1977). Zaman and Chellappah (1970) also studied microfilaremia levels in cats after single and multiple infections with *B. pahangi* in Singapore. Susceptibility varied greatly from animal to animal; in some animals, persistently high microfilaremia was produced, with one animal reaching a level of 1700 mf/20 cmm of blood; in others only low, transitory peaks were produced. Experimental infection of monkeys with *Brugia malayi* produced varying degrees of microfilaemia among the animals (Wong *et al.*, 1977). In endemic areas, human response to infection is also quite variable; patients may be seen showing microfilaemia without disease, microfilaemia with disease, and disease without microfilaremia.

The sequence of events in a susceptible cat or human are depicted in Fig. 7, in which vector I transmits L_3 (third-stage larvae) to host I. In host I there is a prepatent period which is followed by a patent period if the host is susceptible. The patent period lasts for a variable period of time before it is terminated. During the microfilaremic stage, the infection can be transmitted to other animals or back to the same animal. This cyclical transmission maintains the infection in a given community, and, if it is uninterrupted, the animal and/or human reservoir will continue to grow in a widening geographical range. The patent period is followed by a postpatent period during which the microfilariae are absent from the blood stream although adults may be living in the tissues. The mechanism involved in the termination of microfilaremia is not clearly understood. Both antibodies and cell-mediated immunity may have a role.

X. Laboratory Diagnosis

Microfilariae can be demonstrated by obtaining 20–60 μm of peripheral blood at the appropriate time and streaking it on slides which are then dehemoglobinized and stained. This method apparently has disadvantages (Denham *et al.*, 1971) that include negative diagnosis in low microfilaremia and possible loss during fixing and staining. For more accurate diagnosis, concentration techniques are preferred; although the method described by Knott (1939) gives good results, the microfilariae are concentrated with blood cell debris that may obscure the parasites. The most useful concentration method is the membrane filtration technique (Chularerk and Desowitz, 1970). A modification of this technique is used in the Institute for Medical Research, Kuala Lumpur, Malaysia, and is reproduced here by courtesy of Dr. Mak Joon Wah.

1. 1 ml of heparinized blood is diluted with 9 ml of normal saline in a 10-ml syringe.

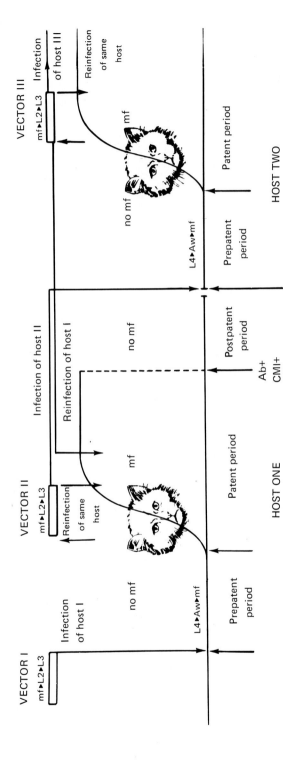

FIG. 7. The sequence of events during infection with *Brugia malayi* in cats, and the possible transmission routes in nature.

2. This solution is passed slowly through the Nucleopore® polycarbamate membrane (5-μm pore size, 25-mm diameter) assembled in a Swin-Lok holder assembly.
3. A further 10 ml of normal saline is slowly passed through the membrane.
4. 5–10 ml of air is then passed through the membrane.
5. The Swin-Lok assembly is carefully detached and the membrane removed. The membrane is placed on a glass slide, and airdried (with a hair dryer).
6. The dried membrane is fixed for 30 sec with methanol, washed by dipping momentarily in water, and then stained with Field's Stain by the following method:
   a. Field's Stain A for 1 sec
   b. Wash in water
   c. Field's Stain B for 1 sec
   d. Wash in water
   e. Field's Stain A again for 1 sec
   f. Wash in water and dry slide
7. The stained membrane is examined directly under the microscope or mounted in a drop of immersion oil with a cover slip before examination. Other body fluids such as chylous urine may be examined by this method.

XI. Distribution in Southeast Asia

A. Thailand

Iyengar (1953) made an extensive survey of filariasis in Thailand and reported the presence of *Brugia malayi* in the peninsular region, a narrow strip of land situated between the Indian Ocean on the west and South China Sea on the east. In this survey, 863 of 4112 persons examined were positive for microfilariae, and 215 had filarial disease. Elephantiasis of the leg, the most common manifestation, was rarely associated with the elephantiasis of the arm. Apart from two cases of hydrocele, genital afflictions involving the penis, scrotum, or testes were not found. These findings concur with those made in other parts of the world which indicate that the incidence of microfilaremia is much lower in persons with filarial disease than in those without. The earliest age at which elephantiasis was observed was 13 years. Nine species of mosquitoes (four *Mansonia* spp. and five *Anopheles* spp.) were incriminated. The infection rates in different vectors ranged between 3 and 17%. Harinasuta *et al.* (1970) studied *B. malayi* infection in southern Thailand and reported the concurrence of infection all along the east coast in the seven provinces of Thailand. In Bangluke canton of Chumporn Province, a microfilarial infection rate of 10.8% was obtained for the nocturnal periodic form. In Chumporn Province as a whole the mean microfilarial and elephantiasis rates were 2.3 and 1.3%, respectively. Elephantiasis was more common in females, with a sex ratio of 1:3. *Mansonia uniformis, M. indiana, M. annulata,* and *M. bonneae* were the main vectors.

The people in this whole area are poor. There are many collections of water with aquatic plants in them. Walking and cycling are the usual means of travel. In wet seasons, many villages become inaccessible even by jeep because of the muddy conditions; in dry seasons, motorized transport to villages can be used.

A nocturnally subperiodic strain of *Brugia malayi* also occurs in southern Thailand (Vasuvat *et al.,* 1966; Guptavanij *et al.,* 1971). Narathivas, Nakarns-rithamaraj, and Chumporn were the provinces investigated. In Chumporn Province the mean microfilarial and elephantiasis rates were 2.3 and 1.3%, respectively. Elephantiasis was more common in females with a sex ratio of 1:3. 1.5 to 4.3% of the domestic cat population were infected with *B. malayi;* these probably acted as the main animal reservoir. It appears that Thailand also has a diurnally subperiodic strain in Chumporn Province (Guptavanij *et al.,* 1971), but the epidemiological aspects of this strain have not yet been determined. Chumporn Province consists mostly of cultivated rice fields, rubber plantations, and fields of other crops. There also are large freshwater swamps with many aquatic plants. The inhabitants, all racially Thai, usually live in houses that are on stilts. Walking and cycling are the main methods of transportation.

Bancroftian filariasis occurs in northern Thailand in areas near the Thai–Burmese border within Kanchanburi Province. The people in this area are mostly nomadic Thai-Karens. Their main occupations are hunting, rice farming, poultry rearing, and gathering forestry products. The area is semiforested and communication is poor. The survey in Sangka-buri district of Kanchanaburi Province, which is in the north of Thailand, revealed a microfilarial rate of 3.6–27.8%. The parasite is nocturnally subperiodic; the mosquito vector, which belongs to the *Anopheles niveus* group, showed an infection rate of 0.22%. Microfilarial rates in the human population are highest among males, with a ratio of 2:1. The youngest person found with microfilaremia was only 2 years old; the oldest 87. Disease manifestations were more common in males, and 8.7% of all persons examined had disease symptoms consisting primarily of hydrocele and funiculoorchitis (94.8%). Chyluria, edema of the legs, and low abdominal pain were found in some cases; there was no elephantiasis.

B. West Malaysia

Peninsular Malaysia has long been known to be endemic for filariasis (Wilson, 1961), and surveys have shown that infection occurs throughout the country in various rural and urban populations (Mak, 1976). It is now known that *Brugia malayi* occurs in two different forms, nocturnally periodic and subperiodic. The periodic form is endemic mostly in the coastal rice field regions and is transmitted chiefly by open swamp species of *Mansonia* and by *Anopheles* spp. such as *A. campestris* (Reid *et al.*, 1962). Natural infections in animals are rare, and the parasite is not regarded as a zoonosis; it is, however, possible to transmit the infection experimentally to laboratory animals such as gerbils. In addition to the Malay population, which is involved in rice farming, the parasite was detected among aborigines and rural Malays living in inland hill areas of Kelantan, Selangor, and Pahang. The lesions produced are mainly localized to the legs; enlargement of upper limbs and scrotum is uncommon, and chyluria does not occur.

The subperiodic strain is localized mainly along the riverine swamp forest regions in the states of Pahang, Perak, Selangor, and Johore. The chief vectors of the subperiodic strain are the swamp forest *Mansonia* spp. As mentioned earlier, subperiodic *B. malayi* has a large animal reservoir, and transmission from man to animal is easy; it is, therefore, a true zoonosis. The clinical manifestations are the same as in periodic *B. malayi*. *Wuchereria bancrofti* also occurs in two forms, urban, found in cities and towns such as Penang and Kuala Lumpur, and rural. The incidence of infection is low, and because of improvement in hygiene and sanitary conditions, transmission is probably at a very low level.

The rural form, the principal type, occurs in the aboriginal populations in Selangor, Negri Sembilan, Johore, Pahang, and Perak. In addition, foci have been found in some offshore islands such as Pulau Tioman and Pulau Aur (both off Johore). The rural strain is transmitted by *Anopheles maculatus, A. letifier,* and *A. whartoni* (Wharton *et al.*, 1963; Cheong and Omar, 1965). In contrast to other parts of Asia, elephantiasis caused by *W. bancrofti* is relatively uncommon. In comparison with other countries of Southeast Asia, the rural population of Malaysia has a higher standard of living. The majority of the rural population is Malay and lives in wooden houses built on stilts. The *kampongs* (villages) form a narrow fringe of cultivated land along the banks of various rivers, locations selected because of the readily available water and fertile soil. At the back of the *kampongs,* there usually are large areas of freshwater swamp forest containing many water plants which support *Mansonia* spp. In addition, water plants such as *Eicchornia* flourish in manmade lakes and excavations such as disused tin mines scattered throughout Malaysia. The communication system is generally good and most of Malaysia is open to motorized traffic throughout the year. In contrast, the aboriginal populations are difficult to manage because of their living conditions, nomadic nature, and inaccessible habitat.

The infection rates vary greatly from area to area. In heavily infected villages and rubber estates, rates may be as high as 36%. In areas where subperiodic *B. malayi* is endemic, the microfilaria rates tend to be higher where leaf monkeys (*Presbytis* spp.) are also infected (Mak Joon Wah, *personal communication*).

Wharton, Laing, and Cheong (1963) found *W. bancrofti* rates of 2 to 18% and *B. malayi* rates of 3 to 30% among the aborigines.

C.   East Malaysia

Zulueta (1957) surveyed Sarawak and found that both *Wuchereria bancrofti* and *Brugia malayi* were present. *W. bancrofti* was found only in some areas of the fourth division; *B. malayi* was detected in flat coastal regions along the large rivers and occasionally in the hills. The racial groups most affected were the Malays and Chinese living on the coast and in the estuaries of the large rivers. The Sea Dayak or Iban, the indigenous people who live in the hills and further inland, are occasionally infected. The prevalence among Malays is usually higher than among the Chinese. This is probably caused by a difference in habits, the Malays being primarily a rural population easily exposed to mosquitoes in their *kampong* houses. The Chinese, mostly traders, are urbanized and live in compact buildings that are well protected against mosquitoes.

In Sabah, surveys made by Barclay (1969) found both subperiodic *B. malayi* and *W. bancrofti* with microfilarial rates of 22.7 and 4.7%, respectively. In a more recent survey, *B. malayi* was also detected by Hii (1978) in the Beaufort district and Kuala Penyu.

D.   Singapore

One of the early surveys for filariasis was made by Danaraj *et al.* (1958) who examined 902 persons, mostly warded patients in the general hospital of Singapore. The microfilarial rates among the three major ethnic groups were Chinese 4.2%, Indians 6.8%, and Malays 5.7%. The higher rates among the Indians were attributed to their frequent visits to the endemic region in India. In contrast, it was felt that the majority of the Chinese and Malay populations acquired the infection in Singapore itself. In 1972, Colbourne and Ng surveyed some selected areas and found a microfilaria rate of 1.9%. It seems very unlikely that any transmission is occurring at present, because eosinophilic lung and other manifestations of filariasis have practically disappeared.

E.   Indonesia

Filariasis in Indonesia is an important public health problem because it has a wide distribution and high infection rates and is often associated with disease. All three species (*Wuchereria bancrofti, Brugia malayi,* and *B. timori*) are endemic. Initial filariasis surveys were made by Brug (1927), and the literature was reviewed by Lie (1970). *W. bancrofti* is prevalent in Western Irian (New Guinea) where it concurs with *B. malayi* on practically all the islands of Timor, Rote, Flores, and Sumba. *W. bancrofti* is endemic in major cities such as Jakarta (Lie and Rees, 1958). *B. malayi* is found mostly in rural coastal regions and low island areas. Both periodic and subperiodic forms occur and can coexist as they do in Bengkulen in South Sumatra (Lie *et al.*, 1960). *W. bancrofti* is associated with elephantiasis and hydrocele in Western Irian, but in Jakarta it seldom causes elephantiasis, although hydrocele is common (Lie, 1970). *B. malayi* is usually associated with recurrent lymphangitis, fever, scarring, and elephantiasis of the lower limbs (Partono *et al.*, 1977). Timor filariasis produces a serious disease consisting of recurring episodes of inguinal and femeral lymphadenitis, abscesses of lymph glands, and also elephantiasis, mainly below the knees (Dennis *et al.*, 1976). As in other parts of Indonesia, the microfilarial rates of *W. bancrofti* are generally lower in the younger age group (1–5 years) and rise gradually to a high level in the 11–20 age group (Lie, 1970). Rates vary from 10 to 16.3% in Jakarta and from 15% in Bengkulen to as much as 26.8% on the island of Pam. For *B. malayi*, the microfilarial rates vary from 0.6–33% in Sulawesi to 44.8% in Bengkulen, Sumatra.

In many parts of rural Indonesia the villages, usually located along roads or rivers, are often surrounded by rice fields or swamps. The houses are constructed of wood or bamboo with roofs of thatched palm leaves. Transportation by roads, available on some islands, is generally poor. Sanitary conditions are unsatisfactory in major cities such as Jakarta, allowing extensive breeding of *C. quinquefasciatus*. In Indonesia, people from Java have been encouraged to transmigrate to other islands. This movement from nonendemic to endemic areas has led to comparative studies of the disease between locals and immigrants. It appears that elephantiasis appears more frequently among the immigrants compared to the natives (Partono *et al.*, 1977). These observations indicate that either there are ethnic differences in pathogenicity or that the individuals who have not been previously exposed to infections tend to develop the lesions more readily.

F. Philippines

Brugia malayi infection has been reported from the islands of Palawan, Tawitawi group of the Sulu Islands, Mindanao, and Eastern Samar (Carbrera and Arambulo, 1973). The vectors are *Mansonia* spp. In Palawan, the breeding areas of *M. bonneae* appear to be deep swamps covered with giant pandanus plants. In Mindanao, *M. uniformis* and *M. bonneae* breed in shallow swampy areas planted with rice. *Mansonia* spp. are attracted to both carabao and human baits. Cats have been found to be infected with *B. malayi* in Palawan. The microfilarial rates in these areas range from 0.46 to 64%.

Wuchereria bancrofti is present on all the major islands, especially Luzon,

Lyte, Samar, Bohol, Palawan, and Mindanao. It is nocturnally periodic, and the main vectors are *Anopheles poecilus* and *A. flavirostris*. The relationship between *A. peocilus* and humans is especially interesting; the mosquitoes breed in water accumulations in the axils of such plants as abaca, banana, and pineapple, and humans working in these plantations are more likely to be exposed to infection. Abaca is grown in plantations that may be at a considerable distance from the workers' homes, and men often sleep on the plantations overnight during the growing and stripping of abaca. The mosquitoes breeding in the plants are attracted to the relatively few men present in these isolated areas, who consequently receive large number of bites. In this situation, filariasis becomes an occupational disease. In the mountain province of Luzon, *A. niveus* is probably involved in the transmission of *W. bancrofti*. The microfilarial rates, as in other areas, increase with age and range from 1.9 to 45%.

Clinical manifestations of *W. bancrofti* infections include elephantiasis of limbs and genitalia, hydrocele, and chyluria. Elephantiasis below the knees and enlargement of lymph glands is seen in *B. malayi* infections.

G.   Indo-Chinese States

Both *Brugia malayi* and *Wuchereria bancrofti* occur in Vietnam. The survey by Millie (1954) in the Red River delta revealed a nocturnally periodic *B. malayi* microfilarial rate of 0.8 to 19.6%. *W. bancrofti* showing nocturnal periodicity was found in Hanoi (2.7%) and in the middle Tonkin region (22.9%). Examination of concentrated blood samples revealed endemic foci of infection with *W. bancrofti* among the Montagnard tribesmen residing in areas north and west of Saigon, and among Cambodians in Du Dop, Song Be, Hon Quan, and Hinh Thank. The prevalence rate in the endemic regions ranged from 5 to 22%. No infection was demonstrated in Saigon or in the Mekong river district (Colwell *et al.*, 1970). Rates of seropositivity in U.S. military personnel were 14% in endemic areas as compared to 3% in apparently nonendemic areas.

In Laos, Tawil (1979) surveyed 27 villages in the Vietiane province; a total of 2339 persons (1372 males and 967 females) were tested using 20-µl blood samples. Only one positive case was detected showing *W. bancrofti* infection. No further information is available from Laos and Cambodia.

XII. Conclusions

Because filariasis is a mosquito-transmitted infection, ecological factors relating to vectors and their interactions with the animal and human hosts are very important. The ecological relationship between animals and man is also important wherever the parasite exists as a zoonosis. The nature of the parasite life cycle is such that the worm burden continues to build up in a given area, because of repeated infection so long as the vector population remains constant or increases. Increases in vector populations, especially of *Culex quinquefasciatus,* have occurred in many places and are directly related to man's behavior. However, not much research has been directed toward the relationship between human ecology and filariasis. That the need for this is obvious has been pointed out by Dunn (1974), who also outlined the type of study required.

In general, filariasis is a disease of the poor and underprivileged. Lower socioeconomic classes are affected in both the rural and the urban areas. A study of a rural area of the Philippines showed that when a crude index of socioeconomic status, reflecting the ownership of land, house, water buffalo, radio, etc., was used, people showing the lowest scores had the greatest chance of having filarial infection and clinical disease (Grove *et al.,* 1978).

In contrast to the increase of filariasis in depressed areas, an improvement in living conditions greatly reduces transmission. In Singapore, clinical filariasis is no longer seen because government housing with sanitary facilities is now available to most Singaporeans. Another example of the natural disappearance of filariasis due to improvement in standard of living is seen in Australia. *W. bancrofti* was probably introduced into northern Australia in 1800 with the importation of labor from the Pacific islands (Cilento and Richards, 1924). Subsequently, the disease became endemic in the coastal areas of Queensland, parts of New South Wales, and the Northern Territory. During the twentieth century, the prevalence rates were as great as 11.5%. After the turn of the century, the prevalence dropped steadily, and by 1949 the disease had become a rarity (MacKerras, 1958; McMillan, 1967). During this period the human reservoir became smaller and smaller until transmission finally ceased. Similarly, a survey in Kresek, West Java (Sri Oemijati *et al.,* 1978) recorded a very low incidence of filariasis compared to the situation approximately 10 years previously. During this period there was no drug treatment, insecticide spraying, nor any dramatic population movement; however, a well-organized irrigation system was developed, and conversion of the swamps to rice fields resulted in the decrease of breeding sites for *Mansonia* spp. mosquitoes and a subsequent decrease in filariasis. Therefore, there is no doubt that economic and educational improvement has a profound effect on the containment and, possibly, the ultimate disappearance of the infection.

Cultural habits may have strange effects on the control of disease. Nelson (1978) postulates that use of western style dress or increased affluence in poor countries of Africa render the disease no longer obtrusive, hence the public health authorities have become increasingly less interested in the disease. To change cultural habits is difficult. Traditionally, rural houses in Southeast Asia have many windows to allow free circulation of air. This in turn allows mosquitoes to come in and rest under furniture, behind doors, and in other dark places. An educational program directed toward the use of mosquito nets, or the alteration of housing so that sleeping rooms at least can be made mosquito-proof, would be very useful.

There seems to be no form of Asian traditional medicine with proven efficacy that could be used in the treatment of filariasis. The "traditional medicine" as practiced in many parts of Asia is often based on unscientific concepts, and without any controlled studies its value cannot be assessed. Diverting scarce resources to training in any practice of traditional medicine is, therefore, undesirable. There is no short cut to the scientific approach to the control of filariasis based on chemotherapy, education, sanitary improvement, and antimosquito measures. The sooner this is realized the better it will be for the people living in endemic regions.

References

Anon. (1977). "A Barefoot Doctor's Manual," pp. 341–343. Running Press, Philadelphia.

Anderson, R. C., Chabaud, A. G., and Wilmott, S. (1976). "CIH keys to the nematode parasites for vertebrates in Commonwealth", pp. 59–116. Agricultural Bureaux, England.

Barclay, R. (1969). Filariasis in Sabah, East Malaysia. *Ann. Trop. Med. Parasitol.* **63**, 473–488.

Beaver, P. C. (1970). Filariasis without microfilaraemia. *Am. J. Trop. Med. Hyg.* **19**(2), 181–189.

Brug, S. L. (1927). *Filaria malayi* n.sp. parasite in man in the Malayan Archipelago. *Far East Assoc. Trop. Med., Trans. Congr., 7th* **3**, 279.

Burton, G. J. (1959). Studies on the bionomics of mosquito vectors which transmit filariasis in India. *Indian J. Malariol.* **13**(⅔), 1–145.

Carbrera, B. D., and Arambulo, V., II. (1973). Human filariasis in the Philippines. *Acta Med. Philipp.* **9**, 160–173.

Cheong, W. H., and Omar, A. H. (1965). *Anopheles maculata*, a new vector of *Wuchereria bancrofti* in Malaysia (Pulau Aur) and a potential vector on mainland Malaya. *Med. J. Malaya* **20**, 74–84.

Chularerk, P., and Desowitz, R. S. (1970). A simplified membrane filtration technique for the diagnosis of microfilaraemia. *J. Parasitol.* **56**, 623–624.

Cilento, R. W., and Richards, R. E. (1924). Filariasis in Australia. *Med. J. Aust.* **1**, 325.

Colbourne, M. J., and Ng, W. K. (1972). An assessment of filariasis transmission in Singapore. *Southeast Asian J. Trop. Med. Public Health* **3**, 40–44.

Colwell, E. J., Armstrong, D. R., Brown, J. D., Duxbury, R. E., Sadun, E. H., and Legers, L. J. (1970). Epidemiologic and serologic investigations of filariasis in indigenous populations and American soldiers in South Vietnam. *Am. J. Trop. Med. Hyg.* **19**, 227–231.

Cross, J. H., Partono, F., Hsu, M. Y., Ash, L. A., and Oemijati, S. (1979). Experimental transmission of *Wuchereria bancrofti* to monkeys. *Am. J. Trop. Med. Hyg.* **28**(1), 56–66.

Curtis, C. F., and Feachem, R. G. (1981). Sanitation of *Culex pipiens* mosquitoes: A brief review. *J. Trop. Med. Hyg.* **84**(1), 17–25.

Danaraj, T. J., Schacher, J. F., and Colles, D. H. (1958). Filariasis in Singapore. *Med. J. Malaya* **12**, 605–612.

Denham, D. A., and McGreevy, P. B. (1977). Brugian filariasis: Epidemiological and experimental studies. *Adv. Parasitol.* **15**, 243–309.

Denham, D. A., Dennis, D. T., Ponnudurai, T., Nelson, G. S., and Guy, F. (1971). Comparison of a counting chamber and thick smear methods of counting microfilariae. *Trans. R. Soc. Trop. Med. Hyg.* **65**, 521.

Dennis, D. T., Partono, F., Purnomo, Atmosoedjono, S., and Saroso, J. S. (1976). Timor filariasis: Epidemiologic and clinical features in a defined community. *Am. J. Trop. Med. Hyg.* **6**, 797.

DeZulueta, J. (1957). Observations on filariasis in Sarawak and Brunei. *Bull. W.H.O.* **16**, 699–705.

Dunn, F. L. (1974). Human behavioural factors in the epidemiology and control of *Wuchereria* and *Brugia* infections. *WHO/FIL* 74/22.

Edeson, J. F. B. (1972). Filariasis. *Brit. Med. Bull.* **28** [No. 1 (Research in Diseases of the Tropics)], 60–65.

Edeson, J. G. B., Wilson, T., Wharton, R. H., and Laing, A. B. G. (1960). Experimental transmission of *Brugia malayi* and *B. pahangi* to man. *Trans. R. Soc. Trop. Med. Hyg.* **54**, 229–34.

Ewert, A. (1967). Studies on the transfer of infective *Brugia pahangi* larvae from vector mosquitoes to the mammalian host. *Trans. R. Soc. Trop. Med. Hyg.* **61**, 110–113.

Faust, E. C., Beaver, P. C., and Jung, R. C. (1976). Animal agents and vectors of human diseases 4th ed., p. 292. Lea & Febiger, Philadelphia.

Gimlette, J. D., and Burkill, I. H. (1930). *In* "The Garden's Bulletin, Straits Settlements: The Medical book of Malayan Medicine" (M. Ismail, trans.). **VI**(3), 105.

Grove, D. I., Valeza, F. S., and Cabrera, B. D. (1978). Bancroftian filariasis in the Philippine villages: Clinical, parasitological and social aspects. *Bull. W.H.O.* **56**, 975–984.

Guptavanij, P., and Harinasuta, C. (1977). The periodicity of *Brugia malayi* in South Thailand. *Southeast Asian J. Trop. Med. Public Health* **8**(2), 185–189.

Guptavanij, P., Harinasuta, C., Sucharit, S., and Vutikes, S. (1971). Studies on subperiodic *Brugia malayi* in Southern Thailand. *Southeast Asian J. Trop. Med. Public Health* **2**, 44–50.

Hamon, J., and Mouchet, J. (1967). *Culex pipiens fatigans* resistance to insecticides. *Bull. W.H.O.* **37**, 277.

Hamon, J., Adam, J. P., and Rickenbach, A. (1964). "*Culex pipiens fatigans* Wied and the Urbanization of West Africa". W.H.O. Seminar on *Culex pipiens fatigans*, Geneva.

Harinasuta, C., Charoenlarp, P., Sucharit, S., Deesin, T., Surathin, K., and Vutikes, S. (1970). Studies on Malayan filariasis in Thailand. *Southeast Asian J. Trop. Med. Public Health* **1**, 29.

Hawking, F. (1979). Diethylcarbamazine and new compounds for the treatment of filariasis. *Adv. Pharmacol. Chemother.* **16**, 129–193.

Hii, J. L. K. (1978). A re-survey of the prevalence of Malayan filariasis in South-west Sabah, Malaysia. *Med. J. Malays.* **33**, 26–29.

Hoeppli, R. (1959). "Parasites and Parasitic Infection in Early Medicine and Science," p. 526. Univ. of Malaya Press, Singapore.

Iyengar, M. O. T. (1953). Filariasis in Thailand. *Bull. W.H.O.* **9**, 731–766.

Katamine, D. (1970). Studies on the periodicity of microfilaria. *In* "Recent Advances in Researches on Filariasis and Schistosomiasis in Japan". Univ. of Tokyo Press, Tokyo/Univ. Park Press, Baltimore, Maryland.

Knott, J. I. (1939). A method for making microfilarial surveys on day blood. *Trans. R. Soc. Trop. Med. Hyg.* **23**, 191–196.

Lie, K. J. (1970). The distribution of filariasis in Indonesia. A summary of published information. *Southeast Asian J. Trop. Med. Public Health* **1**, 366–376.

Lie, K. J., and Rees, D. M. (1958). Filariasis in Indonesia: distribution, incidence and vectors. *Proc. Int. Congr. Trop. Med. Malaria, 6th* **2**, 361–370.

Lie, K. J., and Sandosham, A. A. (1968). The pathology of classical filariasis due to *Wuchereria bancrofti* and *Brugia malayi* and a discussion of occult filariasis. *Proc. Seminar Filariasis*

Immunol. Parasitic Infect. (A. A. Sandosham, and V. Zaman, eds.), pp. 125–133. Southeast Asia Regional Meeting on Parasitology and Tropical Medicine, 3rd, Univ. of Singapore.

Lie, K. J., Soegiarto, C., and Winoto, R. M. P. (1960). Filariasis in Bengkulen, Sumatra. *Penyelidikan diKetjamatan Talang Ampat dan Tais, Berita Departemen Kesihatan Republik Indonesia* **9**, 28–38.

Mackerras, M. J. (1958). The decline of filariasis in Queensland. *Med. J. Aust.* **1**, 701.

Mak, J. W. (1976). Epidemiology of filariasis in Malaysia. *Proc. IMR 75th Anniversary Symposium on Dengue, Filariasis, Malaria and Scrub Typhus*, 6–7th Feb., 1976. Inst. Med. Res., Kuala Lumpur.

McMillan, B. (1967). Is filariasis in the Northern Territory of Australia? *Med. J. Aust.* **2**, 243.

Mille, R. (1954). Nouvelles recherches sur l'incidence des filarioses humaines au Nord-vietnam. *Bull. Soc. Path. Exot. Ses. Fils.* **47**, 339–356.

Nelson, G. S. (1978). "Mosquito-borne Filariasis". *In* Medical Entomology Centenary, Symp. Proc. (1978), pp. 15–25. *Publ. R. Soc. Trop. Med. Hyg.*, London.

Ottesen, E. A., Nancy, R. M., MacQueen, M. J., Weller, P. F., Amos, D. B., and Ward, F. E. (1981). Familial predisposition to filarial infection—not linked to HLA-A or B locus specificities. *Acta Trop.* **38**, 205–216.

Partono, F., Oemijati, S., Hudozo, Joesoef, A., Clark, M. D., Durfee, P. T., Irving, G. S., Taylor, J., and Cross, J. H. (1977). *Brugia malayi* in seven villages in South Kalimantan, Indonesia. *Southeast Asian J. Trop. Med. Public Health* **8**(3), 400–407.

Partono, F., Purnomo, Dennis, D. T., Atmosoedjono, S., Oemijati, S., and Cross, J. H. (1977). *Brugia timori sp.n.* (Nematoda: Filarioidea) from Flores Island, Indonesia. *J. Parasitol.* **63**(3), 540–546.

Purnomo, Partono, F., Dennis, D. T., and Atmosoedjono, S. (1976). Development of the timor filaria in *Aedes togoi:* Preliminary observations. *J. Parasitol.* **62**(6), 881–885.

Ramalingam, S. (1975). Vectors of *Wuchereria bancrofti* and *Brugia malayi* in the South and Southeast Asian regions: their distribution, biology and control. *Ceylon J. Med. Sci.* **24**(1,2), 1–37.

Reid, J. A., Wilson, T., and Ganapathipillai, A. (1962). Studies on filariasis in Malaya: The mosquito vectors of periodic *Brugia malayi* in North-west Malaya. *Ann. Trop. Med. Parasitol.* **56**, 323–326.

Sri Oemijati, F., Partono, H., Hadi, T. T., Clarke, M. D., Gunning, J.-J., and Cross, J. H. (1978). *Brugia malayi* in Kresek, West Java, Indonesia: The effect of environmental changes on filarial endemicity. *Trop. Geog. Med.* **30**, 301–304.

Tawil, N. A. (1979). Microfilaria survey in Vietiane, Laos. *Southeast Asian J. Trop. Med. Public Health* **10**, 483–485.

Vasuvat, S., Guptavanij, P., and Harinasuta, C. (1966). Studies on the periodicity of microfilariae of *Brugia malayi* in Nakornsrithommaraj province. *J. Med. Assoc. Thailand* **49**, 16.

Wharton, R. H. (1962). The biology of *Mansonia* mosquitoes in relation to the transmission of filariasis in Malaya. *Bull. Inst. Med. Res., Fed. Malaya*, 1–113.

Wharton, R. H., Laing, A. B. G., and Cheong, W. H. (1963). Studies on the distribution and transmission of malaria and filariasis among aborigines in Malaya. *Ann. Trop. Med. Parasitol.* **57**, 235–254.

Wilson, T. (1961). Filariasis in Malaya—a review. *Trans. R. Soc. Trop. Med.* **55**(1), 108–129.

Wong, M. M., Guest, M. F., Lim, K. C., and Sivanandam, S. (1977). Experimental *Brugia malayi* infection in the Rhesus monkey. *Southeast Asian J. Trop. Med. Public Health* **8**(2), 265–273.

Yao, K. M. (1975). Mosquito breeding in oxidation ponds. *Proc. Nat. Symp. Waste Water Disposal*, p. 56–61. Univ. of Engineering and Technology, Lahare.

Zaman, V., and Chellappah, W. T. (1970). Microfilaraemia levels in cats after single and multiple infections with *Brugia pahangi*. *Southeast Asian J. Trop. Med. Public Health* **1**(2), 293.

5

Intestinal Capillariasis in the Philippines and Thailand

JOHN H. CROSS

United States Naval Medical Research Unit No. 2
Manila, Philippines

MANOON BHAIBULAYA

Faculty of Tropical Medicine
Mahidol University
Bangkok, Thailand

I. Introduction

Epidemics associated with intestinal helminthic infections are usually uncommon, but in the Philippine Islands in the middle of 1965 an outbreak of the disease now known as intestinal capillariasis or capillariasis philippinensis occurred. For several years this created a challenge to physicians, public health workers, and biomedical scientists.

II. History

A. Philippines

1. SUPERSTITIONS

In the *barrio* (village) of Pudoc West, Tagudin, in the province of Ilocos Sur, Northern Luzon, an increasing number of the population began to experience gastroenteritis characterized by gurgling stomach, abdominal pain, and diarrhea. After 1 or 2 months the symptoms increased, and the afflicted began to die of a wasting illness. The villagers became alarmed and believed that they were all destined to die of the disease they now called "The Mystery Disease of Pudoc." They considered the village to be cursed because of offenses committed against the god which according to legend lived in the nearby Amburayan River.

There were two versions of what had caused the curse on the *barrio*. The most widely accepted explanation was associated with a mango tree. It was said that while some villagers were cutting a large branch from the mango tree two children of the river god had been killed as they passed under the falling branch. In retribution, the river god condemned the village, saying that all who lived in Pudoc West would die of a mysterious disease. The second version said the *barrio* people were doomed because they had killed and eaten a water buffalo that had accidentally washed from the river into a Pudoc West lagoon but had belonged to the river god.

As a result of these superstitions, and the illness and deaths that were being witnessed, some of the *barrio* residents moved to other *barrios,* abandoning their homes and fields (Fig. 1). Others stayed in the *barrio* and, to protect themselves from the evil spell, hung talismans such as rice-hull stuffed dolls and crude bamboo crosses on their houses (Fig. 2). They believed that these would ward off the evil spirits. For further protection, two spiritualists, exorcists, or witch doctors known collectively in the Philippines as *herbularios* from the mountain areas

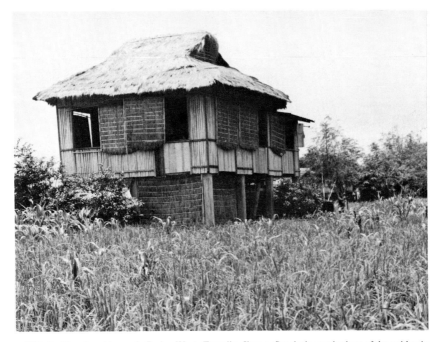

FIG. 1. Abandoned house in Pudoc West, Tagudin, Ilocos, Sur during early days of the epidemic of intestinal capillariasis.

of Central Luzon were hired to rid the *barrio* of the curse. The first step taken by the exorcists was to have erected adjacent to the mango tree (Fig. 3) a small shrine of bamboo and nipa with a bamboo altar. The witch doctors asked the villagers to pay tribute to the river god by placing contributions of money, pigs, chickens, and other food and valuables on the altar. This, they said, "would encourage the river god to lift the curse." However, the contributions disappeared into the pockets and stomach of the *herbularios* overnight, while the illness and death continued. The people were told that if they walked under the mango tree they would die, and consequently, they avoided the tree except to place offerings on the altar at the shrine.

The population in Pudoc West, as in most of the Philippines, is Roman Catholic, yet they continue to believe in the superstitions. The exorcists remained for many months deceiving the people and condemning health workers when they arrived in the area. The villagers realized that the exorcists were not helping but were afraid to challenge them. It was only after one of the witch doctors died of the "mysterious disease" that the people realized that they had been victimized and forced the remaining spiritualist out of the *barrio*.

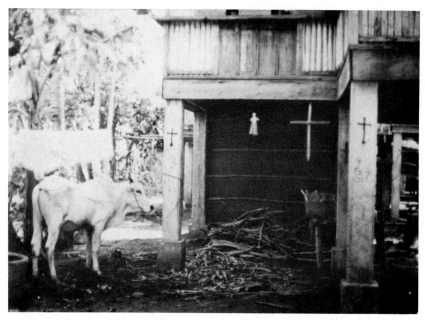

FIG. 2. *Barrio* house adorned with a doll talisman and crosses to ward off the curse cast upon the people by the god of the Amburayan River.

2. EPIDEMIC

Toward the end of 1966, a Catholic missionary priest from the municipality of Tagudin became alarmed by the reports coming from Pudoc West of the numerous deaths. He notified a senator who was a native of Tagudin, who in turn notified the Philippine Ministry of Health in Manila. Medical teams from Manila arrived in February 1967 and, unaware of the nature of the disease, took precautions when they visited the *barrio,* even to the extent of wearing face masks. They found the reports to be correct; a number of people were ill and an unusually high number of people, especially middle-aged men, had died of a chronic enteritis of unknown etiology during the previous 18 months.

The medical team first suspected that the deaths had resulted from an intoxication resulting from the consumption of a sugar cane wine known locally as *basi.* However, samples of the wine subjected to toxological examination were found to be safe for consumption. Bacteriological and other microbiological examinations of blood and stools were carried out, but no pathogens associated with gastroenteritis were found. Supportive or palliative treatment given was of little specific benefit. The etiology of the disease was finally determined at the autopsy

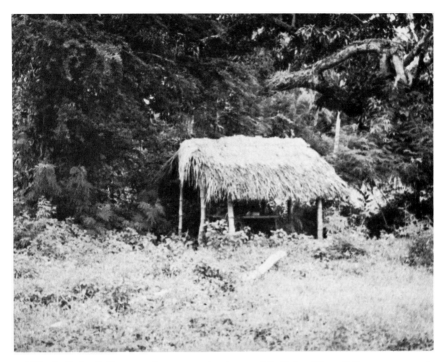

FIG. 3. Shrine built to pay homage to the river god in Pudoc West. Fallen mango tree in background, which legend states killed two children of the river god.

of a fatal case in which a large number of tiny worms, later identified as *Capillaria* sp., were found in the small intestine. About this time eggs, larvae, and adult capillarids were also found in stools of people with symptoms (Dizon and Watten, 1969). In a retrospective study conducted in Pudoc West, Detels *et al.* (1969) found that a total of 229 cases of intestinal capillariasis had occurred between August 1965 and January 1968, an attack rate of 32%. At least 60 people were thought to have died prior to February 1967.

Although the epidemic resulted in international recognition of the disease, the first report of the syndrome and the parasite responsible had been made a few years earlier. The victim was a 29-year-old male school teacher from the municipality of Bacarra, Ilocos Norte, approximately 150 km north of Pudoc West. He had a history of chronic alcoholism, recurrent ascites, emaciation, and cachexia, and had been suffering from an intractable diarrhea for 3 weeks prior to admission at the Philippine General Hospital in Manila. After he died a large number of worms was recovered at autopsy (Salazar, 1980). The parasite was not identified to any known species at the time, and Chitwood *et al.* (1964) made a preliminary report of the case at the First International Congress of Parasitology in Rome. These authors subsequently described the parasite as a new species, *Capillaria philippinensis* (Chitwood *et al.*, 1968).

B. Thailand

The first case of intestinal capillariasis in Thailand, reported in 1972, was an 18-month-old girl who was admitted to a Bangkok hospital with generalized edema (Pradatsundarasar *et al.*, 1973). The child was from Samut Prakarn Province, 25 km south of Bangkok. Following this, Thai physicians became aware of the disease and additional cases were reported in succeeding years.

III. Distribution and Prevalence

A. Philippines

Only one case of intestinal capillariasis was documented from Bacarra, Ilocos Norte, but retrospective investigations revealed that a number of people had died of the disease between 1963 and 1965. The physician who initially treated the school teacher had seen additional patients at about the same time, all with similar symptoms and all of whom had died. The relatives of the deceased were interviewed and the clinical records examined. Approximately 13 persons from three *barrios* had died with symptoms characteristic of capillariasis philippinensis. A stool survey was conducted in one of the *barrios,* Cabulalaan, at the time of the retrospective study (November, 1968), and although intestinal parasites were found in 100% of the population, *Capillaria philippinensis* was not present.

The first cases in the Tagudin area were from Pudoc West. After the disease was recognized, additional cases began appearing in neighboring *barrios* and towns; over 100 cases and 13 deaths occurred during the next few months. The majority of the cases in 1967 came from Tagudin and Bangar, an adjacent town south of Tagudin in La Union Province (Fig. 4). An emergency hospital and the Capillariasis Research Center were opened in Tagudin in June 1967, and cases began to come from other Ilocano provinces in Northern Luzon (Ilocos is the area of Luzon where people speak the Ilocano dialect). Between February and December 1967 there were 1037 parasitologically confirmed cases of intestinal capillariasis of which 77 resulted in death. By the end of 1968, the endemic area extended along the western coast facing the South China Sea from the province

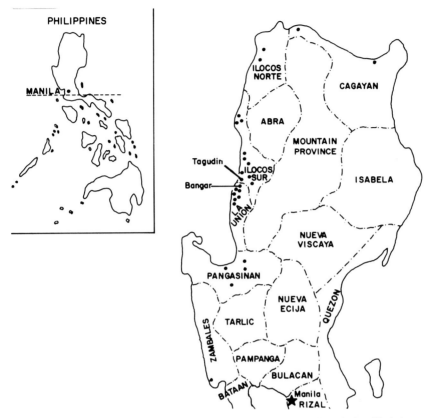

FIG. 4. Map of Northern Luzon indicating provinces and towns where intestinal capillariasis was endemic. Cases are still reported from some of the places indicated by the black dots.

of Pangasinan in the South to Cagayan Province in the north. During the next few years, cases continued to appear in the Tagudin/Bangar area, but in decreasing numbers after effective treatment was established. However, small numbers of cases continued to appear in the north. In 1972, a new focus of infection was found in an Ilocano population living in the area of San Narciso, Zambales Province, 150 km south of Tagudin. A few persons died before the disease was identified but over the next few years 32 patients were successfully treated (Tidball *et al.,* 1978). In 1978, a team conducting a survey for schistosomiasis identified another endemic focus in the municipality of Santiago, Agusan del Norte Province, Mindanao (Carney *et al.,* 1983). A number of people, possibly as many as 18, had died before the cause of the disease was determined.

Very few cases have been seen in the Tagudin area in recent years; most have been from *barrios* near Vigan, the capital of Ilocos Sur, 100 km north of

Tagudin, and from Claveria, Sanchez, Mira, and Buguey in the province of Cagayan. Small epidemics occur in these areas for periods of 18 to 24 months; those infected are treated, and the number of cases subsides. A flare-up will occur in a new or formerly endemic area, and again die out after all those affected have been treated.

The number of confirmed cases of intestinal capillariasis and of deaths from February 1967 until December 1981 is presented graphically in Fig. 5. The disease nearly disappeared in 1972, but since then 21–65 new cases have been seen and treated yearly at the Capillariasis Research Center. Few deaths occur today because the treatment is effective. Those who die are usually persons who are not seen and treated until irreversible effects of the disease have developed. Unfortunately, even 15 years after the initial epidemic physicians fail to recognize the symptoms, and laboratory technicians misidentify the parasite and eggs. Since the disease was first recognized in 1967 and the infections documented, there have been 1806 confirmed cases and 108 deaths. Many others have died of symptoms characteristic of capillariasis philippinensis, but the infections were not parasitologically confirmed.

Throughout the years distribution of the infections among males and females and various age groups has remained constant. Early in the epidemic, it was recognized that twice as many males as females became infected, especially males between 20 and 40 years of age, and this 2:1 ratio has been maintained throughout the years (Fig. 6). The youngest patient was only 2 years of age and the oldest 85.

Figure 7 is a map of the Philippine Islands indicating areas in which cases of intestinal capillariasis have been identified. The majority of the cases have been from the coastal province of Northern Luzon and one area of Northern Mindanao. Since 1970, biomedical surveys have been conducted jointly on most of the main islands by the U.S. Naval Medical Research Unit No. 2 and the Bureau of Research and Laboratories of the Philippine Ministry of Health. Over 20,000 stool specimens have been examined but *C. philippinensis* has not been found except in the endemic areas of Luzon and Mindanao.

B. Thailand

In Thailand only 25 parasitologically confirmed cases of intestinal capillariasis have been recorded, with the patients coming from as many different localities in Central, North, and Northeast Thailand (Fig. 8). However, in mid-1981 an epidemic developed in Sisakis Province in Northeast Thailand. According to a local physician, over 100 persons acquired the disease and 9 died as a result of infection.

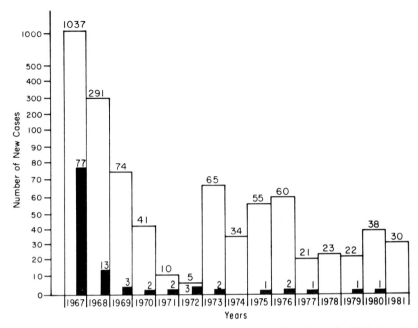

FIG. 5. Age and sex distribution of cases of intestinal capillariasis in the Philippines from February 1967 through December 1981. ■ = Deaths.

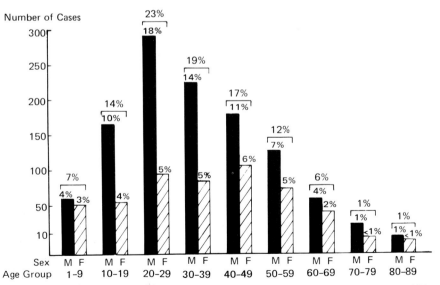

FIG. 6. Parasitologically confirmed cases of intestinal capillariasis and deaths from February 1967 through December 1981. ■ = 1269 Males (70%). ▨ = 737 Females (30%).

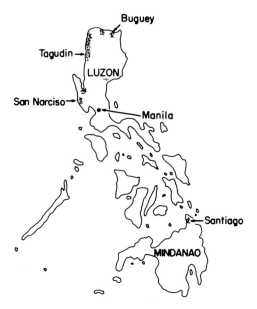

FIG. 7. Map of the Philippine archipelago indicating endemic areas for intestinal capillariasis in Luzon and Mindanao.

C. Japan

Our suspicion that unrecognized capillariasis philippinensis may be occurring elsewhere in the Far East was confirmed by a report from Japan in January 1981. A 28-year-old male restaurant cook who had never left Japan acquired the disease, and was diagnosed and treated (Moriyasu Tsuji, personal communication).

IV.   Climate

A. Philippines

There are two seasons in Northern Luzon, dry and wet. The dry season is from November through May, and the wet season, June through October. Figure 9 presents the average number of new cases of intestinal capillariasis by month as recorded at the Capillariasis Research Center from February 1967 through December 1981; it shows that more cases are seen in the wet months than in the dry season of the year. The bar graph of total cases by month is heavily biased by the

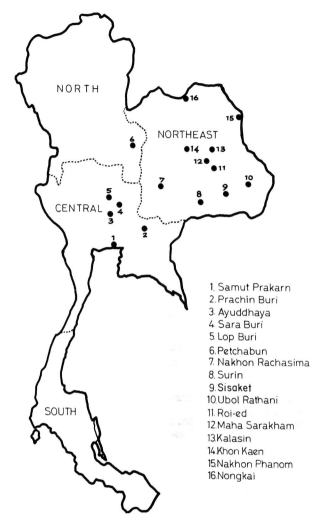

FIG. 8. Map of Thailand indicating villages in which cases of intestinal capillariasis have occurred.

first 2 years with a total of 1328 cases; however, when these 2 years are omitted, the trend is still clear. Further analysis of the data was done by using 12-month moving averages to determine the trend. The moving average was established, and for the wet season the number of cases was above the trend 46% of the time whereas for the dry season the number was above the trend only 28% of the time. This difference is significant with $p < .05$ by the χ-square test.

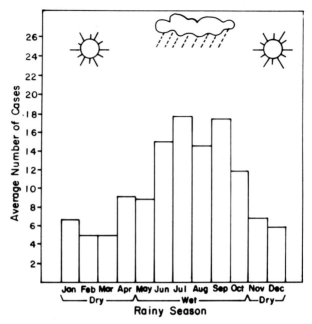

FIG. 9. Monthly averages of cases of intestinal capillariasis from February 1967 through December 1981; more cases were recorded during the rainy season than in the dry season.

B. Thailand

There are also dry and wet seasons in Northeast Thailand, although in the south it rains the year round. Because serious water shortages develop in the northeast during the dry season, most settlements are along the rivers and streams. It is difficult to show a relationship between climate and the disease in Thailand; the cases have been too few and too widespread in distribution, and have occurred during various times of the year except for the epidemic in June, July, and August of 1981.

V. Parasite

Capillaria philippinensis was described as a new species by Chitwood *et al.* (1968). It is one of the smallest nematodes reported in man (Fig. 10). The males are 1.5–3.9 mm in length; width at the head is 3–5 μm, at the stichostome 23–28 μm, and at the cloaca 18 μm. The spicule in the male is 230–300 μm in

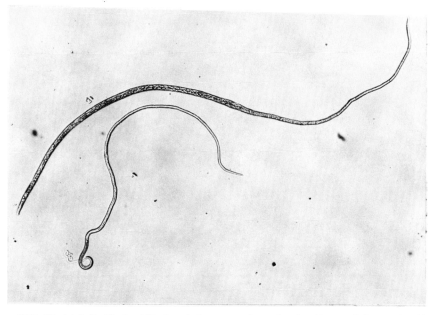

FIG. 10. Adult *Capillaria philippinensis* from man; above, female with eggs, below, male with extended spicular sheath.

length, and the sheath (440 μm) of the spicule is without spines. The anus is subterminal and the tail has ventrolateral expansions which contain two pairs of papillae. Females measure 2.3–5.3 mm in length with widths of 5–8 μm at the head, 25 μm at the widest portion of the stichostome, 28–36 μm at the vulva, and 29–47 μm post vulva. The vulva is salient, without a flap, and located immediately behind the end of the esophagus. The anus is subterminal. Females may contain typical bipolar thick-shelled capillarid eggs or thin-shelled eggs containing embryos or first-stage larvae in the uterus. However, most females contain typical single-cell thick-shelled eggs (in an experimental monkey infection the ratio of oviparous to larviparous females was approximately 200:1). Eggs seen in the feces are peanut-shaped with flattened biopercular plugs, and measure 36–45 by 20 μm (Fig. 11).

VI. Experimental Life Cycle

Early in the Tagudin epidemic, research was directed toward determining the life cycle of the parasite and its means of transmission. At the time, life histories of

larvae reached maximum size after 3 weeks in the fish, and although doubling in length they appeared to remain in the first larval stage; no molting was observed.

Larvae from fish were subsequently fed to monkeys (*Macaca cyclopis, M. fascicularis,* and *M. mulatta*), and patent infections developed in 22–96 days in 23 monkeys. The period of egg production ranged from 1 to 14 months, but monkeys never manifested symptoms of the disease. Daily egg counts were made and pooled data from eight monkeys were computer analyzed. The results indicated an egg production cycle with peak outputs occurring at 22 ± 6 days. In necropsies on monkeys given 30–50 larvae performed 3–4 months after infection, 10,000–30,000 worms were recovered. These findings confirmed previous observations from human autopsies in which autoinfection was suspected because of the presence of larviparous females; all stages of the parasite were found in large numbers (Cross *et al.,* 1972).

A variety of other laboratory, domestic, and wild animals were fed either larvae recovered from fish or the entire fish. Infections did not develop except in a few small wild rats (*Rattus* sp.) which developed short-term patent infections but never suffered ill effects. Mongolian gerbils (*Meriones unguiculatus*), however, when exposed to infection demonstrated patent infections at an average of 27 days and died at an average of 46 days (Cross *et al.,* 1978). As a result of these studies, additional gerbils were used for a series of experiments, and the life cycle of this unique parasite was elucidated. Larvae from fish were given to gerbils by stomach tube; a pair of gerbils was killed each day, the worms collected, and the development of the parasite followed (Table I). The larvae developed into adult males or females in 10–11 days and the female worms started to produce larvae in only 13–14 days. These larvae then developed into second generation adult males and females in 22–24 days and the second generation females produced eggs that passed in the feces 24–35 days postinfection. Similar to the findings in monkeys, most female worms were oviparous but larviparous females were always present. Therefore, internal autoinfection is an integral part of the life cycle both initially and in maintaining the infections (Cross *et al.,* 1978).

In another experiment to determine the reproductive potential, a number of gerbils were given only two larvae. Two gerbils developed patent infection at 29 and 31 days and continued to produce eggs until they died at 46 and 47 days. At necropsy 2520 and 5353 *Capillaria philippinensis* in all stages were recovered from the small intestines.

Infections can be maintained in the laboratory without exposing eggs to fish and feeding larvae from fish to gerbils. Gerbils with patent infection are killed at 30–40 days and about 100 adult worms and larvae, recovered from the small intestine, are given to clean gerbils by stomach tube. Infection can be continually passed in gerbils and some monkeys by this procedure, but other laboratory, wild, and domesticated animals tested were resistant to infection.

TABLE I

Development of *Capillaria philippinensis*
in the Mongolian Gerbil, *Meriones unguiculatus*

Days of infection	Stage of parasite[a]
1–3	L_1
4	$L_1(m)$
5	$L_1(m), L_2(m)$
6	$L_1(m), L_2(m), L_3$
7	$L_2(m), L_3$
8	$L_3(m), L_4$
9	$L_3L_4(m)$; young adults
10	$L_4(m)$; young adults
11	L_4; adults; ♀ egg development
12	Adults; ♀ egg development
13	Adults; ♀ larvae in-utero
14–16	Adults; L_1
17–18	Adults; L_1, L_2
19–20	Adults; L_1, L_2, L_3
21	Adults; L_1, L_2, L_3, L_4
22–24	Adults; L_1, L_2, L_3, L_4; young adults
25–40+	Adults; L_1, L_2, L_3, L_4; young adults
	Most ♀ worms with thick-shelled eggs in-utero
	A few ♀ worms with larvae in-utero

[a]L = Larval stage; m = molting.

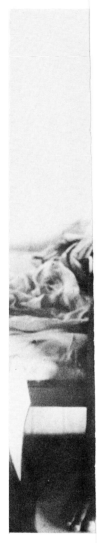

FIG. 13. Adult male Ilocano v

resulting from hypokalem
sections of worms were al
 In some patients jejunal l
ultrastructure of the tissue s
widespread separation of t
jejunal tissue taken at necro

In Thailand, Bhaibulaya *et al.* (1979) tested the susceptibility of nine species of Thai fish to *C. philippinensis* infection and found that six species (*Cyprinus carpio, Puntius gonionotus, Aplocheilus panchax, Gambusia holbrooki, Rasbora borapetenis,* and *Trichopsis vittatus*) could be experimentally infected. The larvae from the Thai fish were cylindrical in shape, bluntly rounded at both ends with a characteristic stichostomal oesophagus. These larvae produced patent infections and death when given to gerbils.

In further studies, Bhaibulaya and Indra-Ngarm (1979) were able to infect two species of fish-eating birds (*Amaurornis phoenicuris* and *Ardeola bacchus*) by feeding them infected fish. The prepatent period ranged from 16 to 30 days and some birds died as a result of the infection. At necropsy of one *A. bacchus* 29 days postinfection, more than 19,000 worms were recovered.

The susceptibility of fish-eating birds to *Capillaria philippinensis* was confirmed in studies conducted in Taiwan in which three species (*Bulbulcus ibis, Nyticorax nyticorax,* and *Ixobrynchus sinensis*) developed infections after being given either larvae from fish or adult and larval worms recovered from gerbil intestines. Some of the Taiwan birds died; on one occasion more than 10,000 worms were recovered from a bird given 26 larvae from fish (Cross *et al.*, 1979).

In man the disease c
early stages with onl
discomfort, and occ:
progresses, the sym
increased borborygr
vomiting, weight lo:
The patients are ini
they experience pro
dehydration or anas
limited to the presen
of the parasite are
potassium, carotene
sugars, and a proteir
in the disease usuall
resulting in heart fa
for some deaths (Da

Seriously ill patie
Philippines. The sy
known by Ilocanos
patients are treated l
The only death in 1:
admission to a Man
treatment for gastrc
treatment. He died t
bowel at autopsy. T
hospital or physiciai

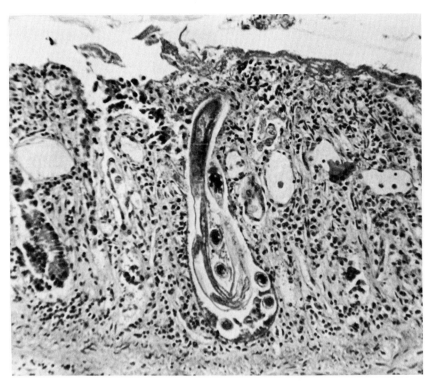

FIG. 14. Histologic section of intestine from a patient with intestinal capillariasis. Note the sloughing of the mucosa, the denuded villi, cellular infiltration, and sections of a worm in a crypt.

pressive degeneration of the cells, mechanical compression, and the presence of a thick layer of electron-dense homogenous material along the oral tip of the parasite. The mechanical separation of the cells by the parasite and microulceration due to parasite secretions are considered responsible for the fluid, electrolyte, and protein loss (Sun *et al.*, 1974).

IX. Diagnosis

A presumptive diagnosis is usually made when a patient from the endemic areas reports a gurgling stomach, abdominal pain, and diarrhea. However, confirmed diagnosis requires finding eggs, larvae, or adult *Capillaria philippinensis* in the stools. Repeated stool examinations may be required in some cases, but generally only one or two are necessary. In some cases in which the parasite could not

A number of autops
have usually occurre
and in the jejunal tis
were estimated in 1
found to be atrophic
and the lamnia prop
and a few eosinophi

be initially demonstrated, the stools usually contained eggs or worms after treatment. Serological tests have been used on an experimental basis (Banzon *et al.*, 1975; Cross and Chi, 1978) but are not considered reliable; they are also unnecessary. The parasite may also be found in jejunal aspiration and jejunal biopsies, but these procedures are usually not required either. In the endemic areas, the symptoms are easily recognized, and stool examinations usually confirm the diagnosis.

X. Treatment

Once the etiology of Pudoc's Mystery Disease was determined, physicians investigating the epidemic treated patients with intravenous fluids and antidiarrhetics; every anthelmintic available at the time was also tested. Some anthelmintics were therapeutically effective but too toxic (*e.g.*, Dithiazanine), and most others were ineffective. Thiabendazole was tested and found effective, but at dosages of 50 mg/kg/day side effects occurred; also, the parasites reappeared in the feces with returning symptoms a few days after the standard 3-day regimen. Relapses were common among those first treated with the drug, and a number of trials were required before an effective treatment schedule was established (Cabrera *et al.*, 1967; Whalen *et al.*, 1969, 1971; Singson, 1969). Thiabendazole was the drug of choice in dosages of 25 mg/kg for 10–17 days, followed by a maintenance dosage of 1 g every other day for 16 weeks.

Relapses

This regimen was used for several years, but relapses occurred in a large number of the patients, most often in those who failed to follow the physician's instructions. Having left the hospital, the patients did not return for follow-up and a new supply of the drug. The patients were then required to remain in the hospital for at least 1 month and were instructed to return for follow-up. However, relapses continued to occur. Singson (1974) reported relapses in 68% of 1219 cases of intestinal capillariasis treated at the Capillariasis Research Center. As the relapses continued, the patients returned for treatment, some as often as 11 times. Fortunately, the drug, although given repeatedly to many, saved lives.

In 1972, mebendazole became available. Although it was found to be effective, relapses continued to occur until an effective regimen was established. Various dosage regimens and schedules were tried and eventually dosages of 400 mg/day for 20 days for patients treated for the first time, and the same dosage for

30 days for relapsed patients, were determined to be the most effective (Singson et al., 1975). Relapses occurred at a very low rate for a few years and in recent years have nearly ceased. One patient has relapsed 16 times from 1967 until 1980; he was treated six times with thiabendazole, seven times with mebendazole (both at varying dosage schedules), twice with flubendazole, and finally with mebendazole again at dosages of 600 mg daily for 49 days followed by 200 mg daily for 30 days and 100 mg daily for 7 months. He has been followed for over 2 years without relapse and is presently in excellent health.

It is believed that relapses result from incomplete elimination of the parasites and that the drug may be more effective against the adult worms than the larval forms. If medication is continuous at high dosages, the adults are eliminated, and when the larvae mature they are subsequently affected by the drug and eliminated; when relapses occurred, thiabendazole or mebendazole had been discontinued too early. This was particularly noticeable in the mebendazole trials whenever the dosages were low or the duration of treatment was short (Singson et al., 1975).

Mebendazole is very effective against Capillaria philippinensis as well as the soil-transmitted nematodes, and side effects are rare although high dosages are given over extended periods.

XI. Transmission

While studies were underway on the management and treatment of the disease and on the life cycle of the parasite, investigations were also being conducted to determine the means of transmission, and the sources and possible reservoirs of infection in nature.

To determine whether a relationship existed between Capillaria philippinensis and other intestinal parasites, stool surveys were conducted among the people living in infected barrios. For example, if a person with C. philippinensis also had echinostomiasis or heterophysiasis, stool samples could provide evidence that either snails or fish were possible sources of infection. The surveys were especially valuable in detecting asymptomatic cases. Although 23 barrios and over 7000 people were examined, no correlation between C. philippinensis and other parasites was evident. Most people (94%) had one, and more often two or as many as 10 different parasites as determined by single stool examinations (Table II). The high prevalence of the soil-transmitted nematodes and intestinal protozoa provides an insight into sanitary practices and conditions, and the presence of the trematode and cestode infections is indicative of eating habits.

TABLE II

Prevalence[a] of Intestinal Parasites (by %) among Human Populations Living in 23 *Barrios* in Northern Luzon Philippines by Age and Sex[b]

	Age						Sex		
Parasites	0–9 (2314)[c]	10–19 (1626)	20–29 (890)	30–39 (833)	40–49 (750)	50+ (1004)	Male (3687)	Female (3730)	Total (7417)
Protozoa									
Entamoeba histolytica	4	5	6	7	8	7	5	7	6
Entamoeba hartmanni	2	5	4	4	4	4	4	3	4
Entamoeba coli	17	30	32	37	32	33	23	32	28
Endolimax nana	4	8	12	15	13	13	7	11	9
Giardia lamblia	14	12	6	6	4	3	11	8	9
Chilomastix mesnili	1	1	2	2	4	2	1	2	2
Helminths									
Capillaria philippinensis	1	2	3	2	3	2	2	1	2
Ascaris lumbricoides	71	69	57	60	55	52	59	67	63
Trichuris trichiura	74	90	86	88	85	84	81	85	83
Hookworm	23	41	41	41	42	46	42	31	36
Strongyloides stercoralis	1	0	1	1	2	2	1	1	1
Taenia spp.	0	0	0	0	2	2	1	1	1
Heterophyid	0	0	1	2	1	1	1	1	1
Opisthorchid	0	0	1	2	1	1	1	1	1
Echinostoma ilocanum	7	10	14	15	17	13	12	11	11
Didymozoid[d]	0	1	0	1	1	1	1	1	1

[a]Percentages to nearest whole number.

[b]Single stool specimens examined by direct and formalin-ether concentration.

[c]The numbers in parentheses refer to the number of persons examined.

[d]Other intestinal parasites found: *Trichomonas hominis, Enterobius vermicularis, Hymenolepis nana, Iodamoeba butschlii,* physalopterids, *Hymenolepis diminuta, Balantidium coli,* and diphyobothriids.

Dietary histories of those with intestinal capillariasis were documented in a search for a possible common source of infection, but none was found. The eating habits of the Ilocanos are quite different from those of Filipinos elsewhere in the archipelago and provide an excellent means for the transmission of parasites. The basic food is not different, consisting of rice, dried fish, and vegetables, usually eaten with the fingers. However, there is a great variety of plant and animal life eaten raw by Ilocanos which is not eaten uncooked by Filipinos in other regions. A dish known as "jumping salad" is very popular (Fig. 15). Eaten raw, this consists of live shrimp seasoned lightly with vinegar, garlic, and chili peppers. Snails may be eaten partially cooked or raw. The large black snail, *Pila luzonica,* is a major source of echinostomid infection among Ilocanos. Squid, fish, crabs, seaweed, and other marine and aquatic life are eaten cooked or

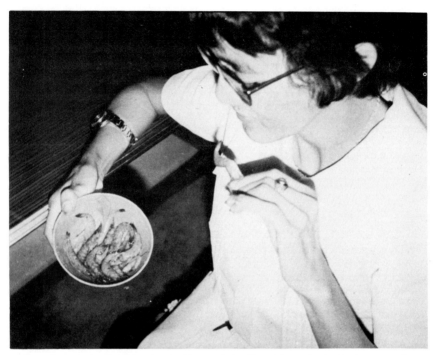

FIG. 15. "Jumping Salad," a favorite Ilocano dish of live shrimp mixed with vinegar, garlic and chili pepper.

uncooked. Larger fish are usually cooked over an open fire or in a pot. The vital organs of goats, cows, and carabaos may be eaten raw, especially while drinking the sugar cane wine (*basi*) or Philippine gin. Finely chopped, raw goat skin with seasoning is also relished. Fluid or juice from domestic animal intestines (Fig. 16), uncooked or lightly boiled, is poured onto rice as flavoring before eating. Dogs, slightly cooked or singed over a wood fire, are eaten on special occasions.

In the light of these findings, all animals that could be obtained were examined for larval and adult stages of *C. philippinensis*. Over 150,000 specimens of marine, aquatic, terrestrial, and aerial animal life in the Tagudin areas, in addition to thousands of samples of market foods, were examined. Many other species of *Capillaria* were found in birds, bats and rodents, but adult *C. philippinensis* was found only in man. A few capillarid larvae were found in fish, but it was not determined at the time if they were *C. philippinensis* (Cross *et al.*, 1970). A number of animals were also examined for the parasite in Thailand but none was infected (Bhaibulaya, 1975).

The Pudoc West lagoons provide considerable food for the villagers. Fish,

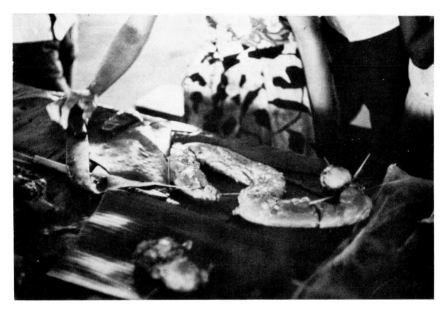

FIG. 16. Juice from the intestines of animals such as these are mixed with rice for seasoning in Ilocano areas of the Philippines. Sold in Tagudin, Ilocos Sur market.

crab, shrimp, clams, and snails are caught in traps made of bundles of tree branches tied together and submerged in the water (Fig. 17). After a few days the bundles are removed from the water and placed into large woven baskets (Fig. 18), and the aquatic life removed (Fig. 19). Fish are also caught in the lagoons by seines or by the illegal use of dynamite.

Fish that were determined experimentally to be intermediate hosts for *Capillaria philippinensis* (*Hypseleotris bipartita, Ambassis miops,* and *Eleotris melanosoma*) are easily collected from the lagoons. In one study, *bagsit* (*H. bipartita*) collected from the lagoons in the area was fed to gerbils which developed *C. philippinensis* infections; this demonstrated the natural transmission of *C. philippinensis* when lagoon fish are eaten raw. *Bagsan* (*A. miops*), when taken fresh from the lagoon, is always eaten raw although it is sometimes dipped into a mixture of vinegar, salt, garlic, and pepper. Some people prefer to bite open the abdomen of the *bagsan* and suck out the intestinal juices. *E. melanosoma* is usually eaten cooked and only rarely eaten raw. The amount of cooking, however, is minimal; the fish is simply placed in boiling water until the skin cracks; this required only 20 sec in a laboratory experiment. *H. bipartita* is highly relished in the raw state, especially in the rainy season when the female is gravid; the people consider the egg-laden females especially tasty.

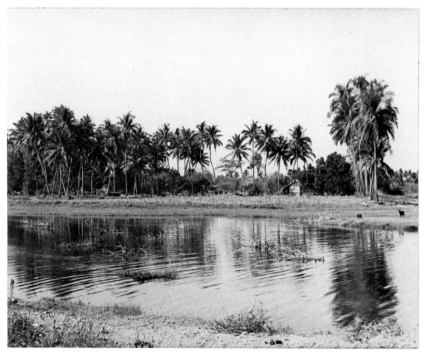

FIG. 17. Lagoon of Pudoc West, Tagudin, Ilocos Sur with tree branches submerged in the water to serve as a trap for aquatic animal life.

XII. Occupation and Habits

A. Philippines

The rural Ilocano men are basically farmers but occasionally fish in the lagoons along the shores of the South China Sea and the Babuyan Channel of northern Luzon. Female members of the family help in the fields during the planting and harvesting, but more often work around the house or weave Ilocano cloth on a loom which is usually located under the house. Boys above 10 years of age may also work in the fields, and the girls help around the house, weave, and help care for the younger children. Many of the teenagers and young adults attend school in Manila or Baguio. The men usually work in the fields during the day, cultivating rice in the rainy season and tobacco in the dry season. It is customary in the Tagudin area for the males to also tend the fish traps in the lagoons, rivers, and streams; this is usually done in the afternoon after working

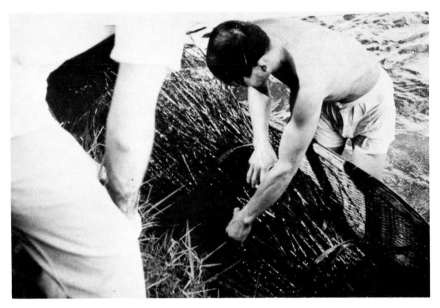

FIG. 18. Bundle of branches used as a trap are shaken in a basket to recover aquatic animal life for eating.

in the fields. While at the water, the men may seine for fish, empty the fish traps, and bathe. At this time in the afternoon they are usually hungry and therefore will eat some of the day's catch of raw fish, shrimp, crabs, or snails. The men then return home, where the rest of the family may eat the day's catch either raw or cooked. The people prefer the aquatic animal life to be freshly caught if eaten raw; if it is not fresh, then it is usually cooked. If the catch is large, it may be brought to the market in the town or a nearby market in a neighboring town to be sold. Market-purchased fish, clams, crabs, and shrimps are usually, but not always, cooked before eating.

Adult males often enjoy gathering in the *barrio* at night to drink *basi* or Philippine gin and eat raw food from the lagoons, or meat or vital organs from domestic animals. On a number of occasions, some of the male patients from the same *barrio* reported drinking and eating together prior to their illness. The eating of raw freshwater fish, more common among Ilocano males than other members of the family, provides one explanation for significant differences between the number of cases of intestinal capillariasis between males and females.

In the endemic area of Santiago, Mindanao, the people have some of the same eating habits as Ilocanos. They enjoy eating some species of uncooked fish from Lake Mainit and the rivers flowing from the lake. They also eat freshwater snails

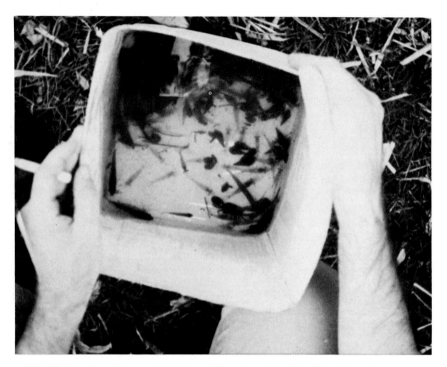

FIG. 19. Container of water with shrimp, fish, crabs, and snails collected from lagoon traps.

and crabs found in the area, consequently acquiring echinostomiasis and paragonomiasis along with heterophyiasis and intestinal capillariasis from fish.

B.   Thailand

In Thailand, most of the people enjoy eating raw food, especially raw meat and freshwater fish. The high prevalence of opisthorchiasis and heterophyiasis (and at times trichinosis) in the northeast is evidence of the practice. Bhaibulaya *et al.* (1979) experimentally infected six species of Thai freshwater fish with *Capillaria philippinensis;* four species of fish (*Cyprinus carpio, Puntius gonionotus, Rosbora borapetensis,* and *Trichopsis vittatus*) are eaten raw (Fig. 20). The fish are prepared for consumption by chopping the entire fish into small pieces and seasoning these with the juice from fermented salted fish, lime juice, and red peppers. Some people, however, chew freshly caught fish.

All Thai patients with intestinal capillariasis have been from rural areas, and the adults have all been farmers and fishermen.

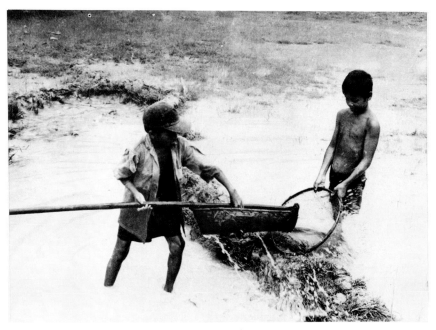

FIG. 20. Thai boy fishing for small fish in Saraburi Province, Thailand.

XIII. Sanitation

Although pit privies and water seal toilets are available in the rural areas of northern Luzon, most Ilocanos, as well as most rural Filipinos, prefer to defecate in open fields. Many people complain of constipation if they are "required to move their bowels in a closet." The habit of indiscriminate defecation is responsible for the high prevalence of intestinal parasites (Table II) and may have played a major role in the 1967–1968 epidemic of intestinal capillariasis. The Pudoc West lagoons, in addition to providing food for the villagers, also provide water for bathing and laundering, and the edges of the lagoons are often used as a latrine. During the epidemic, soiled bed linen from patients was washed in the lagoons and the streams emptying into them. The linens were often soiled with feces, and at times even patients' bedpans were washed in the lagoon. Eggs of *Capillaria philippinensis* were therefore deposited into the waters where fish could become exposed to infection. When soil around infected households was examined, *C. philippinensis* embryonated eggs were also found; eggs could easily be washed into the lagoons by the torrential rains that occur almost daily during the peak of the rainy season.

Domestic animals roam freely around the *barrios* throughout the area, defecating indiscriminately. Carabao, pigs, goats, and chickens are kept under houses, and dogs are everywhere.

Most drinking water originates from open wells or from community pumps. The water is usually neither treated nor boiled prior to drinking. Adults usually bathe in the lagoon or streams; children are bathed in the yards near the water pump.

Sanitary conditions in Thailand are not much different from those in the Philippines. Defecation is indiscriminate, and drinking water is taken from the rivers and streams or from wells.

XIV. Comments

There has been speculation that capillariasis philippinensis is a new disease of man, but considering the eating habits of the Filipinos and Thais in the endemic areas the disease probably is endemic and has gone undiagnosed since the populations began eating raw fish. In Northern Luzon, people have been dying of a gastroenteritis for generations, yet the specific causes were undetermined. Only the simplest laboratory examinations are done at hospitals in the rural Philippines because of financial constraints, and autopsies are almost never performed. Stool examinations for ova and parasites are made, but to the inexperienced laboratory technicians *C. philippinensis* eggs are not too different from those of *Trichuris trichiura*. In early 1967, one embarassed laboratory technician admitted finding *C. philippinensis* eggs in the stools of patients from Pudoc West but identifying them as *T. trichiuria*. Similar conditions prevail in Thailand, and the disease has probably been endemic in both countries for a very long time.

The reasons for the large epidemic in Pudoc West and the Tagudin/Bangar area are not known. It has been postulated, however, that the disease was introduced from Bacarra, Ilocos Norte, the town with the first reported case. The Ilocanos are peripatetic people. They are hard working and industrious, travel-ing widely throughout the Philippines seeking work when there is little at home. (Most of the Filipinos that have migrated to the United States and elsewhere are Ilocanos. They live simply and are conservative and frugal, saving their money to educate the children. They have been likened to the Hakka of China and also have been nicknamed the "Jews of the Philippines.") The introduction of the disease from Bacarra to Pudoc West could have been made by one of the villagers who travelled to Bacarra to find work. After acquiring the infection he would have returned to Pudoc West, and becoming ill, contaminated the area and the lagoon with egg-laden feces. Fish in the lagoon subsequently ingested the eggs, became infected and, when eaten raw by other *barrio* residents, caused more infections. After becoming well established in that *barrio,* the parasite spread to other *barrios* and to towns when fish from lagoons were trapped, or purchased from the markets, and eaten uncooked. Fish from the lagoons also could have migrated to the rivers and streams and to other lagoons, establishing new foci of infection.

There also is speculation about the reasons why the disease almost disappeared from the Tagudin area. At the time of the epidemic, and for months after, thiabendazole was widely used. Most patients received high doses and the drug was readily available in local pharmacies without prescriptions. Anyone with the slightest diarrhea or gastrointestinal upset, fearing the disease, went to a pharmacy and purchased the drug. It was determined early in the epidemic that eggs from patients taking thiabendazole would not embryonate; consequently, eggs passing from persons on treatment were unable to develop. It is believed, therefore, that the widespread use of thiabendazole contributed to the decrease of the disease.

Presently, there are relatively few cases of capillariasis philippinensis being reported in the Philippines. Most of those now appearing are from the Ilocos region of Luzon where the patients still give a history of eating freshwater fish. The cases are more or less sporadic with a few occurring in an area for a year or two and then disappearing. Recent speculation on the cause of these small epidemics voices the suspicion that fish-eating birds may be a natural reservoir of infection. Some birds that can be experimentally infected are known to be migratory, and it is possible that infection can be acquired from fish along the migratory pathways, the birds in turn providing eggs for infection of fish. If the infection is fatal to birds, as has been seen in the laboratory, they may only live long enough to infect a few areas. Once introduced, the infection is established and a localized epidemic occurs. Furthermore, it is likely that only a few fish become infected with the parasite, at least in the farming or more developed areas along the coast. Most Ilocanos enjoy eating uncooked fish, yet less than 1% of the population in the province of Ilocos Sur has become infected. Furthermore, although Thais routinely eat raw fish only a few cases are known. In experimental studies attempting natural transmission in gerbils, a large number of gerbils were fed hundreds of fish over a 2-year period before three animals acquired infections. Over 30,000 fish were examined after the life cycle through the fish was established, but *Capillaria* larvae were found in only 10 fish. Similarly, in Thailand over 8000 fish consisting of 25 different species were examined from Saraburi Province, but none was naturally infected with *C. philippinensis.*

Although it has been shown that a number of different fish in the Philippines and Thailand are able to serve as intermediate hosts, these may not be the most important in the transmission cycle in nature. If the natural reservoir is a fish-eating bird or mammal in sylvatic areas, other species of fish may be more commonly infected. The ability to infect experimentally a diverse variety of fish and several species of fish-eating birds indicates a broad potential source for natural infections and geographic distribution.

C. philippinensis has been reported from man only in the Philippines, Thailand and, more recently, Japan; the parasite becomes a public health problem in population groups which retain habits of eating raw freshwater fish. The parasite probably exists elsewhere in Southeast Asia and the Far East, but remains unrecognized. Many Asian populations eat raw freshwater fish. How many suffer from a gastroenteritis of unknown etiology that could be capillariasis philippinensis? If a careful search were made for the parasite, it might be found elsewhere in Asia.

Control of the disease in humans could be accomplished by eradicating the habit of eating uncooked fish. In practice, however, it would be difficult. Educational campaigns have been tried, but the people paid little attention, and cases still appear. Most rural Ilocanos, even those with some education who realize that certain parasites may be acquired from raw food, retort that "cooking destroys the flavors they relish as well as some of the nutritive value of the food, and furthermore, their ancestors have had these unique eating habits for generations and they seemed to have lived full lives."

Superstition continues to linger among the people in the endemic areas of Luzon. One patient recently seen in a Manila hospital was surprised when he was informed about the disease and its means of transmission. When he first became ill in his *barrio* in Pangasinan Province, he consulted a *herbulario* who burned a pumice stone and, as the smoke rose, told the patient that he had a worm infection acquired from eating raw fish. He paid little attention to this at the time and when his condition continued to worsen, went to Manila. The staff of the Manila hospital became concerned upon hearing this story since the diagnosis had been made much more easily by the *herbulario* than by their modern methods. Of course the *herbulario* may have been well aware of the symptoms since the gurgling stomach and diarrhea, more or less sure signs of the disease, are well known in the Ilocano area.

Acknowledgment

A great many people throughout the years have been involved in the study of intestinal capillariasis in the Philippines. Dr. Carlos Singson and Dr. Tirso Banzon made very valuable contributions as did Dr. J. J. Dizon, Dr. J. Valera, and Dr. E. Zurrudo of the Philippine Ministry of Health. In recent years, Dr. A. Battad and Dr. V. Basaca-Sevilla have supported and encouraged the work. Furthermore, the work could not have been done without the dedication of a large number of technicians from the Philippine Ministry of Health and the NAMRU-2 Laboratory in Taiwan; two who were assigned to the project at the beginning and are still working in Tagudin are Mr. C. T. Lane and his wife Sally (Guevarra) Lane. We wish also to thank the commanding officers of NAMRU-3, Captain R. H. Watten, P. F. D. Van Peenen, K. Sorensen, and W. H. Schroeder, who have continuously given their support and counsel; and Mr. Richard See, NAMRU-2 Biostatistics Department, who provided statistical assistance throughout the years. Funding for the studies came from the Philippine Ministry of Health and the U.S. Naval Medical Research and Development Command for Work Unit MF51.524.0026A. Thanks and gratitude are also extended to Professor S. Vajrasthira, Head of the Department of Helminthology, Mahidol University, for support and for providing facilities to carry out experiments in Bangkok, Thailand.

References

Banzon, T. C., Lewer, R. M., and Yagore, M. G. (1975). Serology of *Capillaria philippinensis* infection: Reactivity of human sera to antigens prepared from *Capillaria obsignata* and other helminths. *Am. J. Trop. Med. Hyg.* **24,** 256–263.

Bhaibulaya, M. (1975). Studies on capillariasis philippinensis in Thailand. I. Epidemiologic survey. *Rep. Thailand Nat. Res. Council,* p. 11.

Bhaibulaya, M., Indra-Ngarm, S., and Anathapruit, M. (1979). Freshwater fishes of Thailand as experimental intermediate host for *Capillaria philippinensis. Int. J. Parasitol.* **9,** 105–108.

Bhaibulaya, M., and Indra-Ngarm, S. (1979). *Amaurornis phoenicurus* and *Ardeola bacchus* as experimental definitive hosts for *Capillaria philippinensis* in Thailand. *Int. J. Parasitol.* **9,** 321–322.

Cabrera, B. D., Canlas, B., and Dauz, U. (1967). Human intestinal capillariasis. III. Parasitological features and management. *Acta Med. Philipp.* **4,** 92–103.

Carney, W. P., Mercado, A. S., Pagaran, I. G., Vergel, A. G., and Cross, J. H. (1983). Intestinal parasites of man in Agusan del Norte, Mindanao, Philippines with emphasis on schistosomiasis. *Southeast Asian J. Trop. Med. Public Health* **11** (*in press*).

Chitwood, M. B., Velasquez, C., and Salazar, N. G. (1964). Physiological changes in a species of *Capillaria* (Trichuroidea) causing a fatal case of human intestinal capillariasis. *Proc. Int. Congr. Parasitol., 1st,* **2,** 797.

Chitwood, M. B., Velasquez, C., and Salazar, N. G. (1968). *Capillaria philippinensis sp. n.* (Nematoda: Trichinellida) from intestine of man in the Philippines. *J. Parasitol.* **54,** 368–371.

Cross, J. H., Banzon, T. C., Murrel, K. D., Watten, R. H., and Dizon, J. H. (1970). A new epidemic diarrheal disease caused by the nematode, *Capillaria philippinensis. Ind. Trop. Health* **7,** 124–131.

Cross, J. H., Banzon, T. C., Clarke, M. D., Basaca-Sevilla, V., Watten, R. H., and Dizon, J. J. (1972). Studies on the experimental transmission of *Capillaria philippinensis* in monkeys. *Trans. R. Soc. Trop. Med. Hyg.* **66,** 819–827.

Cross, J. H., Banzon, T. C., and Singson, C. N. (1978). Further studies on *Capillaria philippinensis:* Development of the parasite in the Mongolian gerbil. *J. Parasitol.* **64,** 208–213.

Cross, J. H., and Chi, J. C. H. (1978). The ELISA test in the detection of antibodies to some parasitic diseases in Asia. *Proc. SEMEMO-TROPMED Semin., 18th,* Kuala Lumpur, Malaysia, pp. 178–182.

Cross, J. H., Singson, C. N., Battad, S., and Basaca-Sevilla, V. (1979). Intestinal capillariasis: Epidemiology, parasitology and Treatment. *In* "Health policies in developing countries". *R. Soc. Med. Int. Congr. Ser.* **24,** 82–87.

Dauz, U., Cabrera, B. D., and Canlas, B. (1967). Human intestinal capillariasis. I. Clinical features. *Acta Med. Philipp.* **4,** 72–83.

Detels, R., Gutman, L., Jaramillo, J., Zurrudo, E., Banzon, T. C., Valera, J., Murrell, K. D., Cross, J. H., and Dizon, J. J. (1969). An epidemic of intestinal capillariasis in man. A study in a *barrio* in Northern Luzon. *Am. J. Trop. Med. Hyg.* **18,** 672–682.

Dizon, J. J., and Watten, R. H. (1969). Preliminary observations on a new disease in man— Intestinal capillariasis. *J. Philipp. Med. Assoc.* **45,** 5–20.

Fresh, J. W., Cross, J. H., Reyes, V., Whalen, G. E., Uylangco, C. V., and Dizon, J. J. (1972). Necropsy findings in intestinal capillariasis. *Am. J. Trop. Med. Hyg.* **21,** 169–173.

Pradatsundarasar, A., Pecharanond, K., Chintanawongs, C., and Ungthavorn, P. (1973). The first case of intestinal capillariasis in Thailand. *Southeast Asian J. Trop. Med. Public Health* **4,** 131–134.

Salazar, N. (1980). Capillariasis philippinensis: Historical perspective. *Int. Congr. Trop. Med. Malar., 10th,* Manila, Philippines, 9–15 Nov. (*in press*).

Singson, C. N. (1969). Human intestinal capillariasis. *Philipp. J. Intern. Med.* **7,** 189–200.

Singson, C. N. (1974). Recurrences in human intestinal capillariasis. *Philipp. J. Microbiol. Infect. Dis.* **3,** 7–13.

Singson, C. N., Banzon, T. C., and Cross, J. H. (1975). Mebendazole in the treatment of intestinal capillariasis. *Am. J. Trop. Med. Hyg.* **24,** 932–934.

Sun, S. C., Cross, J. H., Berg, H. S., Kau, S. L., Singson, C. N., Banzon, T. C., and Watten, R. H. (1974). Ultrastructural studies of intestinal capillariasis *Capillaria philippinensis* in human and gerbil hosts. *Southeast Asian J. Trop. Med. Public Health* **5,** 524–533.

Tidball, J. S., Aguas, J. P., and Aldis, J. W. (1978). A new concentration of human intestinal capillariasis on western Luzon. *Southeast Asian J. Trop. Med. Public Health* **9,** 33–40.

Tsuji, M. *Personal communication.*

Watten, R. H., Becker, W. M., Cross, J. H., Gunning, J. J., and Jarimillo, J. (1972). Clinical studies of capillariasis philippinensis. *Trans. R. Soc. Trop. Med. Hyg.* **66,** 828–834.

Whalen, G. E., Strickland, G. T., Cross, J. H., Uylangco, C., Rosenberg, E. B., Gutman, R. A., Watten, R. H., and Dizon, J. J. (1969). Intestinal capillariasis—a new disease in man. *Lancet* **1,** 13–16.

Whalen, G. E., Rosenberg, E. B., Gutman, R. A., Cross, J. H., Fresh, J. W., Strickland, G. T., and Uylangco, C. (1971). Treatment of intestinal capillariasis with Thiabendazole, Bithionol and Bephenium. *Am. J. Trop. Med. Hyg.* **20,** 95–100.

6

Changing Patterns of Parasitic Infections in Japan

AKIO KOBAYASHI

Department of Parasitology
Jikei University School of Medicine
Tokyo, Japan

I. Introduction

The distribution of parasitic infections in a country may be greatly affected by such factors as climate, biogeography, and cultural and socioeconomic conditions.

Japan (exclusive of Okinawa) reaches from northeastern Hokkaido to southern Kyushu, almost twice the extent of Italy, France, or the United Kingdom as measured along their longest axes. The mainland consists of four islands: Hokkaido, Honshu, Shikoku, and Kyushu, with the territory divided into 47 prefectures (Fig. 1). Most of the country, being located in the temperate zone, has four distinct seasons. In summer the temperature is high in most parts of the country, attaining a monthly average temperature of 25°C or more, with much rain. Conversely, it is cold in winter except in the southernmost part, the Okinawa Islands. The temperature in the mainland varies greatly from region to region, the monthly averages ranging from 7.8 to −5.6°C, according to latitude.

Because certain parasites such as *Wuchereria bancrofti* (larvae), hookworm (eggs), and *Strongyloides stercoralis* (larvae) are susceptible to temperatures of less than 10°C, these parasitic infections are found more often in southern Japan (Sasa, 1966; Tanaka, 1966; Kamegai, 1978). The extensive prevalences of *Ascaris lumbricoides* and whipworm infections, which spread to the most northern parts, are largely due to the high resistance of the eggs to low temperature. The different distributions of *Plasmodium vivax* and *P. falciparum* may be explained by the different sensitivities of those parasites, as well as those of their vector mosquitoes, to low temperatures. *P. falciparum* is known to be more sensitive to low temperatures than is *P. vivax;* the former species cannot develop below 19°C, whereas the latter can develop at temperatures of 16°C and above. *P. falciparum* and its major vector, *Anopheles minimus,* have been observed to be limited to the southernmost islands but *P. vivax* and its principal vector, *A. sinensis,* are widely observed throughout the country even in Hokkaido.

Japan is one of the leading fishing nations in the world, and fish constitute a major part of the Japanese diet. The dietary habits of the people are responsible for the occasional occurrence of certain helminthic infections: metagonimiasis, clonorchiasis, paragonimiasis, gnathostomiasis, anisakiasis, and diphyllobothriasis. Some persons, having a taste for unusual foods such as snake or frog, may contract sparganosis and more rarely mesocestoidiasis.

The agricultural tradition of using night soil as fertilizer cannot be neglected as a factor in the wide prevalence of parasitic infections, particularly of soil-transmitted helminthiases. In Japan, as other East Asian countries, it is customary to use night soil as fertilizer. This custom began in the fourteenth century, and during the Edo era (1603–1867) it was firmly established among the farmers. Around 1700, Edo (as Tokyo was then called) was the largest city in the world with a population of a million, and both Osaka and Kyoto had several hundred thousand inhabitants. The excrement from inhabitants of large cities was carried away by farmers residing in adjacent areas and applied to cultivated fields. Japan's feudal government took a positive attitude to such practices, even issuing an enactment in support of it. Such long-lasting practices may have been useful in keeping the cities clean and enriching farmlands, but they also resulted in a

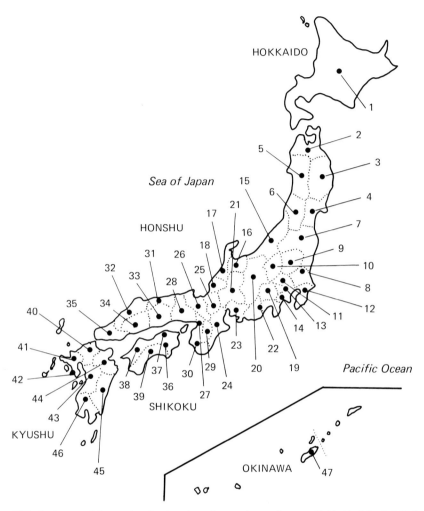

FIG. 1. A map of Japan, showing location of respective prefectures. Hokkaido Island, 1-Hok-kaido; Honshu Island, 2-Aomori, 3-Iwate, 4-Miyagi, 5-Akita, 6-Yamagata, 7-Fukushima, 8-Ibaraki, 9-Tochigi, 10-Gunma, 11-Saitama, 12-Chiba, 13-Tokyo, 14-Kanagawa, 15-Niigata, 16-Toyama, 17-Ishikawa, 18-Fukui, 19-Yamanashi, 20-Nagano, 21-Gifu, 22-Shizuoka, 23-Aichi, 24-Mie, 25-Shiga, 26-Kyoto, 27-Ōsaka, 28-Hyogo, 29-Nara, 30-Wakayama, 31-Tottori, 32-Shimane, 33-Okayama, 34-Hiroshima, 35-Yamaguchi; Shikoku Island, 36-Tokushima, 37-Kagawa, 38-Ehime, 39-Kōchi; Kyushu Island, 40-Fukuoka, 41-Saga, 42-Nagasaki, 43-Kumamoto, 44-Ōita, 45-Miyazaki, 46-Kagoshima; Okinawa Island, 47-Okinawa.

high prevalence of ascariasis, hookworm, and whipworm infections in rural areas over a long period of time.

Urbanization and mechanization of agricultural systems, as reflections of socioeconomic changes, have greatly influenced the patterns of parasitic infections. Knowledge of parasitoses and the people's attitude toward their control have also contributed to a change in prevalences.

II. Soil-Transmitted Helminthiases: *Ascaris lumbricoides,* Hookworm, and Whipworm Infections

There is good reason to believe that ascariasis and hookworm disease were extremely common among Japanese in ancient times. At the end of the nineteenth century, scientific records appeared on the existence of various parasites and their infections in Japan.

A.   Changing Patterns of Soil-Transmitted Helminthiases

From 1918 to 1922, the Government Committee for Investigating Health Problems conducted a systematic survey by stool examination to determine the extent and level of parasitic infections in Japan. Seven villages in seven prefectures were chosen, and results indicated an overall positive rate for parasite eggs of 86.7% for 13,761 persons. The highest prevalences were *A. lumbricoides* (70.1%), hookworm (28.6%), *Trichuris trichiura* (56.9%), and *Trichostrongylus orientalis* (2.9%). Based on these results, the government decided to expand and continue the survey and to conduct a control program. Prefectural governments were requested to perform surveys according to uniform methodology determined by the central government. As a control measure, treatment of infected persons was made a priority with the choice of drugs *ad libitum* among preparations then available. Funds needed for treatment were provided in part by the government. As a result of these operations, the incidence decreased gradually until the end of World War II to a total egg-positive rate of 40%, with *A. lumbricoides* at 35% and hookworm less than 10%.

The early postwar years were a time of great social and economic uncertainty and turmoil. Malnutrition and poor sanitary conditions were widespread. The incidence of *A. lumbricoides* infection increased explosively, the infection rate rising to the 50% level in 1945 and reaching 62.9% in 1949. It was especially

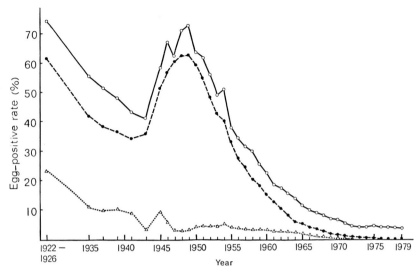

FIG. 2. Yearly changes in results of stool examinations: O———O, total eggs; ●--●, *Ascaris lumbricoides* eggs; △- - - -△, hookworm eggs (Ministry of Health and Welfare).

notable in rural areas where the infection rate often reached 90% or more. Hookworm infection also increased, especially in rural areas where the true rate of hookworm infection was thought to be much higher than that indicated by the statistics (Yanagisawa, 1966).

Faced with this situation, the government consulted specialists about counter-measures against helminthic infections. Periodic mass treatment was suggested and was selected as the basic control measure. Two other measures, night soil control and direct prevention of reinfection, were also considered. Efforts to develop and produce effective anthelmintics were made by scholars and pharmaceutical companies. Studies on the epidemiology of *A. lumbricoides* and hookworm infections were conducted. The Japan Association of Parasite Control (JAPC) was inaugurated voluntarily as a nongovernmental organization whose development and rapidly growing activities are described by Kunii in Chapter 7.

Because of these efforts as well as improvement in living standards, the prevalence rate of *A. lumbricoides* infection decreased gradually but steadily after 1950 to 33.3% in 1955, 15.5% in 1960, 5.3% in 1965, 1.6% in 1970, 0.36% in 1975, and 0.13% in 1979 (Fig. 2). Similarly, the prevalence rate of hookworm infection decreased from 9.6% in 1945 to 0.02% in 1979. Whipworm infections also decreased, but more slowly. Parallelling the prevalence rate, deaths attributed to ascariasis also declined: 2842 occurred in 1951, 548 in 1956, 114 in 1961, and 28 in 1966. The number of deaths attributed to hookworm disease was 1261 in 1951, 480 in 1956, 146 in 1961, and 19 in 1966.

As the prevalence of soil-transmitted helminthiases decreased, "parasite-free schools" began to appear, that is, schools or kindergartens where pupils were shown by stool examinations to be free of parasites. This development began about 1962 in kindergartens and about 1966 in primary and middle schools, becoming more remarkable in later years. For example, in 1972 the proportion of parasite-free schools was 66.3% of 3977 kindergartens, 25.0% of 7432 primary schools, 22.7% of 3428 junior high schools, and 18.4% of 1200 senior high schools (Morishita, 1974).

B.   The Control Program

In designing the control program, studies on the epidemiology of *Ascaris lumbricoides* and hookworm infections were helpful. A number of studies on the seasonal variations of the reinfection and egg density found in various infection sources were reviewed (Yanagisawa, 1966; Morishita, 1972).

The control program for soil-transmitted helminthiases included three measures: periodic mass treatment, night soil control, and direct prevention from reinfection. Periodic mass treatment was regarded as the major thrust, because it was considered to be the most feasible under the circumstances. The program was primarily directed to the control of *A. lumbricoides* infections.

1.   BASIC RESEARCH ON RESPECTIVE CONTROL MEASURES

a.   *Mass Treatment*

i.   Development and Production of Effective Anthelmintics.   In order to achieve repeated mass treatment on a nationwide scale, it was necessary to develop effective anthelmintics and to establish standard therapeutic regimens for mass treatment rather than for individual therapy. There was also an urgent need to produce anthelmintics in large quantities. Pharmacologists and manufacturers contributed by developing and producing effective drugs, and parasitologists tried to establish standard therapeutic regimens. Successful determination of the structural formula of the effective fraction of *Digenea simplex* (Murakami *et al.,* 1953) is a good example of a drug for ascariasis. The anthelmintic active against hookworm, 1-bromo-2-naphthol, is another example (Miura, 1954). Standardization of therapeutic regimens for available anthelmintics was carefully studied (Morishita, 1955; Ishizaki and Komiya, 1963). These contributions coupled with the successful mass production of santonin, 1-bromo-2-naphthol, and other drugs made it possible to perform repeated mass treatment of people with *Ascaris lumbricoides* and hookworm infections.

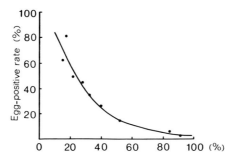

FIG. 3. Relationship between *Ascaris lumbricoides* egg-positive rates and proportions of persons discharging unfertilized eggs alone among the positives (Komiya *et al.*, 1962).

ii. Theoretical Analysis of Effects of Repeated Mass Treatment. The process of reduction of reinfection of *Ascaris lumbricoides* by repeated mass treatment was analyzed theoretically by Komiya (1959). Repeated mass treatment causes two preventive effects against infections. Gradual decrease in total worm burden in a community is the primary effect, and a consequent increase in the ratio of those positive cases discharging only unfertilized eggs is the secondary effect. In this secondary effect, the ratio will be approximately 20% if the total incidence rate is 40–50%, attaining percentages as high as 80% or more if the total incidence rate diminishes to less than 5% (Komiya *et al.*, 1962) (Fig. 3). This means that the proportion of persons actually constituting sources of infection is only 1% although the total incidence rate is 5%. Under such conditions, the eradication of *A. lumbricoides* infection is considered possible. Thus, the secondary effect is helpful in acceleration of the control program toward the ultimate goal of eradication.

It has been suggested (1) that two or three mass treatments per year are necessary and (2) that in Japan such treatments should, for maximum effectiveness, be given in winter and summer when the infection is less prevalent (Kobayashi, 1954; Yajima, 1955). Winter was recommended as the best season for mass treatment for hookworm (Matsuzaki, 1951).

b. Mass Examination

Fecal examinations must be performed for mass treatment, and the fecal examination technique should be sensitive, simple, and cost-effective. A technique devised by Kato and Miura (1954) meets these conditions.

c. Night Soil Control

Parasite eggs in night soil will be killed if kept in a storage tank for a certain length of time. Studies were made on the period required to kill the eggs of

Ascaris lumbricoides and hookworm and whipworm eggs in night soil under different conditions. Based on these studies, construction of *kairyo benjo* (improved latrines) or toilets with separate tank systems for feces and urine were devised. Application of certain ovicidal chemicals to night soil was also studied and a combined use of calcium superphosphate and sodium nitrite (Kozai, 1962) and thiabendazole (Kutsumi, 1967) proved effective. These control measures were rarely applied by farmers, however, because of high cost, nor was killing eggs by adding night soil to compost heaps practiced because it required additional labor.

d.   Elimination of Parasite Eggs from Vegetables

Synthetic detergent is useful for the elimination of *Ascaris lumbricoides* eggs from vegetables (Kobayashi and Kumada, 1957). Other control measures were compared and evaluated by Kozai (1962), Kutsumi (1967), and Uchida *et al.* (1967).

2.   PROGRAM FOR *Ascaris lumbricoides* ERADICATION CAMPAIGN

The following are recommended for *Ascaris lumbricoides* eradication (Komiya, 1962):

a.   In Rural Areas

i.   Communities with Prevalence Rates of More Than 30%.   Mass treatment should be performed three times a year. In addition, night soil should not be used as a fertilizer for the cultivation of vegetables that are eaten raw. The use of synthetic detergent for washing vegetables before consumption, and the habit of keeping hands clean, should be recommended. By continuous efforts, the infection rate is expected to fall to a 30% level after several years, when the program for the second control stage will be started.

ii.   Communities with Prevalence Rates of 5 to 30%.   Mass treatment is required twice a year. Other preventive measures against reinfection are also required as mentioned above.

iii.   Communities with Prevalence Rates of Less Than 5%.   These communities are considered to be in the eradication stage. Thorough treatment of individuals excreting fertilized *A. lumbricoides* eggs and careful application of preventive measures should be made; a follow-up inspection is necessary. Precise fecal examinations are required to detect very light infections and also to determine complete cures.

b. In Urban Areas

Mass treatment may be done twice a year. The use of synthetic detergent for cleaning vegetables may be necessary.

c. Schoolchildren

Mass treatment may be performed twice a year. Health education is necessary.

3. ANALYSIS OF CHANGING PATTERNS OF SOIL-TRANSMITTED HELMINTHIASES

As mentioned above, the prevalence rate of *A. lumbricoides* infection has decreased markedly after the high rates of the early postwar years; it may even be said that the infections have been completely eradicated from most parts of Japan. The changes in patterns of hookworm and whipworm infections are more or less similar; there are several reasons for the successful eradication.

Mass treatment on a nationwide scale caused an increase in production of anthelmintics. For example, santonin output which was only 679 kg in 1948 reached 1 ton in 1949 (dosage for 10 million adults). In following years it increased further, reaching a high of 8.5 tons in 1952. Thus, a sufficient amount of drugs was made available. The successful mass production of kainic acid and the discovery of the synergistic effect of santonin and kainic acid have also contributed to more effective mass treatment. Similarly, development and mass production of 1-bromo-2-naphthol as well as other drugs have contributed to the decrease in hookworm infections. The establishment of the Japan Association of Parasite Control made it possible to achieve extensive mass examination and mass treatment for these infections.

Night soil disposal is another important factor. Night soil was used by farmers as fertilizer extensively in the years 1948–1949 because of a shortage of chemical fertilizer. However, the application of night soil decreased gradually after 1950 and markedly after 1956. Chemical fertilizers were more widely used after 1955, reflecting their increased availability. This trend, which may be a reflection of economic rehabilitation and socioeconomic development, became prominent after 1954 when the first upsurge of economic growth occurred. Industrialization developed rapidly and more manpower was needed in large cities, resulting in a shortage of younger persons in rural areas. A series of such changes discouraged farmers from undertaking such laborious tasks as moving and handling night soil, hence the increase in use of chemical fertilizers. On the other hand, night soil disposal has increased in large cities and towns by enactment of laws. The areas and populations covered by such laws have been expanding yearly, for example, 47% of the total populations in 1955, 56% in 1961, 65% in

1965, 82% in 1970, and 99% in 1975. This trend contributed to the decrease in parasitic infections, particularly since about 1955.

Appearance of synthetic detergents may be another factor. These appeared about 1956, and production increased from 533 tons in 1957 to 2219 tons in 1958, to as high as 110,000 tons in 1968. It may be assumed that the increased output of synthetic detergents and the increasing habit of using detergents to wash vegetables in households have also contributed to the decrease in infections.

III. Endemic Helminthic Infections

From ancient times, certain endemic helmintic diseases, either localized or wide-spread, have been known to seriously affect the Japanese people. Among these schistosomiasis, filariasis, clonorchiasis, and paragonimiasis were the most prominent.

A. Schistosomiasis Japonica

A peculiar disease causing edema and ascites had prevailed in some areas of Japan, but until the beginning of the twentieth century the etiology of the disease was not known. Fujii (1847) first described the symptoms of this peculiar disease in his medical document, "Katayama-ki." Katsurada (1904) incriminated a male worm isolated from the portal vein of an infected cat in Yamanashi as the pathogen of the disease and named it *Schistosoma japonicum.* In the same year, Fujinami (1904) found a female worm in a human autopsy in the Katayama district. In later years, acquisition of the disease by the percutaneous route through contact with water in the endemic areas was clearly documented. In 1913, Miyairi and Suzuki reported that a newly discovered snail, *Oncomelania nosophora,* was the intermediate host.

1. CHANGING PATTERN OF SCHISTOSOMA INFECTIONS

Areas endemic for the disease are (1) the Kofu Basin in Yamanashi Prefecture, (2) the Katayama district in Hiroshima and Okayama Prefectures, (3) the area along the Chikugo River in Fukuoka and Saga Prefectures, (4) the area along the Tone River in Chiba, Saitama, and Ibaraki Prefectures, and (5) the Numazu area in Shizuoka Prefecture. Among these areas, the Kofu Basin was the largest area of snail infestation and estimated number of patients (91 km^2; 65,000 persons),

TABLE I

Prevalence of *Schistosoma japonicum* in Endemic Areas of Japan
from 1948 to 1950[a]

Area	Prefecture	Number examined	Positive for *S. japonicum* eggs	
			No.	%
Kofu Basin	Yamanashi	3055	979	32.0
Tone River area	Chiba	414	32	7.7
	Ibaraki	808	55	6.8
	Saitama	311	17	5.4
Numazu area	Shizuoka	607	40	6.5
Katayama district	Hiroshima	613	172	28.0
Chikugo River area	Saga	502	184	36.6
	Fukuoka	214	156	72.9
		6524	1635	25.1

[a]From Yokogawa, 1974.

followed by the Chikugo River area (68 km^2; 24,000) and the Katayama district (10 km^2, over 11,000) (Okabe, 1964).

Control of the intermediate host snail was considered to be the most effective prevention of this disease. Caustic lime and calcium cyanamide were found to be effective molluscicides and were applied to paddy fields and irrigation ditches. Paralleling a decrease in the snail population density, the incidence of the disease decreased gradually each year in these areas until the end of World War II. For example, in the Kofu Basin, the annual incidence of *Schistosoma japonicum*-infected persons was 7888 in 1910, 5716 in 1924, and 1256 in 1942 (Yokogawa, 1974). In the Katayama district, the number of patients was 2150 in 1920, 810 in 1925, 112 in 1930, 81 in 1935, 33 in 1940, and 12 in 1942 (Okabe, 1964). However, after the war the prevalence of the infection again increased, possibly because of decreased snail population control.

From 1948 to 1952, a joint survey team of U.S. and Japanese scientists conducted an extensive survey of schistosome infections in the endemic areas (Olivier, 1948; Hunter *et al.*, 1951; Ritchie *et al.*, 1951, 1952, 1953). The results, summarized in Table I, indicate that the prevalence of infection among the populations of the areas averaged 25.1%. The Ministry of Health and Welfare initiated a control program in 1957; as a result, the prevalence of *S. japonicum* egg-positive cases in the endemic areas decreased rapidly. For example, in the Kofu Basin the incidence of egg-positive cases was 280 (2.8%) of 10,008 examined in 1955, 170 (2.2%) of 7,731 in 1960, 170 (2.2%) of 7,757 in 1965, 24 (0.2%) of 10,849 in 1970, and 12 (2.4%) of 509 in 1975; since 1978 no

TABLE II

Progress of Prefectural Filariasis Control Program in Japan[a]

Prefecture	1962 Number examined	1962 % positive	1963 Number examined	1963 % positive	1964 Number examined	1964 % positive	1965 Number examined	1965 % positive	1966 Number examined	1966 % positive	1967 Number examined	1967 % positive
Okinawa (Miyako)	—	—	—	—	—	—	66,333	19.16	62,702	4.87	32,541	3.09
Okinawa (Yaeyama)	—	—	—	—	—	—	—	—	—	—	46,590	7.27
Kagoshima	135,557	6.62	167,604	3.94	99,864	4.50	81,503	3.58	61,969	3.16	68,446	1.73
Nagasaki	202,941	1.31	167,950	0.90	138,349	0.64	62,789	0.70	42,611	0.60	44,814	0.58
Kumamoto	—	—	—		41,038	0.27	15,486	0.77	5,382	0.80	10,246	0.45
Miyazaki	—	—	25,040	0.012	3174	0	—		—		—	—
Oita	—	—	25,061	0	22,107	0	—		—		—	—
Ehime	211,244	0.049	65,452	0.15	20,603	0.14	5,411	0.037	—		—	—
Kochi	13,078	0.31	29,933	0.10	10,642	0.11	—		—		—	—
Tokyo	269	0.74	5,683	0.81	2,592	0.42	2,466	0.45	2,399	0	2,250	0
Niigata	—	—	22,513	0	—	—	—		—		—	—

[a]From Sasa et al., 1970.

a. Ryuku Islands

In 1965, the Mf-positive rate was 19.16% in Miyako Island. Drugs were administered to positive cases according to a determined dosage schedule. In the next year, the positive rate was reduced to 4.87%, and further in the third year to 3.09%.

b. Kagoshima Prefecture

The prevalence of filariasis in the main islands of Japan is highest in Kagoshima Prefecture, especially in the islands southwest of Kyushu. The overall positive rate determined by an annual survey was 6.62% in 1962, reduced to 1.73% in 1967. Okamoto (1963) reported that a total of 2222 patients with chyluria visited 202 hospitals in the 5 years prior to the control program. Among them, 1722 were from Kyushu and Okinawa Prefectures. Sato *et al.* (1971), in their observation of outpatients at Kagoshima University Hospital, reported that the number of patients with elephantiasis and hydrocele had decreased by at least one-half in 10 years, and chyluria patients had decreased similarly.

c. Nagasaki Prefecture

This prefecture is the second most important endemic district in the main islands. In 1962, the Mf-positive rate was 1.31%. After 6 years of the control program, it had decreased to 0.58%.

d. Kumamoto Prefecture

In the first survey, the percentage of Mf-positive cases was already low (0.27%). The control program in the following years was directed mainly to infected areas.

e. Ehime Prefecture

Only 33 positive cases were detected in 1958 by a blood survey of 2050 persons. The reduction in the number of positives was remarkable; in 1965 only two positive cases were detected.

f. Other Prefectures

No Mf-positives were detected by surveys in Niigata or in Ōita in 1963, although both districts had been endemic in the past. Only three cases of filariasis were discovered among 25,040 persons in Miyazaki Prefecture, which had also been previously known as an endemic district. These statistics indicate that most of the former endemic areas had become free from infection or that infection had diminished rapidly. In the Izu Islands, where both malayan and bancroftian filariasis had been known, Mf-positive cases were not detected after 1966.

2. THE CONTROL PROGRAM

The National Filariasis Control Program was operational from 1962 to 1969 on the main islands of Japan. The program involved (i) microfilarial blood survey of people in the endemic areas, (ii) mass treatment of Mf-positive cases with di-ethylcarbamazine, and (iii) control of vector mosquitoes, *Culex pipiens pallens*. The program covered 10 prefectures; survey teams were organized by prefectural governors. All inhabitants of endemic areas over 1 year of age were examined for Mf, and Mf-carriers were given diethylcarbamazine. From the results of studies by Wharton *et al.* (1958) and Yamamoto (1965), total dosages were determined to be 72 mg/kg; 3.6 g for adults, 3.0 g for 12 to 15-year-olds, and 18 g for 6 to 11-year-olds. A therapeutic regimen of weekly, daily, or monthly dosages was chosen *ad libitum* by the local government. The cure rates were 68.4–79.7% in Kagoshima Prefecture, 86.7–94.4% in Nagasaki Prefecture, and 89.4–93.5% in Kumamoto Prefecture. About 3 months after completion of the initial course of treatment, the Mf-carriers were reexamined and those who were still positive received another course.

The following mosquito control methods were adopted: survey of mosquito fauna and breeding places, removal of mosquito breeding places with emphasis on sewage ditches near houses, use of mosquito larvicides and natural controls, and residual spraying of insecticides. The above procedures were repeated every year in the affected prefectures, and varying degrees of reduction of the Mf-positive rates were obtained in all control areas. Thus, there was a rapid decrease in filarial infections among Japanese, although occasional infections do occur. In addition to the active control program, changes in the natural environment may have contributed to the successful eradication of filariasis as they did in schistosomiasis, paragonimiasis, and soil-transmitted helminthiases.

C. Paragonimiasis

Until recently, of the five species of the genus *Paragonimus* existing in this country, only *Paragonimus westermani* was known to cause disease in man. However, *P. miyazakii* also is now known to be parasitic in man. Humans may acquire the infection by eating freshwater crabs such as *P. westermani* from *Eriocheir japonicus* and *Potamon dehaani* (Nakagawa, 1915), and *P. miyazakii* from *Potamon dehaani* (Kamo *et al.*, 1961).

1. PARAGONIMIASIS WESTERMANI

Until about 1930, paragonimiasis westermani had been found in various parts of Japan excepting Hokkaido and Aomori Prefecture. The patients were often misdiagnosed as having pulmonary tuberculosis. Accumulated data obtained mainly in the Kyushu and Shikoku areas during 1885–1894 indicated that of 3990 patients with chest diseases, 5% were positive for *Paragonimus* spp. eggs. The development of the skin test antigen (Yokogawa *et al.*, 1955) made it possible to perform extensive surveys. In some endemic areas positive skin test rates between 1.4 and 19.5% for the inhabitants were obtained during 1954–1959, and approximately one-third of the skin test positives excreted *Paragonimus* eggs. Discovery of the effectiveness of bithionol against paragonimiasis (Yokogawa *et al.*, 1961) permitted made mass treatment and resulted in successful cures. Consequently, prevalence of the infection has rapidly decreased to the point of eradication. In 1973 and 1975, however, human cases of paragonimiasis occurred in parts of Kyushu, and it was suspected that the infections had been acquired by eating wild boar meat containing *P. westermani* larvae (Miyazaki *et al.*, 1978). No infections have been reported since 1978.

2. PARAGONIMIASIS MIYAZAKII

Initial outbreaks of human cases of paragonimiasis miyazakii occurred in Kanagawa and Yamanashi Prefectures in 1974 (Yokogawa *et al.*, 1974; Minai *et al.*, 1974; Hayashi, 1975; Kobayashi *et al.*, 1975) and since then more than 60 proven cases have been reported. Most of these patients manifested marked eosinophilia and repeated pleural effusion with or without spontaneous pneumothorax. Eggs were not found in feces or sputum of the patients, who were found to have acquired the infection by eating the small freshwater crab *Potamon dehaani* raw at sea food restaurants, where live crabs were served as a garnish and eventually eaten raw by the customers after they had become inebriated. It was also shown that these crabs were mostly from a particular site along the Ōi River. Two or three series of bithionol treatment were required for a complete cure.

D. Clonorchiasis

Until recently, *Clonorchis sinensis* infections were commonly found in certain areas of Japan. Four years after the first Chinese report of *C. sinensis*, Ishizaka (1878) found the parasite in a human autopsy in Okayama Prefecture. Most research on the life cycle of the parasite (Kobayashi, 1910; Muto, 1918) and on the pathology, symptomatology, therapy, and prophylaxis of the disease was conducted by Japanese researchers. Inoue (1900) identified Okayama, Shiga, and Miyagi as the most important endemic areas of 18 prefectures. In Kiushi village, a well-known endemic focus in Miyagi Prefecture, the infection rate among the inhabitants in 1883 was as high as 55.6% (495 persons examined), and it was 32.9% in 1892. Surprisingly enough, however, a survey conducted 79 years after the initial investigation revealed no patients (Komiya and Suzuki, 1962). In Okayama Prefecture, the prevalence of the disease was also high in past years. From 1886 to 1898, the Prefectural Investigation Committee for Endemic Diseases performed surveys on the inhabitants of five villages and found the infection rate was 30.4–67.2%. Later the average was 16.5% (Ritchie *et al.*, 1951), and recently the infection became negligible. In Shiga Prefecture, Komiya *et al.* (1960) examined a total of 4021 persons in 14 villages for clonorchiasis and found 13.3% (2.5–54.2%) infected. This suggests endemic foci still exist. The total number of persons with clonorchiasis reported by JAPC was 9727 during 1961–1965, 7370 during 1966–1970, 2707 during 1971–1975, and only 54 during 1976–1979.

The decrease in the incidence of clonorchiasis is again remarkable. Although the decrease began much earlier, it is probable that it was accelerated recently by rapid changes in conditions. A diminished population density of the intermediate host snail resulting from pollution of its aquatic habitat by waste materials from factories and agricultural chemicals has contributed to the decline. Land reclamation and greater awareness of the disease may also have contributed to the rapid decrease. Effects of treatment on the patients have been negligible, since effective drugs for clonorchiasis were not available until recently.

E. Metagonimiasis

Metagonimus yokogawai was discovered by Yokogawa in Taiwan in 1911. In the same year the *ayu* fish, *Plecoglossus altivelis,* was found to serve as the second intermediate host (Yokogawa, 1912). In Japan, about 50 species of fish are known to be second intermediate hosts (Komiya and Suzuki, 1966; Kagei and Oshima, 1968). Among these fishes, the *ayu* and white bait, *Salangichthys microdon,* are regarded as the most important (Komiya *et al.*, 1958). A survey of *ayu* for *M. yokogawai* metacercariae in rivers in various parts of Japan indicated that 55 out of 66 rivers harbored infected fish (Kagei and Oshima, 1968). In the southern and western parts of the country, some rivers contained heavily infected fishes. *Ayu* collected from 14 rivers in Kyushu were found to be heavily infected at a rate as high as 90%. The longer period of temperatures over 20°C may be responsible for the higher rates of infection in fish in southern rivers. Although the average prevalence rate of *M. yokogawai* infection in Japanese people has remained at a constant 0.2–0.3% during the past 15 years, high infection rates were found in some endemic areas; for example, 73.9% in Shimane, 57.1% in Yamaguchi Prefecture (Kagei and Kihata, 1972), and 51.4% in Ibaraki Prefecture (Komiya *et al.*, 1958). A correlation was observed between the infection rates in *ayu* and the infection rates among the inhabitants of areas along rivers (Kagei and Kihata, 1973).

F. Echinococcosis

In Japan, both *Echinococcus granulosus* and *Echinococcus multilocularis* have been found. Reports of human cases of *E. granulosus* infection have totaled about 70 since 1881, mostly in the southern parts of Japan, and about 190 human cases of *E. multilocularis* infection have been recorded since the first report in 1928 in the Tohoku district. At present, two endemic foci are known in northern parts of Japan, Rebun Island and the Nemuro district of Hakkaido. On Rebun Island, 32 miles from the island of Hokkaido, no human echinococcosis was known until the first case was reported in 1937. In the 29 years from 1937 to 1965, 127 patients with the disease were found and half of them died. A control program was introduced, but 13 additional cases had been found by 1979. The occurrence of the disease on the island was caused by an introduction of foxes from Simushir Island, Middle Kurils, where both foxes and rats were found to be infected with this parasite. Twelve pairs of red foxes were introduced during 1924–1926 for the purpose of raising foxes to control damage by the vole, *Clethrionomys rufocanus bedfordiae*. Killing of foxes was prohibited for 10 years; accordingly, the foxes multiplied thus establishing the life cycle of *E. multilocularis* in the island (Yamashita, 1973). The initial occurrence of cases was noted about 10 years after the introduction of the foxes, an interval that coincides with the prepatent period of the disease.

In 1965, two cases of echinococcosis multilocularis occurred for the first time at the eastern tip of Hokkaido in the Nemuro district, and since then 24 additional patients have been reported. The occurrence of the disease in this district is also considered to result from the multiplication and spread of foxes that initially migrated from the Kuril Islands and from Yururi Island when the sea iced over (Yamashita, 1973). As a result of the control program, occurrence of new infections has nearly ceased. In Honshu, about 20 human cases have been reported, but these patients probably contracted the infection elsewhere.

IV. Parasitic Infections through Marine and Anadromous Fishes

A. Anisakiasis

Anisakiasis is a disease of the alimentary tract caused by the larvae of the nematode *Anisakis*. Sporadic reports of gastrointestinal eosinophilic granuloma caused by some ascarid larvae have appeared since 1940. Asami *et al.* (1965) were the first in Japan to identify the *Anisakis*-like larvae from two human cases;

these larvae were identical with those reported by Van Thiel (1962). Stimulated by these findings, research on the parasite and anisakiasis has continued actively and reported cases have accumulated (Oshima, 1972). The particular preference of Japanese for eating raw fish makes this parasitosis rather common. Fish inhabiting the northern Pacific, such as cod, trout, salmon, and herring, are the most heavily parasitized with *Anisakis* sp. larvae with a prevalence as high as 70–100% (Kobayashi *et al.*, 1966; Shiraki and Otsuru, 1968). In mackerel (*Pneumatophorus japonicus japonicus*), horse mackerel (*Trachurus japonicus*), and cuttlefish (*Todarodes pacificus*), which seasonally migrate along the islands of Japan, *Anisakis* sp. larvae (Type I) were found with rates from 15 to 50% (Kobayashi *et al.*, 1966; Kobayashi *et al.*, *unpublished*). These three fish species, often eaten raw by Japanese, are considered the most important sources of the infection (Table III).

A definitive diagnosis of anisakiasis prior to surgery and histological examination of tissues is difficult. Clinical diagnosis of proven cases of anisakiasis were reported by Yoshimura (1966) and Ishikura (1969), in which gastric ulcer and tumor were the most frequent diagnoses given for gastric anisakiasis and acute appendicitis for intestinal anisakiasis.

Very recently, another type of anisakiasis caused by *Terranova* sp. larvae, Type A, [identified by Koyama *et al.* (1969) as possibly *T. decipiens*] has been reported (Suzuki *et al.*, 1972). A total of 62 cases of this type had been reported by 1978.

B. Diphyllobothriasis

In Japan, diphyllobothriasis is contracted by the ingestion of anadromous fishes such as trout and salmon that are infected with the larvae of *Diphyllobothrium latum*. Trout caught in Japanese waters on their migratory routes to spawning constitute a major source of the infection, and northern and northwestern parts of Japan have been identified as endemic areas. Occasional human cases of diphyllobothriasis were reported until about 50 years ago, and after a long period with no reports, human cases are again appearing. These cases were mostly found in areas previously known as endemic, such as Aomori, Akita, Niigata, Toyama, Ishikawa, and Fukui Prefectures. Fifty cases were found in Aomori Prefecture in the 12 years prior to 1978 (Yamaguchi *et al.*, 1978); 74 cases occurred in Niigata Prefecture from 1975 to 1978 (Hotta *et al.*, 1978), and 82 cases in Toyama, Ishikawa, and Fukui Prefectures in 1974 and 1975 (Yoshimura *et al.*, 1975). Sporadic cases were also reported in some nonendemic areas such as Nagano, Kyoto, Okayama, and Chiba Prefectures. The significant increase in recent years may be attributed to the increasing habit of eating raw trout, *Oncorhynchus masou,* and to the improved sources of supply for fresh fish. The infection rates of trout with diphyllobothriid larvae were roughly 30–40% during 1919–1939 (Eguchi, 1964). Recent surveys indicate that the infection rates in the fish are essentially the same as those found in earlier investigations. The accumulated data indicate the average infection rates in trout in Yamagata, Akita, Niigata, and Toyama are 54, 36, 32, and 16%, respectively.

V. Other Helminthic Infections

A. Enterobiasis

The prevalence of *Enterobius vermicularis* infections was extremely high before World War II and for some time afterward. Surveys conducted during 1950–1960 reported average egg-positive rates greater than 50%, and often 90–100% of children were infected (Akagi, 1973). Since 1962, when the School Hygiene Act was revised to include pinworm, a nationwide survey has been conducted by JAPC covering all school children at least once each year. Those positive for pinworm eggs are treated with piperazine or pyrvinium pamoate. The egg-positive rates have gradually decreased to 29.3% in 1961, 17.0% in 1966, 8.97% in 1971, 6.93% in 1976, and 5.58% in 1979. Ito and Mochizuki (1969) showed that successive mass treatment was effective for reduction of the positivity rate. A tendency to familial aggregation of infections was pointed out, and age distributions of infection showed two peaks, the first at 5–9 years and the second at 30–39 years for females or 40–49 years for males (Hayashi *et al.,* 1959).

B. Angiostrongyliasis

Angiostrongylus cantonensis is known to cause eosinophilic meningoencephalitis in man. In Japan, the parasite has become established in the Ryukyu Islands and is expanding into the neighboring Islands and to Japan proper (Otsuru, 1978). Nineteen cases of suspected angiostrongyliasis have been identified since 1969. Among these, nine in the Ryukyu Islands were thought to have been caused by eating or handling the giant African land snail, *Achatina fulica,* and the remaining cases by consuming slugs or toad liver as a folk remedy (Sato *et al.,* 1980).

TABLE III

Incidence of Larval *Anisakis* (Type I) in Fishes and Squids[a]

Fishes and squids	Number examined	% positive	Average number of larva-infected fish	Muscle	
				% positive	Average number of larva-infected fish
Fishes inhabiting the northern Pacific					
Theragra chalcogramma (Pacific pollock)	78	99	28.7	80	4.5
Gadus morrhua macrocephalus (cod)	52	94	88.0	0	0
Oncorhynchus masou (masu)	10	100	20.0	40	39.0
Clupea pallasi (herring)	61	71	4.1	2	2.0
Fishes and squids seasonally migrating along islands of Japan					
Pneumatophorus japonicus japonicus (common mackerel)	125	49	3.7	46	3.9
Todarodes pacificus (squid)	101	50	3.3	19	1.5
Trachurus japonicus (horse mackerel)	82	15	1.8	0	0
Cololabis saira (saury)	20	5	1	0	0

	Species					
Fishes migrating ocean with warm current	Sardinops melanosticta (sardine)	20	0	0	0	0
	Lampris regius (moon fish)	2	100	76.5	0	0
	Katsuwonus pelamis (skipjack)	10	90	6.1	0	0
	Sardia orientalis (Japanese bonito)	12	33	1.3	0	0
	Pneumatophorus japonicus tapeinocephalus (spotted mackerel)	20	55	2.5	15	1.7
	Thynus thynus orientalis (tuna)	20	0	0	0	0
Fishes and squids inhabiting Japanese waters without seasonal migration	Oplognathus punctatus (sea bream)	13	0	0	0	0
	Limanda yokohamae (flatfish)	10	0	0	0	0
	Sepia esculenta (squid)	20	0	0	0	0
	Doryteuthis bleekeri (squid)	24	0	0	0	0
	Loligo japonica (squid)	23	0	0	0	0

[a]From Kobayashi et al. (1966), with additional unpublished data.

159

C. Sparganosis

Sparganosis was first reported in Japan in 1881 by Scheube, and since then more than 200 human cases have been reported. Igarashi (1972), summarizing 213 cases, reported that the regions of occurrence in the body, in their order of frequency, were the inguinal or perineum region (35 cases), the abdominal wall or its cavity (35 cases), the eye (28 cases), the chest wall and/or pleural cavity (22 cases), and the thigh (22 cases). The most probable cause of infection is the ingestion of the infected flesh or raw liver of striped snakes as a tonic.

VI. Protozoan Diseases

A. Malaria

In Japan, indigenous malaria caused by *Plasmodium vivax* was prevalent until the beginning of the twentieth century, having spread throughout the middle parts of Honshu, i.e., Toyama, Ishikawa, Fukui, Shiga, and Aichi Prefectures. In 1900, it was estimated that there were approximately 200,000 cases of malaria with 1,000 deaths annually. During 1934–1938, the estimated annual occurrence of cases was 20,000–26,000 (Otsuru, 1977), but after 1938 the disease decreased rapidly.

At the end of World War II, Japan encountered a new problem, "postwar malaria," when 5.84 million persons returned to Japan from abroad. Of these repatriates, approximately 600,000 were reported to have had malaria (Sawada, 1949). On the mainland, the number of patients decreased rapidly and in 1950 only 1,016 cases were reported; fewer than 10 were reported in 1965 and finally, none. The number of new cases infected by the repatriated patients was estimated at 14,000 during 1945–1946, most of which were *P. vivax* infections with a few exceptional cases of *P. falciparum* (Sawada, 1949; Sasa *et al.*, 1949; Otsuru, 1977).

The problem of postwar malaria was most serious in the Yaeyama Islands of Okinawa Prefecture, where malaria was found in half of the population and many died of *P. falciparum* infection. A malaria control program, organized in 1947 as a joint program by Japan and the U.S. Army, utilized residual spraying of DDT. This control measure was soon effective and the infection rate decreased rapidly. However, in 1951 an epidemic that lasted until 1961 occurred among immigrants from adjacent islands (Teruya, 1976).

In recent years, imported malaria has become a new problem (Nakabayashi *et al.*, 1975; Otomo, 1979). The actual number of such cases is not certain. A nationwide survey conducted by a group researching imported malaria reported the number of cases was 470 during the 8 years from 1972 to 1979; *P. vivax,* 278 cases; *P. falciparum,* 134 cases; *P. malariae,* 10 cases; *P. ovale,* 13 cases; 15 cases of mixed infection, and 20 cases caused by an unidentified species. The number of malarial patients fluctuated from 40 to 72 with an average of 59 per year. Most patients with *P. vivax* infections were those who had returned from trips to Southeast Asia; 70% of the patients with *P. falciparum,* and all of those with *P. malariae* or *P. ovale,* had come from Africa.

B. Amoebiasis

Entamoeba histolytica infection has prevailed among the Japanese people at a relatively high rate for many generations, but the prevalence rates were not known. Increased medical concern regarding the existence of *E. histolytica* carriers motivated epidemiological studies beginning around 1930. Surveys conducted from 1926 to 1942 revealed general prevalence rates of 5–10% (Matsubayashi, 1978). After World War II, a nationwide survey carried out by a joint U.S.–Japan survey team indicated a prevalence rate for 18,788 persons that ranged from 1.8 to 11.3% and averaged 7.0%. Therefore, the average postwar prevalence rate has not changed significantly since the prewar period. High infection rates were reported among repatriates (Saito and Takahashi, 1948); Matsubayashi and Tazaki (1954) reported that rats were important reservoir hosts. According to the Ministry of Health and Welfare, the number of cases of human amoebiasis was roughly 200–300 annually during 1953–1959. After 1960 it began to decrease markedly, and in 1966 only 23 cases were reported.

In some countries, human cases of meningoencephalitis caused by free-living amoebae have recently been reported. In Japan one death, of a 27-year-old woman, was caused by *Naegleria* sp. (Nakamura *et al.,* 1979).

C. Toxoplasmosis

Toxoplasma gondii infections have been found in man and animals in various parts of Japan. The prevalence of the dye test antibodies in animals shown by a number of investigators is 56% in goats, 45% in sheep, 40% in cats, 31% in dogs, 24% in swine, 15% in cattle, 5.4% in rats, 1.8% in horses, and 0.9% in chickens (Kobayashi and Nishikawa, 1976). The prevalence rate among Japanese persons varies from area to area, increasing with age. The rates were found to be higher in the southern than in the northern and western parts of Japan; the rates in the eastern and central areas are intermediate. Persons engaging in certain occupations, such as butchers (Tanaka *et al.,* 1958) and abattoir workers

(Kobayashi *et al.*, 1963), were found to be infected at higher rates. A significant correlation in the prevalence rate between man and pigs was also found (Kobayashi, 1977). In Tokyo district, the prevalence rate of positive dye test among pregnant women was found to be 25%, and the seroconversion ratio during pregnancy was estimated at 0.26% (Kobayashi *et al.*, 1974). Cats excreting *T. gondii* oocysts in the feces were 0.9% (Ito *et al.*, 1974), or 1.1% among cats in Tokyo and adjacent areas (Werner and Walton, 1972).

D. Pneumocystis Carinii Pneumonia

Pneumocystis carinii pneumonia has received attention in Japan since the first case was reported (Yoshimura *et al.*, 1961). By 1979, 292 cases had been reported. Yoshida and Ikai (1979) analyzed these cases for predisposing background diseases. There were no cases accompanied by background disease or malnutrition among newborn babies; congenital immunodeficiency is the most frequent contributing factor to *P. carinii* pneumonia in babies less than 4 weeks old. A considerable number of cases of this type of pneumonia in which leukemia is the most important underlying disease appear at 1 to 5 years of age. After age 5, the proportion with leukemia gradually decreased, and preexisting malignant lymphoma, myeloma, and cancer reciprocally increased with age.

VII. Conclusion

This chapter has reviewed the changes with time in various parasitic infections found in Japan. Although some patterns of infection are not entirely clear, the parasitic infections may be classified into the following categories according to their changing patterns.

1. There has been a marked long-term decrease, without showing a particular rise in wartime. Clonorchiasis, filariasis, amoebiasis, and paragonimiasis may be included in this category.
2. Those showing a high prevalence in earlier days and marked decrease recently, with a significant rise during the prewar and early postwar years. Ascariasis, hookworm diseases, trichuriasis, schistosomiasis, malaria, and possibly enterobiasis may be examples.
3. Those showing no significant change. Diphyllobothriasis and metagonimiasis may be included in this category.
4. Those that have received attention comparatively recently as a medical

concern. Toxoplasmosis, anisakiasis and more recently *Pneumocystis carinii* pneumonia and angiostrongyliasis belong to this group.

Although some of these parasitic infections were adopted as target diseases for special control programs and others were not, most diminished rapidly during the last two decades and some have already been eradicated. Single or interdependent factors may have caused these decreases by interrupting the life cycles of the parasites. Rapid rates of economic growth, urbanization, mechanization of agricultural systems, and night soil disposal may be the contributing factors, as were determined for schistosomiasis, clonorchiasis, paragonimiasis, and many other parasitic infections. However, nationwide campaigns for parasite control conducted by voluntary sectors and the government using mass treatment strategy, as described in the section on soil-transmitted helminthiases, enterobiasis, and filariasis, cannot be discounted.

References

Akagi, K. (1973). *Enterobius vermicularis* and enterobiasis. *In* "Progress of Medical Parasitology in Japan" (K. Morishita, Y. Komiya, and H. Matsubayashi, eds.), Vol. V, pp. 233–279. Meguro Parasitological Museum, Tokyo.

Asami, K., Watanuki, T., Sakai, H., Imano, H., and Okamoto, R. (1965). Two cases of stomach granuloma caused by *Anisakis*-like larval nematodes in Japan. *Am. J. Trop. Med. Hyg.* **14,** 119–123.

Eguchi, S. (1964). *Diphyllobothrium latum. In* "Progress of Parasitology in Japan" (K. Morishita, Y. Komiya, and H. Matsubayashi, eds.), Vol. IV, pp. 345–357. Meguro Kiseichukan, Tokyo.*

Fujii, Y. (1847). Katayama disease (with note). *Chugai Iji Shinpo* **691,** 55–56.*

Fujinami, K. (1904). Further discussion of the Katayama disease and its causative parasite. *Kyoto Igakkai Zasshi* **1**(3), 13–25.*

Hayashi, S., Sasa, M., Kano, R., and Sato, K. (1951). Studies on filariasis on Hachijo-Kojima. (2) Discovery of *Brugia malayi,* epidemiological survey and treatment with Hetrazan. *Nisshin Igaku* **38,** 19–22.*

Hayashi, S., Sato, K., Takada, A., Shirasaka, R., Fukui, M., and Sasa, M. (1959). Studies on the epidemiology of pinworm (*Enterobius vermicularis*) in Japan. *Jpn. J. Exp. Med.* **29,** 213–250.

Hayashi, S. (1975). Paragonimiasis miyazakii. *Sogo Rinsho* **24,** 2104–2112.*

Hosaka, Y., Iijima, T., and Sasaki, T. (1957). Studies on the molluscicide field test with Santobrite (sodium pentachlorophenate) and DN-1 (dinitro-*o*-cyclohexylphenol) for *Oncomelania nosophora. Igaku to Seibutsugaku* **44,** 134–141.*

Hotta, T., Chiba, K., Sekikawa, H., Hasegawa, H., and Otsuru, M. (1978). Epidemiological surveys on diphyllobothriasis latum in Niigata Prefecture. (3). *Jpn. J. Parasitol.* **27** (suppl.), 48.*

Hunter, G. W., III, Ritchie, L. S., Kaufman, E. H., Pan, C., Szewczak, J. T., Yokogawa, M., and Ishii, N. (1951). Parasitological studies on the Far East. IV. An epidemiological survey in Yamanashi Prefecture, Honshu, Japan. *Jpn. Med. J.* **4,** 113–124.

*Articles with asterisks are in Japanese.

Igarashi, S., Ikeda, H., Tsujimoto, K., and Miura, H. (1972). A suspected case of *Sparganum mansoni*. *Hifuka no Rinsho* **14**, 197–204.*

Ijuin, T. (1961). Studies on the epidemiology and control of filariasis. 1. Survey on the filarial infection in Self Defense Force of Japan. *Nagasaki Daigaku Fudobyo Kiyo* **3**, 180–187.*

Inoue, Z. (1900). On *Clonorchis sinensis*. *Tokyo Igakkai Zasshi* **14**, 503–562.*

Ishikura, H. (1969). Occurrence of anisakiasis and its clinical presentation. *Saishin Igaku* **24**, 357–365.*

Ishizaka, K. (1878). Records on an autopsy case. *Igaku Zasshi* **40**, 20–26.*

Ishizaki, T., and Komiya, Y. (1963). Treatment of hookworm infection. *In* "Progress of Parasitology in Japan" (K. Morishita, Y. Komiya, and H. Matsubayashi, eds.), Vol. III, pp. 409–480. Meguro Kiseichukan, Tokyo.*

Ito, J., and Mochizuki, H. (1969). Studies on the preventive effect of successive mass treatment with pyrvinium pamoate on pinworm infection in a rural area. *Jpn. J. Parasitol.* **18**, 52–61.*

Ito, S., Tsunoda, K., Nishikawa, H., and Matsui, T. (1974). Small type of *Isospora bigemina*: Isolation from naturally infected cats and relation with *Toxoplasma* oocyst. *Nat. Inst. Anim. Health Q.* **14**, 137–144.

Japan Army Medical Bureau (1913). Distribution of filariasis in Japan. *Gunidan Zasshi* **41**, 332–348.*

Kagei, N., and Oshima, T. (1968). Nationwide epidemiological surveys on the metacercariae of *Metagonimus yokogawai* in "Ayu", *Plecoglossus altivelis*, in Japan. *Jpn. J. Parasitol.* **17**, 461–470.*

Kagei, N., and Kihata, M. (1972). Present status of parasitic infections in Japan. *Nihon Iji Shinshi* **2522**, 27–30.*

Kagei, N., and Kihata, M. (1973). Epidemiological studies on metagonimiasis: Correlation between the metacercaria incidence in "Ayu" *Plecoglossus altivelis* and egg-positive rates in the residents. *Jpn. J. Parasitol.* **22**, 218–221.*

Kamegai, S. (1978). The prevalence and geographical distribution of medical parasites in Japan. *In* "Progress of Medical Parasitology in Japan" (K. Morishita, Y. Komiya, and H. Matsubayashi, eds.), Vol. VI, pp. 279–471. Meguro Parasitological Museum, Tokyo.

Kamo, H., Nishida, H., Hatsushika, R., and Tomimura, T. (1961). On the occurrence of a new lung fluke, *Paragonimus miyazakii* n. sp. in Japan. (Trematoda: Troglotrematidae). *Yonago Acta Med.* **5**, 43–52.

Katamine, D. (1962). Clinical and pathological studies on bancroftian filariasis. *In* "Progress in Parasitology in Japan" (K. Morishita, Y. Komiya, and H. Matsubayashi, eds.), Vol. II, pp. 81–100. Meguro Kiseichukan, Tokyo.*

Kato, T., and Miura, M. (1954). Comparison of some stool examination methods. *Jpn. J. Parasitol.* **3** (suppl.), 35.*

Katsurada, F. (1904). Determination of the source of parasitic disease in Yamanashi and the other prefectures. *Tokyo Iji Shinshi* **1371**, 18–22.*

Kobayashi, A. (1954). Studies on the mode of *Ascaris* infections in Gunma Prefecture. (1) On seasonal change of the infection. *Kitakanto Igaku* **3**, 194–199.*

Kobayashi, A., and Kumada, M. (1957). The effect of several syndets on the elimination of *Ascaris* ova attached to vegetables. *Jpn. J. Parasitol.* **6**, 491–498.*

Kobayashi, A., Ishii, T., Koyama, T., Kumada, M., Komiya, Y., Kanai, T., Fukazawa, T., Koshimizu, K., Saito, K., Onoda, T., and Hanaki, T. (1963). Studies on *Toxoplasma gondii*. (V) Incidence of *Toxoplasma* antibodies in abattoir workers, pluck handlers, ham-making workers and normal residents. *Jpn. J. Parasitol.* **12**, 126–135.*

Kobayashi, A., Koyama, T., Kumada, M., Komiya, Y., Oshima, T., Kagei, N., Ishii, T., and Machida, M. (1966). A survey of marine fishes and squids for the presence of Anisakinae larvae. *Jpn. J. Parasitol.* **15**, 348–349.*

Kobayashi, A., Kumada, M., Sakuma, F., Akita, M., and Omura, T. (1974). Survey of pregnant women and their newborn infants for *Toxoplasma* infection, with special reference to frequency of the congenital transmission. *Jpn. J. Parasitol.* **23,** 383–390.*

Kobayashi, A., Suzuki, S., Horiuchi, K., Yokogawa, M., and Araki, K. (1975). Four human cases of paragonimiasis miyazakii. *Jikeikai Med. J.* **22,** 127–135.

Kobayashi, A., and Nishikawa, H. (1976). Toxoplasmosis, its diagnostic method and epidemiology. *Rinsho to Saikin* **3,** 241–248.*

Kobayashi, A. (1977). Studies on toxoplasmosis. *Tokyo Jikeikai Ikadaigaku Zasshi* **92,** 614–633.*

Kobayashi, H. (1910). Studies on *Clonorchis sinensis. Jpn. J. Bacteriol.* **178,** 49–51.*

Komiya, Y., Ito, J., and Yamamoto, S. (1958). An epidemiological survey of *Metagonimus yokogawai* in Kasumigaura district. *Jpn. J. Parasitol.* **7,** 7–11.*

Komiya, Y. (1959). Epidemiology of *Ascaris* infection. *Yakuji Nippo* 2595, 2607, 2609, 2610, 2612, 2613.*

Komiya, Y., Suzuki, N., Kumada, M., Fukushima, T., and Kozai, I. (1960). On the distribution of *Clonorchis sinensis* around the Lake Biwa areas, Shiga Prefecture. *Jpn. J. Parasitol.* **9,** 162–166.*

Komiya, Y., and Suzuki, N. (1962). Distribution and epidemiology of *Clonorchis sinensis. In* ''Progress of Parasitology in Japan'' (K. Morishita, Y. Komiya, and H. Matsubayashi, eds.), Vol. II, pp. 347–392. Meguro Kiseichukan, Tokyo.*

Komiya, Y. (1962). To eradicate round worm. Its theory and practice. A pamphlet, pp. 1–50. Japan Association of Parasite Control, Tokyo.*

Komiya, Y., Kozai, I., and Suzuki, R. (1962). The increase of the ratio of those expelling only unfertilized eggs of *Ascaris* as the rate of the positive for *Ascaris* eggs among the local social groups diminishes and the utilization of this fact to the eradication program of ascariasis in Japan. *Jpn. J. Parasitol.* **11,** 45–52.*

Komiya, Y. (1964). The prevention of schistosomiasis japonica. In ''Progress of Medical Parasitology in Japan'' (K. Morishita, Y. Komiya, and H. Matsubayashi, eds.), Vol. I, pp. 245–274. Meguro Parasitological Museum, Tokyo.

Komiya, Y., and Suzuki, N. (1966). The metacercariae of Trematodes belonging to the Family Heterophyidae from Japan and adjacent countries. *Jpn. J. Parasitol.* **15,** 208–214.*

Koyama, T., Kobayashi, A.,Kumada, M., Komiya, Y., Oshima, T., Kagei, N., Ishii, T., and Machida, M. (1969). Morphological and taxonomical studies on Anisakidae larvae found in marine fishes and squids. *Jpn. J. Parasitol.* **18,** 466–487.*

Kozai, I. (1962). Re-evaluation of sodium nitrite as an ovicide used in the night soil. (IV). On the field trial with Na nitrite–Ca superphosphate mixture and the effect of its application upon *Ascaris* and hookworm infections among people in treated rural areas of Saitama Prefecture. *Jpn. J. Parasitol.* **11,** 400–410.*

Kutsumi, H. (1967). Field trials of Thiabendazole as an ovicide in the control of helminth infections. (III). Epidemiological analysis of the effectiveness in the control of *Ascaris* infection. *Jpn. J. Parasitol.* **16,** 15–27.*

Matsubayashi, H., and Tazaki, H. (1954). Protozoa parasitic to *Rattus rattus norvegicus. Eisei Dobutsu* **4** (special issue), 1–5.*

Matsubayashi, H. (1978). *Entamoeba histolytica. In* ''Progress of Medical Parasitology in Japan'' (K. Morishita, Y. Komiya, and H. Matsubayashi, eds.), Vol. VI, pp. 5–56. Meguro Parasitological Museum, Tokyo.

Matsuzaki, G. (1951). Prevention of *Ascaris* and hookworm infections. *Rinsho Igaku* **37,** 212–223.*

McMullen, D. B., Ishii, N., and Mitoma, Y. (1948). Results of screening tests on chemicals as molluscicides. *J. Parasitol.* **34** (suppl.), 33.*

Minai, N., Chiba, H., Kutsumi, H., Yokogawa, M., and Araki, K. (1974). Human cases with

Paragonimus miyazakii which occurred recently in Yamanashi Prefecture. *Jpn. Soc. Parasitol., East Japan Regional Meeting, 34th, (unpubl.).* *

Miura, K. (1954). Studies on chemotherapy against hookworm disease. On the effect of 1-bromo-2-naphthol. *Jpn. J. Med. Sci. Biol.* **7**, 265–273.

Miyairi, K., and Suzuki, M. (1913). A contribution to the development of *Schistosoma japonicum. Tokyo Iji Shinshi* **1836**, 1–5.*

Miyazaki, I., Terasaki, K., and Iwata, K. (1978). Natural infection of muscle of wild boars in Japan by immature *Paragonimus westermani* (Kerbert 1878). *J. Parasitol.* **64**, 559–560.

Morishita, K. (1955). A general view of anthelmintics for ascariasis. *Shinryo* **8**, 585–594.*

Morishita, K. (1972). Studies on epidemiological aspects of ascariasis in Japan, and basic knowledge concerning its control. *In* "Progress of Medical Parasitology in Japan" (K. Morishita, Y. Komiya, and H. Matsubayashi, eds.), Vol. IV, pp. 3–153. Meguro Parasitological Museum, Tokyo.

Morishita, K. (1974). Outcome of the parasite eradication campaign. *Yobo Igaku.* **80**, 18–26.*

Murakami, S., Takemoto, T., and Shimizu, Z. (1953). Studies on the effective principles of *Digenea simplex*. 1. Separation of the effective fraction by liquid chromatography. *J. Pharm. Soc. Jpn.* **73**, 1026–1028.*

Muto, S. (1918). On the first intermediate host of *Clonorchis sinensis. Jpn. J. Pathol.* **8**, 228–230.*

Nakabayashi, T., Otomo, H., Ebisawa, I., and Ishizaki, T. (1975). Present situation of the imported malaria. *Koshu Eisei Joho* **5**, 1–4.*

Nakagawa, K. (1915). A preliminary report on the discovery of the intermediate host of the human fluke. *Tokyo Iji Shinshi* **1910**, 464–469.*

Nakamura, T., Kobayashi, M., Wada, H., Tsunoda, Y., Arai, K., and Omata, K. (1979). An autopsy case of primary amoebic meningoencephalitis. *Shinkei Kenkyu no Shimpo.* **23**, 500–509.*

Okabe, K. (1964). Biology and epidemiology of *Schistosoma japonicum* and schistosomiasis. *In* "Progress of Medical Parasitology in Japan" (K. Morishita, Y. Komiya, and H. Matsubayashi, eds.), Vol. I, pp. 185–218. Meguro Parasitological Museum, Tokyo.

Okamoto, K., Asechi, S., and Nagata, K. (1963). Recent trend of distribution and treatment of chyluria patients in Japan. *Nippon Iji Shinpo* **2052**, 12–15.*

Olivier, L. (1948). A note on schistosomiasis in eastern Japan. *Am. J. Trop. Med.* **28**, 867–875.

Omori, N. (1962). On the vector mosquitoes of bancroftian filariasis with special reference to the role of *Culex pipiens pallens. In* "Progress of Parasitology in Japan" (K. Morishita, Y. Komiya, and H. Matsubayashi, eds.), Vol. II, pp. 35–65. Meguro Kiseichukan, Tokyo.*

Oshima, T. (1972). Anisakis and anisakiasis in Japan and adjacent area. *In* "Progress of Medical Parasitology in Japan" (K. Morishita, Y. Komiya, and H. Matsubayashi, eds.), Vol. IV, pp. 305–393. Meguro Parasitological Museum, Tokyo.

Otomo, H. (1979). Recent trend toward malaria. *Koshu Eisei* **43**, 865–869.*

Otsuru, M. (1977). The imported malaria in Japan, with special reference to the present situation and therapy. *Nippon Ishikai Zasshi* **77**, 117–125.*

Otsuru, M. (1978). *Angiostrongylus cantonensis* and angiostrongyliasis in Japan, with those of neighboring Taiwan. *In* "Progress of Medical Parasitology in Japan" (K. Morishita, Y. Komiya, and H. Matsubayashi, eds.), Vol. VI, pp. 227–274. Meguro Parasitological Museum, Tokyo.

Ritchie, L. S., Hunter, G. W. III., Kaufman, E. H., Pan, C., Nagano, K., Yokogawa, M., and Szewczak, J. T. (1951). Parasitological studies in the Far East. (V) An epidemiologic survey in Okayama Prefecture. *Jpn. Med. J.* **4**, 307–314.

Ritchie, L. S., Hunter, G. W., III., Pan, C., Yokogawa, M., and Szewczak, J. T. (1952). Parasitological studies in the Far East. (VI) An epidemiologic survey on Kyushu Island, Japan. *Jpn. J. Med. Sci. Biol.* **5**, 299–310.

Ritchie, L. S., Hunter, G. W., III., Pan, C., Yokogawa, M., Nagano, K., and Szewczak, J. T.

(1953). Parasitological studies in the Far East. (VIII) An epidemiologic study on the Tone River area, Japan. *Jpn. J. Med. Sci. Biol.* **6**, 33–43.

Saito, M., and Takahashi, R. (1948). Therapy and epidemiological investigation on so-called cyst carrier of *Entamoeba histolytica*. *Koshu Eiseigaku Zasshi* **4**, 208–211.*

Sasa, M., Takahashi, H., Kogo, T., and Oshima, H. (1949). An epidemic of tropical malaria observed in Hokkaido. *Sogo Igaku* **6**, 340–343.*

Sasa, M. (1962). Distribution of bancroftian filariasis in Japan. *In* "Progress of Parasitology in Japan" (K. Morishita, Y. Komiya, and H. Matsubayashi, eds.), Vol. II, pp. 1–34. Meguro Kiseichukan, Tokyo.*

Sasa, M. (1966). Epidemiology of human filariasis in Japan. *In* "Progress of Medical Parasitology in Japan" (K. Morishita, Y. Komiya, and H. Matsubayashi, eds.), Vol. III, pp. 389–436. Meguro Parasitological Museum, Tokyo.

Sasa, M., Kanda, T., Mitsui, G., Shirasaka, A., Ishii, A., and Chinzei, H. (1970). The filariasis control program in Japan and their evaluation by means of epidemiological analysis of the microfilaria survey data. *In* "Recent Advances in Researches on Filariasis and Schistosomiasis in Japan" (M. Sasa, ed.), pp. 3–72. Univ. of Tokyo Press, Tokyo.

Sasaki, T. (1958). Cementing ditches of the habitat of *Oncomelania* as a control measure of schistosomiasis japonica. *Jpn. J. Parasitol.* **7**, 545–559.*

Sato, H. (1966). On the treatment of filariasis. *In* "Progress of Medical Parasitology in Japan" (K. Morishita, Y. Komiya, and H. Matsubayashi, eds.), Vol. III, pp. 513–527. Meguro Parasitological Museum, Tokyo.

Sato, H., Otsuji, Y., and Maeda, T. (1971). Filariasis. *Naika* **27**, 438–444.*

Sato, Y., Takai, A., and Otsuru, M. (1980). *Angiostrongylus cantonensis* and angiostrongyliasis. *Proc., Sino–Japanese Seminar on Parasitic Zoonoses*, pp. 88–93.

Sawada, T. (1949). The Postwar Malaria. *Nihon Naikagakkai Zasshi* **38**, 1–14.*

Shiraki, T., and Otsuru, M. (1968). On the Anisakinae larvae found in marine fishes of northern Japan. *Jpn. J. Parasitol.* **17** (suppl.), 642.*

Suzuki, H., Onuma, H., Karasawa, Y., Obayashi, M., Koyama, T., Kumada, M., and Yokogawa, M. (1972). *Terranova* (Nematoda: Anisakidae) infection in man. (1) Clinical features of five cases of *Terranova* larva infection. *Jpn. J. Parasitol.* **21**, 252–256.

Tanaka, H., Kojima, S., and Maitani, T. (1958). Study on toxoplasmosis. (1) Toxoplasmin test of the families keeping pet dogs and of the butchers in Niigata City. *Igaku to Seibutsugaku* **47**, 238–242.*

Tanaka, H. (1966). Genus *Strongyloides*. *In* "Progress of Medical Parasitology in Japan" (K. Morishita, Y. Komiya, and H. Matsubayashi, eds.), Vol. III, pp. 591–638. Meguro Parasitological Museum, Tokyo.

Teruya, H. (1976). Postwar changes in major infectious diseases in Okinawa. *Okinawa Kogaikenkyujoho* **9**, 175–217.*

Uchida, A., Nozue, S., Ogura, K., Uchida, F., and Ito, Y. (1967). Measures taken to prevent and exterminate *Ascaris* infection in rural district. (2) Study of factors for *Ascaris* infection. *Report of Institute of Rural Medicine, Chiba Medical School*, 267–272.*

Van Thiel, P. H. (1962). Anisakiasis. *Parasitology* **52** (suppl.), 16–17.

Werner, J. K., and Walton, B. C. (1972). Prevalence of naturally occurring *Toxoplasma* infections in cats from U.S. military installations in Japan. *J. Parasitol.* **58**, 1148–1150.

Wharton, R. H., Edeson, J. F. B., Wilson, T., and Reid, J. A. (1958). Studies on filariasis in Malaya: Pilot experiments in the control of filariasis due to *Wuchereria malayi* in East Pahang. *Ann. Trop. Med. Parasitol.* **51**, 191–205.

Yajima, T. (1955). Studies on the natural infection of *Ascaris* in man. *Jpn. J. Parasitol.* **4**, 23–29.*

Yamaguchi, T., Yamashita, M., Yoshida, H., Inamura, E., and Shimawaki, K. (1978). On the human cases of diphyllobothriasis in Aomori Prefecture. *Nippon Iji Shinpo* **2820**, 29–31.*

Yamamoto, H. (1965). Studies on epidemiology of filariasis. (3) Comparative studies on the effect of diethylcarbamazine on the microfilarial carriers administered at different doses and intervals. *Jpn. J. Parasitol.* **14**, 169–181.*

Yamanashi Prefectural Association of Schistosomiasis Control (1977). Struggle against the endemic disease. pp. 1–330.*

Yamanashi Prefectural Institute of Health (1981). *Personal communication.*

Yamashita, J. (1973). Echinococcus and echinococcosis. *In* "Progress of Medical Parasitology in Japan" (K. Morishita, Y. Komiya, and H. Matsubayashi, eds.), Vol. V, pp. 67–123. Meguro Parasitological Museum, Tokyo.

Yanagisawa, R. (1966). The epidemiology of hookworm disease. *In* "Progress of Medical Parasitology in Japan" (K. Morishita, Y. Komiya, and H. Matsubayashi, eds.), Vol. III, pp. 287–366. Meguro Parasitological Museum, Tokyo.

Yasuraoka, K., Hosaka, Y., and Komiya, Y. (1968). Some laboratory investigations Yurimin P-99 as an experimental molluscicide. *Jpn. J. Parasitol.* **17**, 376–381.

Yokogawa, M., Oshima, T., and Suguro, T. (1955). Intradermal test for paragonimiasis. (I) *Jpn. J. Parasitol.* **4**, 276–281.*

Yokogawa, M., Yoshimura, H., Okura, T., Sano, M., Tsuji, M., Iwasaki, M., and Hirosa, H. (1961). Chemotherapy of paragonimiasis with bithionol. (II) Clinical observations on the treatment of bithionol. *Jpn. J. Parasitol.* **10**, 317–327*

Yokogawa, M., Sano, M., Tsuji, M., Kojima, S., Iijima, T., and Ito, Y. (1969). Treatment of schistosomiasis japonica with niridazole. *Ann. N. Y. Acad. Sci.* **1960** (Art. 2), 933–946.

Yokogawa, M., Araki, K., Saito, K., Momose, T., Kimura, M., Suzuki, S., Chiba, N., Kutsumi, H., and Minai, M. (1974). *Paragonimus miyazakii* infections in man first found in Kanto district, Japan. *Jpn. J. Parasitol.* **23**, 167–179.*

Yokogawa, M. (1974). Epidemiology and control of schistomiasis japonica. *In* "A Symposium on Epidemiology of Parasitic Diseases" (M. Sasa, ed.), pp. 83–99. International Medical Foundation of Japan, Tokyo.

Yokogawa, M. (1976). Review of prevalence and distribution of schistosomiasis in Japan. *Southeast Asian J. Trop. Med. Public Health* **7**, 137–143.

Yokogawa, S. (1912). Additional note on a new heterophyid worm which has *Plecoglossus altivelis* as intermediate host. *Tokyo Iji Shinshi* **1776**, 1–3.*

Yoshida, Y., and Ikai, T. (1979). *Pneumocystis carinii* pneumonia: Epidemiology in Japan, and cyst concentration method. *Zentralb. Bakteriol. Parasitenkd. Infektionskr. Hyg. Abt. 1: Orig. A* **244**, 405–410.

Yoshimura, H., Hirano, T., Okajima, H., Uchida, N., Kato, S., and Kono, M. (1961). An autopsy case of intestinal plasmacellular pneumonia supposed to be caused by *Pneumocystis carinii*. *Igaku no Ayumi* **38**, 158–160.*

Yoshimura, H. (1966). Larva migrans by *Anisakis* larva causing eosinophilic phlegmon of human digestive tract. *Minophagen Med. Rev.* **11**, 105–114.*

Yoshimura, H., Kondo, K., Onishi, Y., Moriya, S., and Kamimura, K. (1975). Diphyllobothriasis in Hokuriku district. *Nippon Iji Shinpo* **2693**, 22–25.*

7

Parasite Control Activities in Japan: Government–Expert–Private Sector Partnership

CHOJIRO KUNII

Japan Association of Parasite Control
Hoken Kaikan Bekkan
Ichigaya, Shinjuku-Ku
Tokyo, Japan

I. Introduction

In Japan, parasitic diseases, particularly ascariasis and hookworm, have long been occupational diseases of farmers. Until the 1940s, farmers comprised a majority of the Japanese population; therefore, the debilitation caused by parasitic infections, particularly hookworm, was a major public health problem (Table I). A primary cause was the traditional use of night soil as a fertilizer. Human feces containing parasite eggs were spread on the fields and, as a result, farmers were infected either by emerging hookworm larvae as they worked barefoot in the fields or by eating contaminated fresh vegetables or pickles, long-standing staples of the Japanese diet.

Mass examination or treatment to control parasites was almost nonexistent.

TABLE I

Geographical Distribution of Hookworm Infection[a]

Place	Number examined	Infection rate (%)	Examination method	References
Saitama Prefecture	419,967	42.9	Concentration	Matsusaki (1942)[b]
Saitama Prefecture	1,036	62.4	Concentration	Komiya et al. (1952)
Gunma Prefecture	3,285	36	Concentration	Ministry of Interior (1929)
Tokyo	1,347	21.4	Direct smear	Nakagawa et al. (1951)
		47.0	Sedimentation	
Okinawa	1,360	63.4	Direct smear	Sasa et al. (1957)
		86.0	Floatation	
		97.0	Culture	
Amami Islands	2,006	90	Direct smear, brine floatation, and filter-paper culture	Sasa et al. (1958)
Hachijo Island	9,970	24.3	Direct smear	Nishida (1958)
		83.8	Floatation	

[a]From Yanagisawa, 1966.
[b]Data were obtained from surveys conducted from 1924 to 1929.

Instead, people would periodically take medicines to deworm themselves. Extract of degenea or Santonin was the most commonly used anthelmintic. These drugs were made available to the public through household medicine distributors based in Toyama Prefecture in northwestern Japan. In the case of hookworm disease, symptoms such as shortness of breath were often mistaken for heart disease; as a result, patients developed serious anemia because of delay of specific treatment. In such cases, 7–10 days of hospitalization were required, which imposed considerable expense. Farmers feared hookworm disease, calling it "blue-in-the-face" disease (in reference to the pallor caused by hookworm anemia), and "at-the-foot-of-the-hill" disease (because of its capacity to cause shortness of breath, which made it very difficult to climb stairs and hills) (Table II).

Following World War II, populations in metropolitan areas such as Tokyo and Osaka were also found to be highly infected with *Ascaris lumbricoides* and hookworm because of the deterioration in the standard of living, food shortages, etc. People were forced to live in small, unsanitary houses, and soap was lacking, as were anthelmintics. To make up for food shortages, people in cities planted vegetables in small home gardens, using night soil as fertilizer. These factors multiplied parasitic infections among family members. Other major infection sources were the children who brought back to their homes infections from rural areas where they had been evacuated during the war. Thus, in the early postwar years parasitic infections had increased to levels as high as

TABLE II

Signs and Symptoms in Hookworm Disease[a] Detected among 101 Japanese Patients[b]

Anemia	Pallor (44)[c], palpitation of the heart (29), shortness of breath (21), oedema (3), tinnitus (2)
Digestive disturbance	Abdominal pain (30), loss of appetite (24), full feeling in stomach (11), pyrosis (8), nausea (6), full feeling in bowels (3), vomiting (2)
Neuromuscular system	Headache (15), dizziness (15), weakness in extremities (11), languor (10), stiffness of shoulder (4), oppression of the chest (1)
Other	Change in nail (38), loss of weight (8), light fever (5), pain on sternum (1)

[a]Mostly *Ancylostoma duodenale.*
[b]From Matsusaka, 1931.
[c]Number in parentheses equals number of patients.

60–70% in both urban and rural populations, and health problems caused by parasites became more serious. Symptoms of hookworm disease such as anemia, shortness of breath, light fever, and stomach pain were common, as were stomachaches, appendicitis, and malnutrition resulting from ascariasis. In those years, it became a popular practice among medical practitioners to prescribe anthelmintics. Parasite-related symptoms disappeared soon after deworming, and physicians developed reputations for being skilled. In spite of the high prevalence of parasites, the Ministry of Health and Welfare (MOHW) of the Japanese government took no effective countermeasures. The government considered it more important to control more harmful and life-threatening diseases such as tuberculosis, dysentery, and typhus. Under the circumstances, the general public simply accepted conditions as they were, thinking it impossible to escape from parasites. Parasitism was called a ''national disease'' because of this sociocultural and historical background.

II. Tokyo Parasite Control Association

The Tokyo Parasite Control Association (TPCA) was established in June 1949 as a voluntary organization with technical support from Professor Makoto Koizumi and his staff at the Department of Parasitology, Keio University School of Medicine. The TPCA initiated activities in parasite control education, mass examination, and mass treatment for schools, enterprises, and communities (cities, towns, and villages). Although it charged 10 yen for a stool examination (the average monthly salary then was around 20,000 yen), the TPCA was able to gain enthusiastic support of many people and from the Tokyo Department of Health because of the immediate and visible effects of deworming.

TABLE III

Results of the Stool Examination for Schoolchildren[a]

		Number positive (%)				
District[b]	Number examined	*Ascaris lumbricoides*	*Trichuris trichiuria*	Pinworm	Hookworm	Combined infection (%)
Chuoh	9620	5611 (58.3)	239 (2.48)	6 (0.06)	12 (0.12)	5868 (61.0)
Minato	9782	7096 (72.5)	253 (2.59)	16 (0.16)	20 (0.20)	7385 (75.5)
Shinjuku	1544	1209 (78.3)	38 (2.46)	4 (0.26)	3 (0.19)	1254 (81.2)
Musashino	5011	3912 (78.0)	160 (3.19)	8 (0.16)	16 (0.32)	4096 (81.7)

[a]Tokyo Parasite Control Association, 1949.

[b]These are some of the districts actually covered. At that time Chuoh and Minato districts represented central Tokyo, while Shinjuku and Musashino districts represented suburbs or farming areas.

As the TPCA's activities expanded, its efforts were publicized through radio and newspapers (TV had not yet been introduced) and the Association became known throughout the country. Inspired by the TPCA's activities, similar voluntary organizations were established by medical departments of universities together with volunteer groups in such cities as Osaka, Okayama, Fukuoka, Gunma, Sendai, Matsumoto, Kagoshima, and Yokohama. In the first year of its establishment, the TPCA conducted parasite examinations for schoolchildren in the Tokyo metropolitan area, using the direct smear method. The results are as seen in Table III.

III. Government Attitude

The Japanese government first enacted a law on parasite control, entitled "The Parasite Control Act," in 1931. Because the act stipulated that "health and feces examinations may be ordered by a governor of . . . a prefecture (a mayor in the case of a city as designated by Cabinet Order . . .) when he deems it necessary for the prevention of parasitosis," the act was not effective. Although parasite examination and treatment were conducted by government health centers upon request at a nominal charge, people preferred to go to drug stores or medical practitioners. After the war, the government issued simple directives to health departments of prefectural governments and health centers on the "Mass Treatment of *Ascaris* Infection" in 1949 and the "Mass Treatment of Hookworm Infection" in 1952.

In the meantime, the voluntary parasite control movement began to have such an impact on the government that the MOHW established a Council on Parasite

TABLE IV

Effects of Repeated Mass Treatment for Hookworm Infection among 212 Villagers
(37 Households) in Japan (1954–1956)[a]

	1954			1955				1956		
	Aug	Oct	Dec	Mar	June	Aug	Dec	Mar	July	Dec
Number positive	135	69	58	24	15	12	6	8	6	6
% positive	63.7	32.5	27.4	11.3	7.1	5.7	2.8	3.8	2.8	2.8

[a]From Yanagisawa, 1957.

Control in 1949 with the aim of studying and discussing important issues relating to parasite control. The Council was composed of experts from the Japanese Society of Parasitology and the officers in charge of the MOHW and the Ministry of Education. At its meetings a very interesting argument was raised among members regarding mass treatment as conducted by the TPCA. The argument was posed that even with repeated mass treatment, reinfection would occur as a result of unsanitary living conditions and, therefore, that mass treatment would be futile. Experts countered by insisting that if mass treatment were regularly conducted (at least twice a year) in a given area, the number of fertile parasite eggs would gradually decrease and reinfection rates in the area ultimately would be greatly reduced (Table IV).

Because the environment in Tokyo was contaminated, these arguments could not help but attract the interest of the people concerned. In those days 25% of human waste was channeled into the sea, 25% into sewage systems, and the remaining 50% carried away to neighboring farming areas for use as fertilizer. This created a vicious cycle in that a large quantity of parasite-contaminated vegetables was returned to Tokyo from those areas. The MOHW wished to direct the discussions of Council members toward establishing a national parasite control organization.

IV. Establishment of Japan Association of Parasite Control

The Japan Association of Parasite Control (JAPC) was established in 1955 as a private organization through the efforts of experts from the Japanese Society of Parasitology and 10 voluntary organizations in Tokyo, Osaka, Aichi, Kanagawa, Miyazaki, Fukuoka, Yamaguchi, Hiroshima, Okayama, and Nagano Prefectures. The organizations had previously initiated parasite control activities with

TABLE V

Schedule of the 1969 Training Course for Parasite Laboratory Technicians Sponsored by JAPC

Day	0900–0930	0930–1000	100–1200
1	Orientation	Opening ceremonies	Lecture: Sensitivity of the fecal smear techniques for various helminth eggs
2			Lecture: Problems relating to the identification of various helminth eggs
3			Lecture: Method for EPG examination, Culture Technique for hookworm eggs, and blood examination method for Microfilariae
4			Lecture: Theory and practice of Concentration Technique
5			Lecture: Degeneration process and viability test of *Ascaris* eggs
6			Lecture: Special examination techniques: Perianal Swab Method; Sputum Examination Method
7			Holiday (study and preparation for examination)
8			Examination (written test and practice drill) for certifying qualified parasite laboratory technicians

the technical support of university departments of parasitology or prefectural institutes of health which functioned as research institutes under the jurisdiction of health departments of prefectural governments.

The JAPC served as the headquarters for these associate member organizations. The office was located within the Tokyo Parasite Control Association as the JAPC could not afford its own fulltime staff. The JAPC allocated a small budget to cover administrative costs, which fell far below actual needs; the deficit was covered by the TPCA. MOHW officials served on the JAPC governing board, but no government subsidy was provided.

The objectives of the JAPC were (1) to strengthen and expand the activities of the 10 founding branches by exchanging information, facilitating mutual liaison, improving techniques, conducting publicity campaigns, etc., (2) to help establish similar associations in other prefectures, (3) to conduct training for parasite laboratory technicians in order to develop examination techniques, to study drug effects, and to produce educational materials such as films, slides, charts, posters, and pamphlets in cooperation with the Japanese Society of Parasitology, (4) to conduct fundraising drives for the purpose of constructing laboratories and installing modern facilities, (5) to lobby the MOHW for a positive policy on parasite control through providing information or submitting proposals, and (6) to cooperate with the Japanese Society of Parasitology.

In line with these objectives, a monthly newsletter entitled *Kiseichu Yobo*

TABLE V (*continued*)

1200–1300	1300–1600	1600–1700
Lunch	Practice: Thick Smear Technique and its sensitivity	Demonstration: The first intermediate host of Trematoda and cercariae
Lunch	Practice: Identification of various helminth eggs	Demonstration: The second intermediate hosts of Trematoda and metacercariae
Lunch	Practice: Egg-Count Technique and Egg Culture Technique	Demonstration: Hookworm and other larvae
Lunch	Practice: Concentration Technique	Demonstration: Nematoda
Lunch	Practice: Distinguishing live eggs from dead ones contained in soil, improved latrines, and tank of night soil treatment plant	Demonstration: Trematoda and Cestoda
Lunch	Free discussion	Certificate awards
	Holiday (study and preparation for examination)	
Lunch	Announcement of examination results	

(Parasite Control) was published and distributed to schools, health centers, and health departments of cities, towns, and villages. In addition, an annual national conference, training, block-level lecture meetings, and production of films and other educational materials were instituted one after another (Tables V and VI). In the initial stages, JAPC branches had no reserve funds and had to borrow rooms at university laboratories or government health institutes to serve as their offices. As the demand for parasite examination and treatment, particularly for schoolchildren, increased to very high levels among the general public, they were gradually able to become self-reliant. JAPC branches cooperated with each other under the guidance of the headquarters for further expansion of activities. The number of branches increased year by year; the financial base became more solid; the annual number of examinations rose to 13 million in the peak year (1967); and parasitic infection rates steadily declined over the years (Table VII, Fig. 1).

The activities of this nationwide movement were based on the following principles:

1. Disseminating the concept of preventive medicine. Parasite control is considered a part of preventive medicine, a field in which Japan still lags. Parasitic infections are found mostly in farmers, children, and the urban poor. In view of this fact, it should be emphasized that parasite control is a social movement from

TABLE VI

Number of Trainees Certified in the JAPC Training Course
(1963–1979)

Course	Year	Number of trainees	Number of trainees certified (%)
1st	1963	28	25 (89.3)
2nd	1964	40	35 (87.5)
3rd	1965	39	34 (87.2)
4th	1966	25	23 (92.0)
5th	1967	40	40 (100.0)
6th	1969	32	27 (84.4)
7th	1970	40	34 (85.0)
8th	1971	37	36 (97.3)
9th	1973	29	29 (100.0)
10th	1976	32	32 (100.0)
11th	1977	18	18 (100.0)
12th	1979	21[a]	0[a]
Total		381	333 (87.4)[b]

[a]The 12th training course was conducted for beginners only and trainees were not certified.

[b]Certified trainees represent 92.5% of all trainees, from 1st through 11th courses.

TABLE VII

Results of Stool Examinations Conducted by JAPC

Year[a]	1961	1963	1965	1967
Number examined	9,612,765	11,484,401	12,720,315	13,020,773
% parasitized	16.2	12.9	8.7	6.3
Ascaris lumbricoides	9.1	6.0	3.7	2.5
Hookworm	1.6	2.1	1.4	0.9
Trichuris trichiura	6.0	5.3	3.8	2.7
Trichostrongylus orientalis	0.3	0.3	0.2	0.1
Clonorchis sinensis	0.01	0.02	0.01	0.01
Metagenimus yokogawai	0.1	0.3	0.2	0.2
Schistosoma japonicum	(22)[b]	(0)	(147)	(110)
Paragonimus westermani	(52)	(158)	(54)	(22)
Hymenolepis nana	—[c]	—	(363)	(184)
Diphyllobothrium latum	—	—	—	—
Strongyloides stercoralis	—	—	—	—

[a]Actual examination results are recorded annually.

[b]Number in parentheses shows numbers of cases. Other figures represent percentage of infection.

[c]Data are not available.

the standpoint of social justice, human rights, and humanism. The staff of parasite control organizations should be thoroughly trained regarding this basic concept.

2. Respecting scholars and improving techniques. Parasite control is, in a sense, an academic mission. Without academic support, staffs cannot promote the movement with confidence and pride. Therefore, training and study to acquire advanced techniques should be conducted continuously.

3. Modernizing facilities. Parasite control organizations should endeavor to acquire their own laboratories and offices as soon as possible, and to equip them with modern facilities. For this purpose economizing on expenses and raising funds should be strongly emphasized.

4. Avoiding bureaucracy. Parasite control organizations were created without government aid, but as a result of determination of the people. Therefore, activities should always be imaginative, energetic, and unselfish in order to best serve the people.

Along with the growth of activities, some creative ideas regarding new techniques developed at the branch level. These included

1. The Kato Method, now known worldwide as the Cellophane Thick Smear Method. It was developed in 1961 by Dr. Katsuya Kato, then a medical technician at the Aichi branch, to improve the efficiency, accuracy, and economy of mass examinations.

TABLE VII (*continued*)

1969	1971	1973	1975	1977	1979
10,856,507	9,540,876	7,789,605	4,112,870	3,159,392	2,727,820
3.7	2.14	1.31	1.20	0.82	0.52
1.4	0.72	0.38	0.27	0.22	0.09
0.4	0.23	0.19	0.11	0.05	0.02
1.9	0.98	0.51	0.33	0.20	0.11
0.04	0.03	0.01	0.004	0.003	0.001
(924)	(780)	(819)	(102)	(0)	(14)
0.2	0.09	0.12	0.23	0.35	0.27
(62)	(11)	0.001	(0)	(0)	(0)
(10)	(17)	(0)	(6)	(25)	(0)
(354)	(34)	(12)	(1)	(28)	(11)
—	—	—	(18)	(8)	(5)
—	—	—	(361)	(361)	(337)

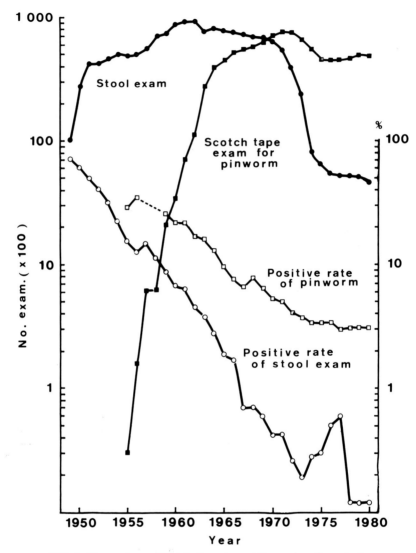

FIG. 1. Changes in parasitic infection rates and the number of examinations.

2. Coizumin (a compound of Santonin and kainic acid). The Tokyo branch developed Coizumin as a new anthelmintic for the treatment of *Ascaris lumbricoides* infections to meet a shortage of modern drugs. Registered as an authorized drug in 1956, Coizumin was used as an effective, inexpensive drug

over a 10-year period in Japan. During this period pharmaceutical companies eagerly produced the drug.

V. Government Policy and Programs

After the JAPC gained recognition by the government for its activities, it was asked to draft guidelines on parasite control. Responding to this request, Professor Y. Komiya, permanent director of the JAPC, drafted guidelines that were adopted by the MOHW as directives: "Essentials of Mass Treatment of *Ascaris* and Hookworm Infections" (June 1958) and "General Essentials of Parasite Control" (June 1959). These essentials played an important role in determining the direction of parasite control in Japan. Major points of these directives are that (1) at the initial stage the target parasites of control programs should be limited to *Ascaris lumbricoides* and hookworm, which are the most prevalent infections in Japan, (2) cities, towns, and villages throughout Japan should periodically conduct mass examination and treatment, (3) attention should be given to sanitary disposal of night soil and cultivation of parasite-free vegetables, and (4) parasite control education should be widely conducted.

Stimulated by the MOHW's commitment, the Ministry of Education enacted a School Hygiene Act in 1958 (as early as 1897 a school hygiene act had been established for the purpose of prevention of infectious diseases; however, with changing conditions, the act became outdated and another act, under the same title, was enacted in 1958). The act stipulated that parasite control should be conducted as part of regular annual health checkups for schoolchildren; this served as a driving force to further strengthen the nationwide parasite control program. By this enactment, the government covered examination and treatment fees for parents, and the demand for parasite examination and treatment increased. Accordingly, the amount of work entrusted to JAPC branches grew rapidly.

In 1963, the MOHW launched a special program for hookworm control. The objective of the program was to control hookworm in selected highly infected agricultural prefectures by allocating funds for 3 years. In the first year, Ibaraki, Saitama, Chiba, and Niigata Prefectures were selected. In the following 2 years, the program included nine prefectures: Akita, Okayama, Miyazaki, Fukushima, Ehime, Kochi, Tochigi, Yamanashi, and Shimane. This special program was enthusiastically welcomed by farmers, who helped the JAPC movement to expand. In addition to the control program for soil-transmitted helminths, the government designed a 10-year plan to control schistosomiasis in 1957. Through such efforts as lining irrigation ditches with concrete, the vector snail has been almost eradicated. In 1962 the government also began a Filariasis Control Program in the southern islands under the jurisdiction of eight prefectures: Kagoshima, Kumamoto, Nagasaki, Miyazaki, Oita, Kochi, Ehime, and Tokyo. The program succeeded in completely eradicating filariasis.

VI. Factors Contributing to the Decrease in Parasitic Infections

Parasitism in Japan, which once prevailed at extremely high rates, has decreased year by year nearly to the point of eradication. In the following sections, factors contributing to the decline in the parasitic infection rates will be discussed.

A. Nationwide Implementation of Parasite Control Programs

As outlined above, the JAPC struggled at the forefront in the battle against parasites. In terms of technical assistance, the Japanese Society of Parasitology added its support to these efforts. The government helped facilitate the promotion of parasite control, jointly undertaken by voluntary organizations and experts, through establishing a parasite control policy, conducting special control programs, and establishing a parasite control week. The teamwork of a tripartite body composed of government, technical experts, and the private sector has resulted in progress toward the common goal of parasite control, with a division of roles according to the characteristics of each sector. The government health centers (1 per 100,000 population on the average; around 700 in number in the 1950s) also played an important role, but they served mainly in the mountainous or remote areas of the country which required more funds to cover. More manageable areas, in terms of finance and geography, were left to voluntary organizations.

B. Distribution of Chemical Fertilizer

After the war, the government promoted the mass production of chemical fertilizer and its distribution in order to increase food production. The government's efforts were successful, and the use of night soil as fertilizer finally ended. Around 1955, in accord with these developments, the authorities in urban areas did their best to solve the problem of human waste disposal.

C.   Improved Quality of Life and Dissemination of Health Information

The standard of living, which dropped to an unprecedented low after defeat in World War II, improved year by year, and by 1955 had reached prewar levels. An abundance of soap and synthetic detergents became available to individual families, which remarkably improved the sanitary conditions of the people. At the same time, health education in schools or through the mass media helped enhance the people's understanding of health. By then, community organizations had begun to conduct various health programs, and the services themselves worked as a catalyst to inspire people to the awareness of good health. Such changes contributed to the dramatic decline in parasitism.

VII.   Preventive Medicine

Since around 1965, as infection rates decreased, the JAPC emphasis has shifted from parasite control alone to preventive health services which range from parasite examinations to examinations for anemia, bacterial infections (e.g., dysentery bacillus and *Salmonella*), cancer (stomach, lung, uterus, and breast), and urinary and other infections. This shift has hastened the modernization of examination facilities and the training of medical technicians in new techniques. The MOHW and health departments of local governments have provided financial assistance for these additional activities.

As part of this shift, the Japan Association of Health Service was established in 1966. Its activities are divided into two categories, mass health examinations and health education. When medical problems are determined, the client is referred to medical institutions such as hospitals, whereas a person found in good health is introduced to health promotion-related organizations in such areas as sports, nutrition, and recreation. Preventive health services are thus provided in cooperation with other institutions, and in accordance with the national slogan, "Early detection and early treatment of diseases." At present the Japan Association of Health Service has 33 branches, or almost one branch in every prefecture, all of which originated from parasite control associations. The branch staffs total 2400 and the total annual income for 1980 reached 15 billion yen (approximately

US$75 million), and activities continue to further expand within a completely self-reliant system (Fig. 2).

VIII. International Cooperation in Parasite Control

Because the parasite control movement was successful in Japan, the JAPC developed plans to contribute its experiences to neighboring countries in Asia. A proposal to the Japanese government suggested the initiation of cooperative parasite control programs with neighboring Asian countries such as Okinawa which was then under the control of the U.S. government and Taiwan and Korea, through the Overseas Technical Cooperation Agency (presently the Japan International Cooperation Agency). These programs also achieved rapid success. The JAPC then suggested extending cooperation to other Asian countries, but it was not possible to promote parasite control by itself to other Asian countries because parasite control was often one of the lowest priority items.

In 1974, the author conceived the Integrated Family Planning-Nutrition-Parasite Control Program, based upon his experiences and observations in the parasite control and family planning movements of Japan. The primary objective of the Integrated Program is to make family planning more acceptable to people by adding a health component or parasite control (mainly of soil-transmitted helminths) and, in association, nutrition to the existing unifunctional family planning program. Of numerous health items, parasite control was selected as an appropriate partner for family planning for a variety of reasons. Control of soil-transmitted helminths is easy to implement and easy for people to understand; it has immediate and visible effects, and therefore pleases people. Parasite control has relevance to all members of a family and can stimulate the interest of the entire community so that it is easy to elicit community participation. Parasite control can also be considered an entry point for health education, maternal and child health, family planning, environmental sanitation, and other development programs; its effects extend well beyond the area of medical treatment.

After long, in-depth discussions with family planners and parasitologists both at home and abroad, the Japanese Organization for International Cooperation in Family Planning (JOICFP—a nonprofit, voluntary organization engaged in international cooperation in the field of population and family planning) established a pilot project in Taiwan in 1975 with the technical support of JAPC and the parasitologists. Funds were made available by a local donor agency, and one year after its inception the Taiwan project showed results. It was reported that acceptance of family planning in the project area greatly increased, and that

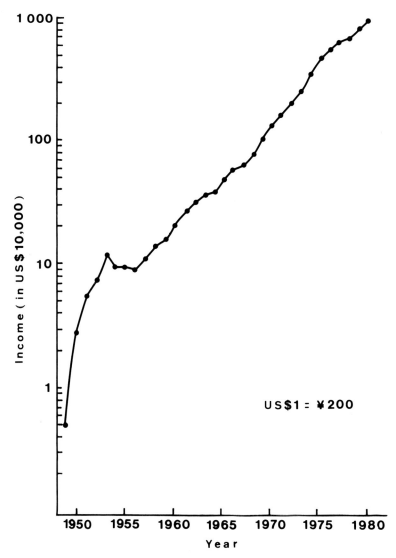

FIG. 2. Increase in income from parasite and other health examinations.

people's confidence in the government health workers and organization had also increased. This stimulated neighboring countries, specifically Indonesia, Korea, the Philippines, and Thailand, to initiate similar projects in 1976. The International Planned Parenthood Federation and the United Nations Fund for Population Activities provide funds, while JOICFP acts as the executing agency for these national projects. After these successes, the Integrated Program expanded further to other countries. At present there are 12 participating countries; the aforementioned 5 countries plus Bangladesh, Brazil, Colombia, Malaysia, Mexico, Nepal, and Sri Lanka.

As in the case of Japan, a tripartite group composed of government, technical experts, and the private sector is taking a vital role in implementing each country's projects, forming a national steering committee as the highest policy-making body. So far, in most countries parasite control has been one of the low priority programs of the government. Therefore, the introduction of the Integrated Program has served as a great impetus to generate the interest of both the authorities concerned and the general public in parasite control, and gradually but steadily it has been proved an effective entry point not only for family planning but for the attainment of primary health care. To promote the Integrated Program more effectively, a group of parasitologists from various Asian countries, which meets annually, has been formed to conduct research on such essential subjects as infection sources and routes, seasonal variation in infection, minimum effective drug dosages, and the efficacy of indigenous drugs. Some of the trials and results have been compiled in the *Collected Papers on the Control of Soil-transmitted Helminthiases* published in 1980 by the Asian Parasite Control Organization.

IX. Conclusion

The parasite control movement in Japan was initially only a small voluntary effort, but over the years it has grown into a comprehensive preventive health services organization, and has established cooperative programs with other countries. These developments have been achieved with the collaborative efforts of government, technical experts, and the private sector, with the private sector functioning in a pioneering role. However, the real impetus to carry on parasite control successfully was furnished by people who felt the need for parasite control and who participated actively in the control program.

References

Komiya, Y., and Aizaki, T. (1952). On the hookworm prevalence in Saitama Pref. *Koshu Eisei* **1**, 33–36.*

*The references with asterisks are in Japanese.

Matsusaki, G. (1942). Epidemiological observation on the helminth infection among inhabitants in a rural village especially on hookworm infection. *Keio Igaku* **22,** 759–768.*

Matsusaka, M. (1937). [Cited from Matsusaki, G. (1966).] Hookworm disease and prevention. *In* "Progress of Medical Parasitology in Japan" (K. Morishita, Y. Komiya, and H. Matsubayashi, eds.), Vol. 3, pp. 188–282. Meguro Parasitological Museum, Tokyo.

Ministry of Interior (1929). [Cited from Yanagisawa, R. (1966).] The epidemiology of hookworm disease. *In* "Progress of Medical Parasitology in Japan" (K. Morishita, Y. Komiya, and H. Matsubayashi, eds.), Vol. 3, pp. 188–282. Meguro Parasitological Museum, Tokyo.

Nakagawa, T., Osada, M., Ishino, K., Ueki, K., Asami, K., and Kimura, S. (1951). Parasitological survey in Hinohara village, Tokyo-to. *Kiseichugaku Zasshi* **1,** 47–51.*

Nishida, H. (1958). Epidemiological study on the helminth infection in Hachijo Island. 1. Helminth species found by the stoool examination in all inhabitants in the island. 2. Symptoms of hookworm patients and effect of anthelmintic treatment. 3. Geographical distribution of *A. duodenale* and *N. americanus.* 4. On the familial aggregation of helminth infection and correlation among parasite infections. *Tokyo Iji Shinshi* **7,** 25–33.*

Sasa, M. (1958). Practice in parasitological examination techniques, the direct smear technique, floatation technique and culture technique, 2nd ed. Univ. of Tokyo Press, Tokyo.

Sasa, M., Tanaka, H., Abē, Y., Uchiyama, H., Ismui, K., and Takikiku, K. (1958). Helminthic fauna in Amami Islands. 1. On the recovery of parasitic helminth eggs by the direct smear, brine floatation and culture methods. *Kiseichugaku Zasshi* **7,** 357–362.*

Tokyo Parasite Control Association (1949). Parasite infection rates in Tokyo metropolitan area. *Kiseichu Yobo*, No. 1.*

Yanagisawa, R. (1957). Hookworm studies in view of public health. *Jpn. J. Parasitol.* **6,** 237–256.*

8

Human Ecology and the Distribution and Abundance of Hookworm Populations

G. A. SCHAD
Department of Pathobiology
School of Veterinary Medicine
University of Pennsylvania
Philadelphia, Pennsylvania

T. A. NAWALINSKI
Division of Parasitology
SmithKline Animal Health Products
Philadelphia, Pennsylvania

V. KOCHAR
Department of Sociology and Anthropology
University of Hyderabad
Hyderabad, India

I. Introduction and General Ecological Background

Hookworm infection is largely confined to the moist tropics and subtropics, because the eggs and free-living larvae of *Necator americanus* and *Ancylostoma duodenale* require a warm, moist, external environment in which to embryonate, hatch, and develop. This global generalization has significant exceptions where large-scale manmade ecological changes permit the establishment of infection in areas otherwise unsuitable. For example, ancylostomiasis is an important disease in areas of Egypt which without irrigation would be much too dry for the parasite's survival; it was once well established in several foci in cool temperate areas of northern Europe, where unsanitated mines and the first tunnels through the Alps created habitats that were sufficiently warm and moist for free-living larval development. Such examples demonstrate the major role that human ecology can play in controlling the global distribution and abundance of these parasites.

Natural ecological variation within the normal ranges of these worms will affect their abundance regionally and, consequently, the degree of hookworm infection in the human population. If ecological factors (e.g., moisture and soil type) are generally favorable, the abundance of hookworm larvae in the soil can be significantly influenced by human decisions concerning the environment, such as whether natural vegetation remains or what plants are cultivated in its place. Extensive natural vegetation usually implies a hunter–gatherer culture with sparse, mobile populations; in this situation hookworms are rarely an important problem (Heyneman, 1977).

In contrast, coffee, tea, rubber, and jasmine plantations (but usually not tobacco, pineapple, or cotton) are often sites of heavy hookworm transmission and a high prevalence of disease. Because plants vary in their ability to shade the soil and thus conserve the moisture required for larval survival, they may exacerbate or mitigate the public health problem. Clearly, under conditions of extensive plantations and other one-crop agriculture, the choice of crop can have an important regional influence on the degree of hookworm endemicity.

Water management also affects the occurrence and abundance of hookworm; irrigation generally favors hookworms, but excess water is detrimental because larval development fails in water-logged oxygen-deficient soils. Thus, cultivation of rice and jute in flooded fields limits transmission of these parasites (Cort *et al.,* 1926; Chandler, 1928).

Other agricultural practices, particularly those that contribute to the widespread fecal pollution of crops, also enhance transmission. The use of inadequately composted human feces as fertilizer has long been associated with serious levels of hookworm infection, especially in parts of the Orient. Even when feces are not used deliberately, heavy fecal pollution of crops such as tea, cacao, and coffee occurs when large groups of laborers are in the field from dawn to dusk with few, if any, sanitary facilities available (Chandler, 1925, 1926; Cort *et al.*, 1922a,b; Cort *et al.*, 1923a,b).

Human Ecological Factors Determining the Distribution and Abundance of Hookworms

1. DEFECATION: CUSTOMS, PRACTICES, AND HABITS

Because people are the only important definitive hosts of *Ancylostoma duodenale* and *Necator americanus,* hookworm disease can be an important problem only where they pollute the soil with their feces. Unfortunately, this practice is still common in many rural tropical and subtropical areas, where the prospects for sanitation are limited not only by poverty but also by preference for defecating in the open rather than in latrines.

In traditional Hindu societies, human feces are repugnant not only for the universally accepted reasons but also are considered personally defiling in a ritualistic sense (Kochar, 1975, 1977a, 1979a). Under these circumstances, and in the widespread lack of understanding of the germ theory of disease, it is virtually impossible to maintain latrines in an acceptable condition, and fouled structures rapidly fall into disuse.

On the other hand, very simple structures and naturally occurring squatting places are extensively used as latrines in rural areas of Burma, Bangladesh, and elsewhere in southern Asia, helping to limit the transmission potential of the hookworm eggs entering the environment. In Burma, bamboo platforms, each with a simple superstructure to screen the user from sight, extend over steep banks and adjacent water courses. In the low-lying delta lands of Bangladesh, similar structures keep the small amount of available high ground occupied by villages relatively free of fecal pollution. In the drier, deltaic areas in West Bengal, steep banks are again favored defecation sites, but platforms are rarely built over them; natural overhangs (e.g., trees and roots), over either a steep slope or flat ground, may serve as elevated squatting places. Feces accumulate in heaps, limiting development of hookworms because hookworm eggs within such decomposing fecal accumulations do not yield infective larvae. For this reason, proper composting of human excreta, particularly with the addition of urine, will result in the death of hookworm eggs and will produce a safe fertilizer.

Obviously, defecation habits, important in seeding the environment with hookworm eggs, are also important in the acquisition of infection. Several leading authorities (Chandler, 1929; Cort, 1941; Beaver, 1961) stress that most people become infected when stationary in fecally polluted areas, as during defecation. Thus, the degree of avoidance or nonavoidance of previously fouled sites in selecting a place to defecate becomes a matter of epidemiological significance. The literature abounds with examples from many cultures indicating that little care is taken to avoid polluted areas. Indeed, although clearly identifiable feces are not stepped on, little avoidance occurs after their incorporation into the soil, when they become invisible and odorless. This is particularly so when the people do not associate feces with disease.

There are some areas such as India, however, where a strong desire to avoid human feces exists; successful avoidance depends on knowing where fecal pollution has occurred. The aggregation of feces in socially accepted and generally recognized defecation grounds makes avoidance possible by most people during most activities. In contrast, where defecation is promiscuous, leading to spatially unpredictable pollution, conscious avoidance becomes impossible when individual deposits become visually obliterated.

When feces are aggregated in specific areas set aside for defecation, most members of the population will be at risk of exposure to infection only when they defecate; thus, people can avoid casual and work-related exposure to infection. The few whose work brings them into contact with defecation grounds will at least be aware of the fecal pollution whether or not visible evidence remains.

The daily risk of exposure at defecation can be reduced further by aggregation of feces within the defecation grounds, making it possible to avoid the specific loci where individual fecal masses have been deposited. If a fecal deposit is visible, this avoidance is easily achieved. However, because of the burying action of dung beetles and rain, a deposit disappears rapidly and combines with the soil so that evidence of its presence is subtle (at least to the untrained eye), appearing as a mound of loose earth. If deposited originally on the leaf-covered ground under a grove of trees or bamboo, this fecal locus is defined further by a circular clear area (a plaque) which stands out in the otherwise continuous carpet of leaves and which remains even after rain has compressed the mound of loose earth. Eventually, the mound becomes flattened with one or more holes representing tunnels of dung beetles. These subtle signs persist for several weeks; if the observer knows where the area has been polluted, he/she can even avoid the exact sites of former fecal deposition. Indeed, there is objective evidence that Bengali villagers do avoid these spots (Section II,E). The Bengali terms for a site of dung beetle activity and for a fecal deposit are identical, indicating that the original nature of an obliterated deposit is known.

Although loci of probable soil infestation can be recognized and avoided, individuals refusing to conform to behavioral norms or lacking normal visual acuity may be exposed to frequent and heavy infection from the clustering of soil infestation occurring in defecation grounds. This may explain the increased worm burden observed among the elderly in West Bengal.

2.   OCCUPATION

Although many authors have associated hookworm infection with agricultural occupations involving soil contact, it is not necessarily these particular occupations that predispose to infection but rather the rural life style with inadequate facilities for the safe disposal of human excrement. When fecal pollution of the soil is concentrated near homes and around villages, all persons are almost equally at risk; indeed those away from home tilling the land may be protected from heavy infection by their regular, prolonged absence from the areas of maximal soil infestation (Chandler, 1929). Ancylostomiasis may also occur in an urban setting if sanitary facilities are lacking; unpaved streets, alleys, and patches of vacant land provide defecation sites for people with an unsophisticated and essentially rural concept of appropriate behavior.

However, agricultural work can have an important influence on the prevalence and intensity of hookworm infection. We have already described how particular crops are associated with varying intensities of hookworm infection because of the different ecological conditions they create and the specific management practices associated with them.

If ecological conditions permit uniform larval development and survival, the infection to which an agricultural labor force is exposed will depend on (1) the distribution and density of fecal pollution and (2) the timing and duration of contact with infested soil. The fecal input may be planned and narrowly distributed, as when a crop is fertilized with night soil, or it may be caused by incidental defecation on agricultural land, in which case fecal distribution and density will vary with diverse human behavioral factors.

Cort et al. emphasized the great danger of housing agricultural laborers along the edge of the plantations where they have to work (Cort, 1941; Cort and Payne, 1922a). This was notable in Trinidad, where feces accumulated between the rows of sugar cane behind the workers' housing so that they were exposed to infection not only during defecation but also when going to and from, and during, work.

Coffee pickers may be exposed to very heavy infection. They remain in the groves for continuous, prolonged periods because picking is a weekly activity for several months; this results in extensive and intensive soil pollution (Cort et al., 1923a,b), and by the end of the harvest season larval populations are uniformly dense and infection correspondingly heavy.

Laborers on tea estates are also subjected to heavy infection (Napier, et al., 1937; Rice, 1927) because they spend long hours far from latrines in the tea gardens where soil pollution is accepted. During the harvest season, every bush is plucked weekly and systematically, precluding avoidance of, and insuring prolonged contact with, polluted ground.

Heavy hookworm infection has been perhaps nowhere more certain than in the districts of China where the mulberry tree is grown to provide leaves for silk-worm culture. The epidemiology of hookworm disease in these areas was described dramatically by Cort et al. (1926a). Intense transmission is fostered by the need to force leaf growth over a short period of time during the warm, rainy part of the year; human feces are added to freshly cultivated soil around the base of each tree; and the urgent need for fertilizer results in the use of fresh excrement laden with viable eggs after the supply of old, well-composted feces (in which most hookworm eggs have died) has been exhausted. Combining the fresh feces with recently worked soil at precisely the time when weather conditions are ideal creates perfect culture conditions for hookworms, guaranteeing a large population of infective larvae.

When the laborers return and harvest the leaf crop after 2–4 weeks, moving systematically around each tree, prolonged contact with virtually every inch of the heavily infested soils is ensured. Unusually severe cases of hookworm dermatitis occurring precisely at this time provide evidence for massive larval invasion.

In some cultures particular kinds of agricultural work are done by members of one sex. Tea leaves, for example, are most often picked by women, and so they may be more heavily infected than men. In contrast, if infection is likely to occur during plowing or other heavy labor usually done by men, infection is likely to be heavier in males. There is considerable danger in assuming such associations too readily because experimental investigations of the effects of host sex on helminth infections have shown there are also sex-related differences in susceptibility; females are usually more resistant than males. Indeed, our data from India show that females are less heavily infected than males; as this difference is apparent even among young children (Nawalinski et al., 1978a), it is unlikely that it results from infection acquired during agricultural pursuits.

Any occupation that increases contact with fecally polluted soil during warm, moist conditions probably predisposes to infection. We have already indicated that unsanitated mines have been sites of intense transmission, and hookworm disease has been reported from such diverse underground operations as coal mines in Europe, gold mines in California and South Africa (Hodgman, 1934), and phosphate mines in arid parts of North Africa (Becmeur et al., 1950). Troops in combat, living close to the earth and lacking sanitary facilities, are exposed to numerous infections including soil-borne nematodiasis. Even when they are well protected with heavy footwear, contaminated soil and mud contacting unprotected parts of the body can cause hookworm infection.

Hookworm infection associated with recreational activities has been described on a number of occasions. In northern India, a game called kabaddi, played on an open field, involves members of one team throwing members of the other to the ground. An outbreak of severe ancylostomiasis followed such a game played on a muddy field that had been contaminated with feces at some time previously (Koshy *et al.*, 1978).

The possibility of water-borne ancylostomiasis remains in some doubt, but in at least one incident infection seems to have occurred while the subjects were swimming because itching and other symptoms suggestive of hookworm dermatitis began while they were still in the water. This was followed in a few days by a severe, life-threatening, prepatent ancylostomiasis; the diagnosis was confirmed by finding extraordinary numbers of young worms in the feces after anthelmintic treatment. In this instance, torrential rains apparently had carried very large numbers of ancylostome larvae into a small bay from an adjoining, heavily polluted valley (Ashford *et al.*, 1933a,b).

The attending physicians described these incidents and published their findings because the infections were very heavy and the patients had unusual symptoms of special medical interest. Had smaller numbers of parasites been involved, the diagnosis might not have been made; perhaps investigations into the mode of infection would not have been conducted and the information would not have reached the literature. It is possible, therefore, that water-borne infection may not be as rare, and occupational groups associated with water may not be as protected, as is generally assumed. Ghadirian *et al.* (1979), for example, thought that rice farmers in Iran are particularly at risk, acquiring these infections in flooded fields. However, no evidence was provided to support the suggestion.

3. FOOD HABITS

Hookworms are rarely considered to be food-borne parasites. Most textbooks convey the impression that they invariably enter the body percutaneously and in fact *N. americanus* does; *A. duodenale*, however, is able to establish successfully after oral entry, as has been shown in experimental subjects (Kendrick, 1934). Food-borne ancylostomiasis is widely recognized in the Orient, where an allergic response to orally acquired larvae (known as *Wakana* disease in Japan) is associated with eating the small, young leaves of Chinese cabbage and radish (Matsusaki, 1966).

It has also been suggested that human hookworm infection can be meat-borne (Schad *et al.*, 1980); they observed that *A. duodenale* larvae migrated to the somatic musculature of several swine, rabbits, and a calf, where they survived for at least several weeks. Lambs and chickens were partially or totally resistant to infection. These preliminary observations suggest an entirely new route of infection whose significance requires further investigation.

Some foods have anthelmintic properties, although none sufficiently strong to be valuable chemotherapeutically. As we know very little about the long-term effects of weak anthelmintics on hookworms, it is possible that food habits could directly influence worm burden. Certain foods (e.g., onions and garlic) adversely affect the development of the free-living stages in feces (Bastidas, 1969); presumably, diets rich in these foods would have an adverse effect on the parasite's reproductive success.

4. CULTURE AND RELIGION

The degree to which people avoid fecal contact depends on aesthetic, hygienic, and/or cultural considerations. Aesthetic considerations are undoubtedly those which most often inhibit such contact. Hygienic considerations (i.e., associations with disease) also inhibit contact, but how completely and consistently depends on the level of understanding of disease transmission.

In some cultures, human feces are avoided not only for the reasons given but also because contact with them is considered defiling. In Hindu and Muslim cultures of Asia, the act of defecation is considered defiling and elaborate ablution practices are necessary to ritually purify the defiled individual. These beliefs and practices reinforce the abhorrence on aesthetic and hygienic grounds and usually result in almost complete avoidance of fecal contact, even where defecation outdoors causes at least some contact to be inevitable.

Among both Hindus and Muslims in rural India it is essential that one achieve a certain personal sacredness, perceptible by others, to maintain one's social status (Kochar, 1979a). Purity is one aspect of this sacredness, and a cleansing act must be performed after defecation or contact with fecally polluted places. Furthermore, impurity is considered contagious and contact with defiled objects, places, or persons must be avoided. Thus, in traditional Indian society, ablution and a change of clothing follow defecation; food crops are not fouled with human excreta, and contact with fecal pollution is generally avoided.

Additionally, regularity with respect to defecation is considered a virtue, and daily bowel movements at the correct time and place, invariably followed by ablution and often by a bath and change of clothes, is generally expected behavior. In fact, this sequence in whole or part has become a daily ritual. Kochar (1979a) states that a popular Bengali text on the daily rituals of a religious Hindu household begins with detailed instructions concerning defecation, even specifying the direction in which to face. He outlines the typical routine as found in our investigations:

> Defaecation every day early in the morning is considered desirable and in fact about 30% of adults complete the act before 6 A.M. Ablution must be done immediately after defaecation by entering a pond or other water body (since Bengalis do not usually carry water with them like in other parts of North India) and by rubbing the peri-anal skin with water in squatting posture. This is followed by rubbing of hands with soil as [a] purificatory act. The termination of defilement is symbolized by taking by hand a mouthful of water and spitting it out. Many also

prefer to take a bath as a continuation of this ritual. In any case, clothes worn during defaecation have to be changed. If bathing is not intended, most adults change from their normal
"clean" clothes before going for defaecation. The high castes are required to loop their sacred
thread around their right ear (as a sign of defilement) until after they have purified themselves.
The ablution must be performed with left hand. Rural Bengalis scrupulously avoid the use of
left hand for eating or handling any cooked food material since it is defiled. These norms are
followed with high conformity. The ritual norms emphasize early socialization of habits
associated with defaecation. Children are reprimanded for not following the correct procedures. Defaecation, contact with faeces, or even a visit to "polluted" defaecation ground,
are deemed to pollute a person and would normally require some purificatory ritual. However,
these norms are followed with modifications suited to person, time and routine. Polluted fields
are not avoided in the same manner as the bamboo groves are.

This culturally based aversion for human feces may not be shared by other
groups. Rural Chinese, for example, value feces as fertilizer and conserve them;
defecation or work that involves night soil is not perceived as defiling and no
purification rituals are required. The Chinese therefore have been at risk of
hookworm infection during agricultural work to an extent that is unusual under
Indian conditions.

Within India itself, Hindus and Muslims in Bengal show pronounced differences in intensity of hookworm infection (Nawalinski *et al.,* 1978a) as well as
in the prevalance of other helminthiases (Chernin, 1954a; Chowdhury *et al.,*
1968a,b). No explanation for this difference is readily apparent, but presumably
it is determined by culturally based behavioral differences that control rates of
exposure.

II. The Ecology of Interacting Human and Hookworm Populations in Rural West Bengal

A. Parasitological Background

It is thought (W.H.O. 1964) that the prevalence and mean intensity of hookworm infection usually vary directly. Therefore, the epidemiology of ancylostomiasis in gangetic West Bengal, where prevalence exceeds 80% although
hookworm burdens are low and disease infrequent, has long held a special
fascination for parasitologists (Chandler, 1926, 1928; Chernin, 1954a,b;
Chowdhury *et al.,* 1968a,b). Realizing that this enigmatic prevalence/intensity
relationship had persisted for at least 40 years in the absence of treatment and
sanitation, Schad *et al.* (1971, 1973, 1975), Kochar *et al.* (1976), and Nawalinski *et al.* (1978a,b) suggested that the parasite populations were being regulated

by natural factors and initiated a multidisciplinary investigation to determine the epidemiology and population ecology of hookworm infection in this area. A highly quantitative life table approach was adopted, strongly influenced by the well-known investigations of Hairston (1962); it provided information that can be broadly characterized as follows:

1. Density and structure of adult worm populations
2. Number of hookworm eggs entering the environment
3. Time and place of defecation
4. Ecological descriptions of the defecation grounds
5. Hatching, development, and survival of free-living stages
6. Distribution and abundance of infective larvae
7. Human behavior and exposure to infective larvae
8. The dynamics of infection as reflected in fecal egg count

In this chapter, we will present selected parts of the investigation, particularly those that involve human ecology.

B. Physiographic, Climatic, and Demographic Background

The research was conducted in an old delta region of gangetic Bengal lying about 40 miles northwest of Calcutta (Fig. 1). Like Calcutta, this area has sharply demarcated seasons, with the monsoon rains beginning in mid-June, decreasing through September, and ending in early October; March through May is hot and dry (Table I).

The low-lying deltaic plain has a few sluggish rivers, many irrigation ditches, canals, and innumerable man-made ponds (tanks), mostly associated with habitations (Fig. 1). The general flatness is interrupted by excavations for sand and clay and by the mounds of earth dug from ponds, canals, and ditches. The cropland consists of extensive treeless areas divided into small plots by low earthen ridges (bunds) that also serve as dikes for irrigation and as raised pathways. These plots are planted with rice, jute, and sugar cane. In the dry season, irrigated land is planted with vegetables (potatoes, eggplant, cabbage, and okra); land that cannot be irrigated is left in rice stubble that is often grazed by cattle, sheep, or goats. Villages with bamboo and banana groves, palms, and occasional shade trees contrast sharply with the areas of open cropland (Fig. 1).

Our investigations were based on the earlier work of Chowdhury and Schiller (1968b). They chose Bandipur Anchal because it was one of the few areas in Bengal maintaining adequate demographic records. We also used these data to select sample populations for our investigations.

The study area included 12 villages with a total population of 6268. It was

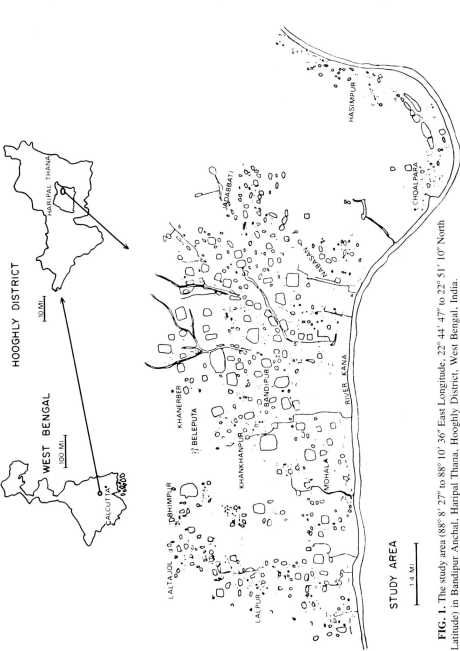

FIG. 1. The study area (88° 8′ 27″ to 88° 10′ 36″ East Longitude, 22° 44′ 47″ to 22° 51′ 10″ North Latitude) in Bandipur Anchal, Haripal Thana, Hooghly District, West Bengal, India.

TABLE I

Selected Meteorological Data for Calcutta, India, 1881–1940[a]

Month	X̄ Daily maximum temperature (°F)	X̄ Monthly rainfall (in.)	X̄ Days >0.1 (in.)
Jan	80	0.4	0.8
Feb	84	1.2	2
Mar	93	1.4	2
Apr	97	1.7	3
May	96	5.5	7
June	92	11.7	13
July	89	12.8	18
Aug	89	12.9	18
Sept	90	9.9	13
Oct	89	4.5	6
Nov	84	0.8	1
Dec	79	0.2	0.3

[a]From Tables of Temperature, Relative Humidity and Precipitation for the World, Part V. Asia. British Meteorological Office, London, 1966. (Reproduced with the permission of the Controller of Her Britannic Majesty's Stationery Office.)

about ¾ mile in width and extended 3 miles along the north side of the Kana River (Fig. 1). The width of the area was chosen so that we could detect any effect on hookworm transmission caused by distance from the river. This seemed plausible because many of the more distant fields are not irrigated in the dry season, remaining in rice stubble. The study area was selected from the larger areas studied by Chowdhury and Schiller (1968b) so that our field station in Bandipur Village would be centrally situated and so that all villages were generally accessible by jeep or bicycle even during the monsoon season. Of the population about 89% were Hindu and 11% Muslim. A detailed survey of our entire sample population indicated that 22% belonged to households classified as nonagricultural; 35%, owner-agricultural; 19%, part-time agricultural; and 25%, nonowner, full-time agricultural labor.

C. Samples and Methods: Parasitological

Two parallel longitudinal investigations of the prevalence and intensity of hookworm infection were conducted. The first involved persons of all ages and was designed to provide seasonal and group-specific information on parasite burdens and on the number of hookworm eggs entering the environment daily.

Our basic random sample of 750 people in 100 households was weighted to assure adequate representation from each village. This sample, which was thought sufficient to provide 600 regular participants during successive, approximately bimonthly rounds of fecal examination, represented about $\frac{1}{10}$ of the population. It was also used for the anthropological phase described in Section II,D.

During the first round of fecal examinations, treatment was offered to about 16% of those who cooperated; assuming some refusals, about 10% of the sample would be cleared of their infection thus becoming available for longitudinal observation in parallel with those left untreated. The extra work involving the treated group (i.e., extra pretreatment and posttreatment egg counts, treatment per se, and posttreatment worm recovery) extended the first round of fecal examinations through 5 months. As each of the other rounds was completed in about 2 months, the entire sample was examined four times in 1969 and five times in the first 10 months of 1970.

A second independent sample of children through 10 years of age was selected to study the dynamics of hookworm parasitism in a group consisting substantially of uninfected or lightly infected individuals. When 90% of a population is parasitized, most of those who have never been infected will be children; among them, rates of acquisition of worms may be studied without considering acquired immunity. Furthermore, both acquisition and loss are most readily apparent in the uninfected or lightly infected segments of the population. The results of this investigation and details of sample selection have been reported by Nawalinski *et al.* (1978a,b).

In the first year of study, 560 children were examined bimonthly; 320 children were added in the second year. An average of 320 (302–383) were cooperative per round in the first year, and 417 (395–445) in the second, with an average overlap of 63%.

All feces were examined by a quantitative modification of the Kato technique using a 50-mg sample of well-mixed feces (Martin and Beaver, 1968).

D. Sample and Methods: Anthropological

A subsample consisting of half the main sample of 100 households was drawn randomly for detailed anthropological investigations; 49 households with 352 persons actually participated. The anthropological investigations may be categorized as follows.

1. Census: all 100 sample households were covered initially to obtain basic demographic data for both the parasitological and the anthropological investigations.

2. Monthly survey of defecation habits: the time and location of every stool passed by all members of the subsample households during the 24 hr preceding the interview were recorded monthly. The location of each of 4395 stools from 352 subjects was verified and recorded on enlarged land use maps.

3. Monthly survey of defecation grounds: each month, one person from each subsample household was requested to physically identify his or her stool. Observations of 448 stools included the degree of fecal pollution around the identified stool, its distance from the nearest stool, the average density of pollution within the defecation ground, and a time–motion simulation of the distances covered from house to trail to pond, etc.

4. Direct observation of defecation behavior: from a discreet distance of at least 150 yards, 200 unidentified subjects were observed at 19 sites over a total of 42 hr to document the sequence of activities and movement to and from the defecation grounds. Accurate time records were also obtained from reliable subjects who were taught the use of a stopwatch.

5. Land use and stool distribution studies: enlarged village maps were used for marking the location of all observable human stools during two different seasons in representative villages.

E. Prevalence and Intensity of Hookworm Infection in Rural Gangetic West Bengal

1. PARASITOLOGICAL OBSERVATIONS

Figure 2 (Nawalinski *et al.*, 1978a) shows that the prevalence of infection in rural Bengali children increases rapidly with age so that more than half of all 5-year-old children were infected; by the eleventh year, prevalence reached 90% with a mean fecal egg count of about 3000 EPG among those infected. Both prevalence and intensity of infection were greater in boys than in girls ($p < .025$).

Prevalence of hookworm infection increased much more rapidly among Muslim than among Hindu children, exceeding 90% by age 4 and becoming almost 100% among children older than age 7 (Fig. 3). Among Hindus, prevalence did not approach 90% until the children were 9 years old. There was little difference in the overall mean fecal egg count of the two religious groups, but the difference was significantly greater in Muslims than in Hindus in 9 of the 10 age cohorts (sign. test, $p = .11$). It is interesting that we also found significantly higher prevalences of other soil-borne helminths (i.e., *Ascaris lumbricoides* and *Trichuris trichiura*) in Muslims than in Hindus. These observations suggest that human behavioral factors related to culture or socioeconomic status have a

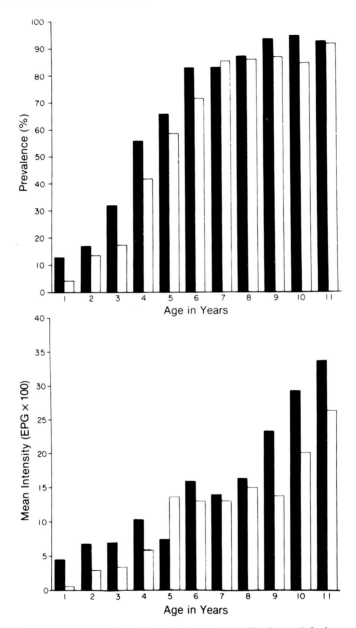

FIG. 2. Prevalence (upper graph) and intensity (lower graph) of hookworm infection among rural Bengali children, by age and sex; mean of 11 bimonthly rounds of stool examination (■ = male, □ = female) (from Nawalinski *et al.,* 1978a).

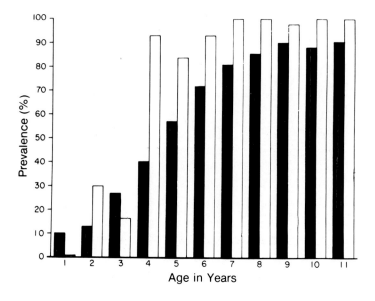

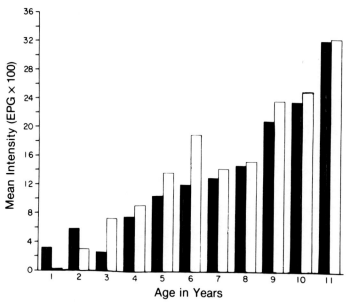

FIG. 3. Prevalence (upper graph) and intensity (lower graph) of hookworm infection among rural Bengali children, by age and religion; mean of 11 bimonthly rounds of stool examination (■ = Hindus, □ = Muslims) (from Nawalinski *et al.*, 1978a).

marked effect on the rate of acquisition of hookworms and other soil-borne helminths.

Data from our basic sample showed that prevalence increased rapidly with age and reached 90–100% among adults (Fig. 4). The rapid rate of worm gain observed in the study of children was not maintained through adulthood. In fact, in men the intensity of infection remained relatively constant from young adulthood through middle age. A similar pattern was seen in women, who may have had a slight net loss of worms. In the oldest age group (over 54) the intensity of infection increased again. Kochar (1975, 1979a) used these same data in evaluating the effect of various human factors on the intensity of infection.

2. ANTHROPOLOGICAL OBSERVATIONS

> It is evident, if the defecation areas are usually the only important sources of infestation, and exposure during the act of defecation the most important time of infestation, that the details of the defecation habits are of very great importance.*

a. Defecation Grounds

About 9% of the sample households had latrines but few people use them; only 0.8% of all stools were passed in latrines. In rural Bengal, certain plots of land are recognized socially as defecation grounds. Households situated in wooded areas often have an adjacent bamboo grove which is used as a site for defecation. Nearly 15% of our subjects had a bamboo grove beside the house; another 10% had another nearby shaded habitat (banana, brush, etc.) used for defecation. Of 195 defecation grounds surveyed, 73% were in bamboo and other shaded habitats and 23% were fields. Unlike permanent defecation grounds in shade, those in fields are temporary and transitory. Fallow as well as planted lands are included in the designation "fields," but land planted with a food crop is not considered pollutable and only rarely is a stool deposited in such a site. During the dry season, a special class of defecation ground (*hegomath*) forms in fallow fields. These *hegomath*s are characterized by a very dense concentration of stools.

b. Defecation Behavior

As mentioned earlier, contact with feces or a defecation ground defiles a Hindu. However, when a villager enters a defecation ground for some other purpose, he will not be unduly concerned about feces around him and a purification ritual rarely follows. Regular, early morning defecation is considered desir-

*From Asa Chandler, "Hookworm Disease," p. 195. Macmillan and Co. Ltd., London, 1929.

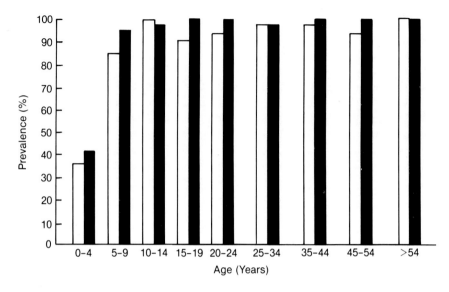

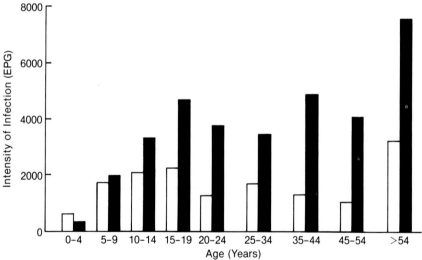

FIG. 4. Prevalence (upper graph) and intensity (lower graph) of hookworm infection in rural Bengali villagers by age and sex; mean of 9 rounds of stool examination (■ = male, □ = female) (from Schad *et al.*, 1975).

able, but this habit is more common among persons of high caste (67%) than among low castes (38%), and more common among Hindus (40%) than among Muslims (24%). In general, 25–30% defecate before 6 AM and 50% before 9 AM.

Fields were used regularly by 80% of agricultural families and 45% of non-agricultural families. Interrogations over 1 year revealed that 43% of all stools are passed in fields, 22% in bamboo, and 39% in all other fully or partly shaded habitats.

On the basis of the time and motion simulation, about 95% of our subjects walked 3 min or less to a defecation ground; 82% walked less than 2 min within the defecation ground; 96% walked less than 4 min (average 1.4 min) in selecting a site, which took about 6 sec to reach from the track; 17% of the subjects took less than 1 min and 72% less than 4 min (average 3 min) to defecate. Ablution is performed immediately after defecation: 41% took less than 1 min and 83% less than 4 min (average 2.5 min) to enter the water. In this part of India with its ubiquitous tanks, canals, and ponds, ablution occurs while standing in water.

c. Avoidance Behavior

Table II shows that avoidance of other stools by villagers while defecating was increasingly equivocal as feces became incorporated with the soil with only evidence of dung beetle activity remaining to mark the location. These "traces," which are least likely to be avoided, constitute the real danger, because fresh and partly turned stools would be too recently passed to yield infective larvae. This equivocation was emphasized by Kochar (1979a).

However, the interaction between man and hookworms when examined on the most relevant scale for the interaction of humans and hookworm larvae (i.e., the length of a human foot) shows that human behavior is protective. As seen in Table III, irrespective of age or sex only 2% of stools were deposited within 6 in. of a trace of feces and only 12% within 12 in. Most stools (67%) were deposited 16 in. or more from a fecal trace, indicating that even those loci on which stools per se were no longer visible were repellent. This is consistent with our recoveries of hookworm larvae in which few clusters of larvae were found within an annulus around a fresh stool equivalent to a human foot in width (Table IV).

Furthermore, because it is not precisely known where the feet of the subject were placed during defecation, even traces within 12 in. do not necessarily imply an infective contact; Although Kochar (1975, 1979a) has interpreted these data otherwise, they are consistent with the relatively strict fecal avoidance so thoroughly stressed in Hindu culture.

d. Use of Defecation Grounds; Hookworm Habitat and Transmission

Of the stools identified during monthly interviews of persons included in our anthropological subsample, about 75% were deposited in defecation grounds. Of these deposits, 72% were in shaded habitats where transmission most often occurs during activities associated with defecation. Of the remaining 28% identi-

TABLE II

Distance to the Nearest Partly Turned, Fully Turned, and Trace Fecal
Deposits from Each of 380 Subject-Identified Stools

Distance	Partly turned		Fully turned		Trace	
	Number	%	Number	%	Number	%
<3 ft	112	30	162	43	225	59
3–6 ft	58	15	80	21	84	22
>6 ft	210	55	138	36	71	19
Total	380	100	380	100	380	100

fied in various nonshaded areas, 80% were in fields where transmission would
not necessarily be limited to times of defecation (Kochar, 1975).

Based on this information and on the amount of time villagers spend at various
tasks that might expose them to infection, it can be calculated that for persons
who plow fields or harvest jute the activity-specific period at risk is about 3 hr
per transmission season, or about 45 min per month (June 15–October 15). For
persons who cut bamboo or collect fuel (the latter often are the aged), the
respective figures are 41 min and 54 min per month. For these occupations,
Kochar (1975, 1979a) reasoned that the increased exposure should be reflected in
increased worm burdens, and expected this to be reflected in increased fecal egg
counts among agriculturalists, particularly the nonowner agriculturalists (i.e.,
parttime and fulltime agricultural workers) doing the most menial tasks.

Thirty percent of all feces are deposited in shaded sites that provide a more
favorable habitat for hookworm transmission than their unshaded counterparts;
direct sunlight is ovicidal and larvicidal, and stools are more aggregated in the
shaded sites. Only 23% of persons defecating in bamboo encountered low densities of fecal pollution (<5 stools/100 ft^2). Open habitats contain 43% of all
feces; except during part of July and August, they provide an unfavorable hab-

TABLE III

Percentage of Stools Deposited by Males and Females at Various Distances from Nearest Fecal Trace

Distance (in.)	Males (n = 184)				Females (n = 117)				Both sexes
	11–19	20–44	≥45	All ages	11–19	20–44	≥45	All ages	
<6	2	3	0	2	0	3	4	3	2
6–11	12	10	20	14	6	23	5	10	12
12–15	18	10	24	18	23	10	22	19	19
>16	68	77	56	66	71	64	69	68	67

TABLE IV

Number of Gauze Pads Examined for Hookworm Larvae
and Frequency Distribution of Larvae Recovered per Pad[a,b]

	Number of gauze pads			Number of infective larvae per sampling pad							
Year	Total	Negative	Positive	1–2	3–4	5–6	<10	<20	<50	<100	>100
1969	1224	1150	74	37	14	10	1	4	4	3	1
1970	1704	1595	109	75	10	6	5	4	6	1	2
Both years	2928	2745	183	112	24	16	6	8	10	4	3

[a]The soil surface in an annulus 30.54 cm wide was examined for infective larvae. The width was based on the length of the average adult foot. Within each sampling annulus, 10.6% of the surface area (i.e., 516 cm^2) was sampled by the damp gauze pad technique developed by Beaver (1953. *Am. J. Trop. Med. Hyg.*, **2**, 102).
[b]From Schad *et al.* (1975).

itat. Additionally, feces are generally less aggregated; 51% of people defecating in fields encountered <5 stools/100 ft^2.

During the transmission season, 62% of all feces are deposited in fields; about 70% of these stools are passed in jute fields. This increases the risk of infection both for the person defecating and for the laborers who harvest jute. Polluting fields planted with nonfood crops (jute) negates some of the advantage of defecating in the fields. If people changed their defecation habitat from bamboo to open sites just before the transmission season (June–October) as 30–40% do, this would further restrict the abundance of hookworm populations. Most of the hookworm eggs in feces passed in fields before 10 AM (i.e., 56% of feces passed in fields or 24% of all feces) are *not* likely to survive. In fact, the average level of infection in a village (with two exceptions, Bandipur and Beleputa) is inversely correlated with the percentage of feces passed in fields (Fig. 5). Interestingly, these two villages represent polar contrasts with respect to a variety of other factors likely to influence hookworm transmission and resistance to infection (see next section).

e. Occupation and Intensity of Infection

Figures 6 and 7 show the relationship between occupation and hookworm infection. It is noteworthy (Fig. 7) that only 113 of 704 subjects in our entire sample population belonged to occupational subclasses that would experience maximal exposure to infection including that due to agricultural work. The occupations having the greatest involvement with the soil had the heaviest infections. This is a normal expectation, and Kochar (1975, 1979a) has interpreted these findings as indicating that epidemiologically important amounts of infection are acquired during agricultural pursuits, thus refuting Chandler's conclu-

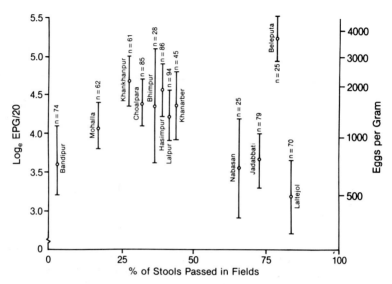

FIG. 5. The intensity of hookworm infection in rural Bengali villagers by village and degree of concentration of stools in fields (from Kochar, 1975).

sion that work in the fields far from the dense fecal pollution around settled areas was, in fact, protective (Chandler, 1929).

Closer examination of the data suggests that a more subtle explanation of the observed differences is required. If exposure to infection in the fields during agricultural activities was largely responsible for the differences between occupational groups, this difference should occur only in groups of working age. Figure 6 shows that the difference is apparent even in young children who are not involved in agricultural work, which suggests that work-related differences in exposure are not the crucial factors determining the between-group differences. If agricultural involvement per se does not provide an explanation, What does? We suggest that a combination of much more subtle factors associated with the overall life style of these groups controls the additional amount of infection observed in the various classes of agriculturalists.

Additional evidence for this interpretation of the data has already been presented: we indicated earlier that two villages did not fit the overall trend showing a decrease in intensity of infection associated with the increasing use of fields for defecation (Fig. 5). Bandipur showed the lower mean level of infection, although a large proportion of the stools was deposited in shaded sites favoring hookworm transmission, whereas Beleputa had the higher mean level of infection although more than 75% of the residents' stools were passed in fields. Of particular relevance to the argument presented is the fact that those villages represent extreme contrasts in education, caste, socioeconomic status, and local ecology as

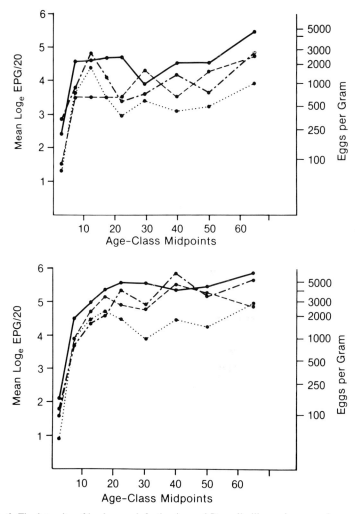

FIG. 6. The intensity of hookworm infection in rural Bengali villagers by sex and occupation of the family head. Upper graph presents data for females, lower graph for males. Family occupation: ——— = agri-labor; —·—· = part-agri; - - - - = owner-agri; ········ = non-agri (from Kochar, 1975).

well as in work-related involvement with the soil. Indeed, this unorthodox interpretation of our observations is also suggested by the data for females shown in Fig. 6 (upper graph). Although few females participate in agricultural labor, their mean levels of infection also varied with "family occupation," suggesting that involvement with soil per se does not determine the level of infection.

The most compelling evidence for the association between occupation and

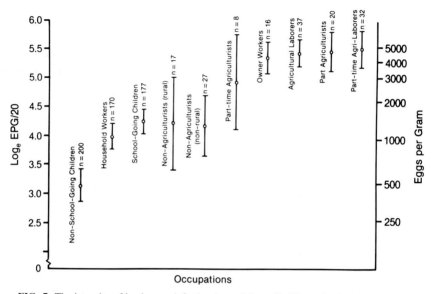

FIG. 7. The intensity of hookworm infection in rural Bengali villagers by individual occupation (from Kochar, 1975).

intensity of infection is presented in Fig. 7, but here too occupation is confounded with other factors. For example, nonschool children have the lowest fecal egg counts, but this category includes many young preschoolchildren whose low egg counts partly reflect insufficient time to have accumulated large numbers of worms. The remaining occupational categories can be combined into two groups, nonagricultural and agricultural workers. Although the former have lower mean egg counts than do the latter, it is also true that the former are largely constituted of children and women, who may well harbor fewer adult worms than do men although exposed to similar levels of transmission. In this connection, the data presented earlier are particularly relevant. As shown in Fig. 2, throughout childhood girls have lower mean egg counts than do boys although it is doubtful that the sexes are differentially exposed to infection as children.

F. Explanations of the Observed Prevalence/Intensity Relationships

It has been suggested that the high prevalence of light infections, so characteristic of much of rural Bengal (Chandler, 1928; Chernin, 1954a,b; Chowdhury and Schiller, 1968b), might be determined largely by transmission and be explicable in ecological terms.

1.   ECOLOGICAL EXPLANATION (SCHAD, 1966)

> The abundance of available, infective larvae approaches zero for most of the year. During the long dry period (October to mid-June), the few larvae which develop after an occasional rain are aggregated, but are rarely on the surface where contact with man is probable. During the monsoon, conditions for larval development and survival are somewhat better, but the soil becomes and remains waterlogged. This water-logging, however, permits formation of sheets of surface water in which larvae, eggs, or both can be carried passively or move actively, to be redeposited when the surface water drains. Redeposition yields a non-aggregated pattern of distribution. Thus, human contact with a few larvae becomes highly probable, but contact with many larvae remains very improbable.
>
> In the brief moist period after the monsoon when soil moisture conditions may be ideal, it is probable that aggregated larval populations form within the immediate area adjoining fecal deposits. If larval dispersal on the surface of the soil cannot take place, it is possible that man escapes infective contact because he deliberately avoids visible (evidence of) pollution.

Subsequent efforts to explain the enigmatic prevalence/intensity relationship by Schad *et al.* (1975) and by Kochar (1975, 1979a) are firmly rooted in this original purely ecological hypothesis.

2.   THE ECOLOGICAL–SOCIOCULTURAL–IMMUNOLOGIC SYNTHESIS (SCHAD *ET AL.*, 1975)

This synthesis is based on our multidisciplinary investigations in India, some of which have been reported previously in greater detail (Schad *et al.*, 1973, 1975; Kochar, 1975, 1977a,b, 1979a,b; Kochar *et al.*, 1976; Nawalinski *et al.*, 1978a,b).

a.   *The Distribution and Abundance of Infective Larvae*

Infective larvae were consistently recovered from the soil surface during the monsoon period, June to October, but not after the soil became dry in November or December (Schad *et al.*, 1973). Experimentally seeded plots also failed to yield infective larvae during the dry intermonsoon period (Schad, 1965, 1966). These observations indicate that for 6–7 months annually larvae rarely, if ever, survive on the soil surface where they would be in a position to infect man.

Because our monthly soil surface samples were taken within an annulus around a freshly passed stool used as a reference point, they indicate actual larval contact with the feet while our subjects defecated. A frequency distribution of the

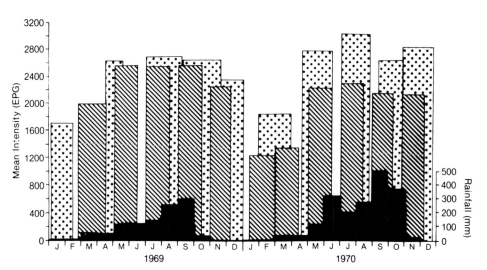

FIG. 8. Seasonal variation in the intensity of hookworm infection in two sample populations of Bengali villagers. One sample was constituted of children only whereas the other was constituted of persons of all ages. The figure also shows the seasonal distribution of rainfall (▒ = EPG, all ages (n = 734); ▨ = EPG, children (n = 560, 1969; 880, 1970; ■ = rain fall) (from Schad *et al.*, 1975).

recoveries of infective larvae based on this focal method of sampling (Table IV) shows that 86% of the positive samples contained 10 or fewer larvae, and only very rarely were dense populations (>100 larvae) found.

From these sets of data, we deduce that (1) the villagers rarely, if ever, encounter hookworm larvae during the dry season; (2) they encounter them frequently during the monsoon; and (3) at any single encounter, the average person will contact only a few infective larvae.

b. The Dynamics of Infection as Reflected in Fecal Egg Counts

A marked seasonal variation in worm burden as judged by fecal egg counts was observed (Fig. 8). The mean egg count varied significantly ($p < .005$) from a midmonsoon peak (2700 epg) to an intermonsoon nadir (1850 epg), then to a second peak (3050 epg) during the following monsoon season. The concurrent investigation of children showed a similar seasonal pattern, with some age-cohorts being net losers of worms year to year (Fig. 9). This annual loss of adult worms must act as a major regulatory mechanism of the hookworm population.

Data from the investigation involving villagers of all ages also showed that the intensity of infection did not increase with age from 15–19 through 45–54 years and, in fact, it may have declined slightly among females (Fig. 4); it increased again in the aged.

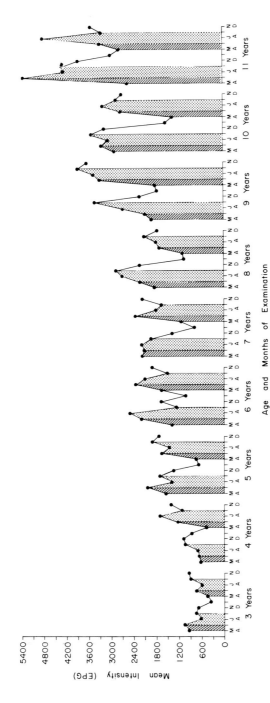

FIG. 9. Seasonal variation in the intensity of hookworm infection among age cohorts of rural Bengali children. Each curve shows the mean fecal egg count by 11 bimonthly rounds of stool examination, beginning in March/April, 1969 and ending November/December, 1970 (▨ = hot dry season; ▦ = rainy season) (from Nawalinski *et al.*, 1978b).

Anthropological investigations of the time and place of defecation and of human behavior in fecally polluted habitats indicated that there was no increase in the use of footwear or decrease in contact with fecally polluted soil that could account for this decrease in worm gain, nor was there a decrease in the frequency of bowel movements that might reduce the number of infective contacts. A study of the distribution of human feces showed that fecal pollution is restricted largely to areas recognized as defecation grounds and that most of the population has little contact with these areas except during activities related to defecation. Therefore, we cannot account for the failure of worm burdens to increase after young adulthood by a change in the rate of exposure, although the increase in the aged may be explained in these ways: they are traditionally given tasks that could bring them into more frequent contact with fecally polluted soils, or there may be a decreased ability or desire among the aged to avoid fecally polluted soils.

c. *Proposed Explanation of the High Prevalence of Light*
    Infections

Our data suggest that the hookworm populations of man in West Bengal are regulated by a seasonal loss of worms in all age groups and by a failure to gain worms from one year to the next during adulthood. A constellation of ecological and human behavioral factors interacts so that man is exposed frequently to low-grade invasions. This rate of infection, known as "trickle infection," probably provokes an effective host resistance so that the average villager sustains a low worm burden. In laboratory investigations of the related hookworm *Ancylostoma caninum,* frequent exposure to small doses of hookworm larvae was very effective in protecting dogs against a heavy challenge infection (Miller, 1965).

The concentration of feces in recognized defecation grounds and the culturally-based avoidance of these areas limits frequent, casual contact with larvae; consequently, most exposure to infection occurs at the time and place of defecation. Even then, there is little or no risk for 6–7 months during the dry part of the year. After the onset of the monsoon, contact with larvae is frequent, but, as we showed, larvae will usually be encountered as individuals or in small aggregates (Table IV). Dense populations of infective larvae must occur directly on the sites of old stools, and unpublished data (Schad, 1965, 1966) indicate that they do; however, human behavior is again protective as such sites are recognized as fecally polluted even after the stools per se have disappeared. This presumably explains why our samples only rarely contained large numbers of larvae. Furthermore, should they contact such a site after repeated low-grade exposures, most individuals may be resistant.

We suggest that the postmonsoon loss of worms is caused by increased host resistance following several low-grade invasions during the monsoon season, and the failure to gain worms during most of adult life may be attributable to increased resistance following repeated infections during childhood and adolescence.

3.   THE SOCIOCULTURAL MODEL (KOCHAR 1975, 1979A)

In his most recent statement concerning the regulation of hookworm populations in Bengal, Kochar (1979a) states that

The existing epidemiological pattern of high prevalence and low intensity can be partly explained by the following concurrent factors:

1. A uniformly high probability of contacting some hookworm larvae because of localized soil infestation, absence of latrines, nonuse of shoes at the time of defecation, and equivocal avoidance of stools.
2. A uniformly low probability of contact with larvae through nonlocalized infestation and dispersion of stools in clusters of low to moderate densities, and restricted activities in defecation grounds.
3. A uniformly low probability of larval development and penetration success due to climatic conditions limiting the development of hookworm eggs and larvae (in open fields particularly), squatting time, and short duration between defecation and ablution in water bodies.
4. Other common factors enhancing the probability of hookworm success by small degrees, such as adverse foot conditions during wet season, use of shaded habitats for defecation, and agricultural activities in polluted fields.
5. A relatively high risk among agricultural laborers and their families due to a combination of social and ecological conditions under which they live and work.
6. Relative prevalence (sic) of a variety of "protective factors" vis-a-vis hookworm infection (Table V).
7. A demographic preponderance of low risk population (children and non-working females).
8. A high awareness of, and anxiety about, subclinical ailments leading to early positive health action within the folk culture context (including popular anthelmintics of unknown efficacy).

Kochar reasons that if sociocultural factors (Table V) are important in regulating hookworm populations, much of the variation in the intensity of hookworm infection should be accounted for by the proper model. In his general socioepidemiological model (Fig. 10), 18 variables included in a binary multiple regression analysis were found to account for 62.7% of the variance in the intensity of hookworm infection among our villagers (Table VI). Because a large fraction of the variance had been accounted for, he concluded that sociobehavioral factors are important in regulating hookworm infection. Kochar also concluded that transmission in defecation areas is not as important as others had suggested (Chandler, 1929; Cort, 1941; Beaver, 1961; Schad *et al.,* 1975) because the parameters defined as "defecation factors" accounted for only 18% of the variance. Although he agrees with the authors cited that focal transmission in defecation grounds is the most important single mode of infection, as already

TABLE V

Sociocultural Factors Predisposing Bengali Villagers toward, and Protecting Them from, the Risk of Hookworm Infection[a]

Risk factors	Protective factors
Universal practice of soil pollution	Latrines and "simple latrines"
Universal equivocal avoidance of stools in selecting a squatting place	Strict avoidance of stools in selecting a squatting place
Universal practice of going barefoot	Use of footwear during activity in infested areas
Prolonged or frequent activities in defecation areas	Restricted frequency or duration of activities in defecation areas
Soil pollution restricted to localized defecation areas increasing the larval populations per unit area	Diffused soil pollution decreasing the larval populations per unit area
Defecation in shaded habitats increasing the chances of survival of larval populations	Defecation in open habitats decreasing the chances of survival of larval population
Pollution of fields under jute crop	Universal avoidance of pollution of fields under crops
Fewer defecation grounds (small area per person)	Many defecation grounds (large area per person)
Absence of trails or pollution on trails	Presence of trails and avoidance of pollution on trails
Poor socialization of defecation habits	Strict socialization of defecation habits
Irregular ablution or delayed ablution	Universal practice of ablution soon after defecation
Nonrecognition of risks; nonrecognition of early symptoms of high infection	Recognition of risks of infection and recognition of early symptoms of high infection

[a]From Kochar (1979a).

noted he sees the observed correlation as a matter of increasing mobility and interaction with fields with a substantial amount of transmission attributable to diffuse soil infestation in the fields.

4. COMPARISONS WITH OTHER AREAS

The literature suggests that in many areas where there are, or were, high prevalences of heavy infection, ecological and behavioral factors interact so that many infective larvae are contacted at individual exposures. It is noteworthy that heavy infections have often been associated with particular kinds of agriculture that favor abnormally high numbers of larvae, and with human behavior that increases the risk of massive exposure (Cort, 1942). The exchange of worms between indigenous and nonindigenous peoples in some areas of the world where heavy infections have been prevalent also merits consideration. In the southern

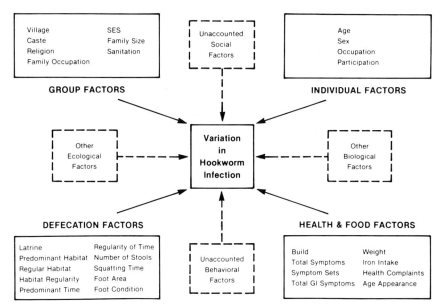

FIG. 10. Factors considered in a socioepidemiological model proposed to account for the variation in the intensity of hookworm infection in a population of rural Bengali villagers (SES = socioeconomic status; ■→ = factors examined in the present analysis; ⌐⌐→ = factors not examined in the present analysis) (Kochar, 1975).

United States, the European immigrant controlled hookworm infection less effectively than did the African (Henderson, 1957; Andrews, 1942a,b). It is less clear whether a cross-susceptibility to infection occurs when two human populations, both presumably originally harboring their own strains of hookworm, come to reside in areas favorable for the propagation of larvae; in the Caribbean both Asians and Africans introduced regional strains of hookworms and both failed to muster adequate host resistance.

III. Implications for Control

It is probable that in the coevolution of host–parasite relationships, a parasite's life history parameters and pathogenic characteristics evolve so that in particular ecological contexts host populations are only rarely exposed to overwhelming parasitism (Hoagland and Schad, 1978). Meanwhile, host populations will be adapting so as to limit the parasite's abundance and to resist the effects of levels of infection expected under average ecological conditions. Human cultural adap-

TABLE VI

Contribution of 18 Selected Sociobehavioral Factors to the Level
of Hookworm Infection Observed in Bengali Villagers,
as Determined by a Binary Multiple Regression Analysis

Variables	Reduction in r^2	Rank
Group factors	$(r^2 \times 100)$	
Village	12.7	1
Family occupation	5.9	4
Caste	7.9	2
Religion	3.6	8
Socioeconomic status (SES)	0.5	14
Subtotal	30.6	
Individual factors		
Age	4.5	5
Occupation	1.9	9
Sex	1.2	11
Subtotal	7.6	
Defecation factors		
Squatting time	6.1	3
Stools (number per day)	4.3	6
Foot conditions	4.3	6
Regular habitat	1.8	10
Habitat regularity	1.1	12
Defecation time (time of day)	0.2	16
Other variables	0.3	15
Subtotal	18.1	
Health factors		
Total symptoms	3.9	7
G.I. symptoms	0.7	13
Iron intake	1.8	10
Subtotal	6.4	
Total (all variables)	62.7	

tations will enhance biological mechanisms of resistance, and patterns of behavior perceived as protecting against disease will become part of the cultural heritage passed on to succeeding generations.

In rural Bengali culture we have observed human behavioral characteristics that protect against the acquisition of heavy hookworm infection, and others that increase exposure to infection (Table V) (Kochar, 1975, 1979a).

The established protective characteristics that are already part of Bengali culture should be emphasized, at least initially, in any organized program of health education directed against hookworms. The authors have difficulty reaching a consensus regarding the degree with which Bengalis actually avoid fecal pollution once the stool per se becomes invisible (the soil at the point of pollution remains infective). However, we do agree that traditional Hindus would desire in principle, if not in practice, to avoid such a "defiled" locus. This, then, provides a point of attack for the health educator; these traditional views can be reinforced by stressing the traditional basis for avoidance of fecal pollution as well as the health benefits.

The dense accumulation of feces in fallow fields during the dry season (forming *hegomaths* or fouled land) is highly desirable for hookworm control, since the temperatures attained within stools exposed to direct sunlight are rapidly lethal to hookworm eggs. In the absence of more sanitary methods for fecal disposal, the use of *hegomaths* should not be discouraged, although to the health administrator with a sophisticated urban orientation this may seem less than satisfactory. In our study area, latrine programs, desirable as they might seem to the outsider, would be of little immediate use. Some households have latrines but people do not use them, and without maintenance they rapidly become repugnant. In Hindu societies the problem of maintenance can be particularly difficult, because such work can only be done by members of certain castes; in our study area, suitable people were already fully occupied in other menial but more acceptable forms of labor and were not available for latrine maintenance. This illustrates the unexpected and sometimes largely incomprehensible difficulties associated with introducing new concepts and technologies in traditional social settings, and supports the suggestion that one should try initially at least to work within those settings and reinforce their positive characteristics.

Schad (1979) has suggested that until widespread eradication of helminths such as hookworms is possible in undeveloped countries, it may be desirable to encourage persistence of low-grade, well-tolerated infections which stimulate acquired resistance to superinfection. If a parasite is reintroduced into an area from which it was eradicated, local populations could be particularly vulnerable to previously nonpathogenic levels of infection. Thus, disease rather than mere infection could occur and an important new focus of clinical parasitism would be established where none existed before.

IV. Relevance for Socioeconomic Development

Hookworm infection is the second most prevalent human helminthiasis. More than 900 million people harbor these worms, which in common with the other geohelminths *Ascaris lumbricoides* and *Trichuris trichiura* are often associated with malnutrition and chronic ill health throughout vast areas of the tropical world. Little precise information exists concerning the socioeconomic costs of gastrointestinal parasitism and malnutrition, but there can be little doubt that such parasitisms represent an important burden for rural tropical and subtropical populations.

We have already indicated that major ecological changes such as widespread irrigation of arid lands, or extensive changes in vegetative cover such as in plantation agriculture, can greatly increase the prevalence of hookworm infection. Thus, although malaria and schistosomiasis have received virtually all the recent attention, ancylostomiasis has undoubtedly increased and will continue to increase as more land is brought under irrigation and cultivation in undeveloped countries lacking sanitary facilities.

Rural crowding in the absence of needed changes will also increase the prevalence of hookworm disease through both an increase in the density of fecal pollution and a probable decrease of iron intake, so that light or moderate infections presently well tolerated will be sufficient to produce hookworm anemia (Ball, 1966). Crowding and rural development without health education could exacerbate any tolerable hookworm problem by fostering social changes which tend either to minimize the effects of indigenous protective factors or to maximize the effects of indigenous risk factors. With little understanding of hookworms and the factors favoring their transmission, poorly educated people could easily abandon taboos which have provided protection against infection, seeing them only as discredited or outmoded customs and beliefs. Indeed, the growing belts of unsanitated squatter habitation surrounding most tropical cities are rife with infection, including hookworm.

The costs of hookworm infection to tropical and subtropical societies, which cannot be stated precisely, urgently need careful investigation. Although good anthelmintics are available and hookworms can be easily controlled, the fact that 900 million people harbor them indicates that we have not controlled them and that new investigations directed to new or improved methods are urgently required. The omission of hookworms from the World Health Organization list of the six most important tropical diseases has severely limited hookworm research. Urgent new work must be done to quantify the burden of ancylostomiasis and then to provide cost–benefit data for the range of strategies already available for controlling hookworms. In traditional societies, health education techniques which use and encourage established protective social practices and customs will prove among the most cost effective.

References

Andrews, J. M. (1942a). New methods of hookworm disease investigation and control. *Am. J. Public Health* **32,** 282–288.

Andrews, J. M. (1942b). Modern views on the treatment and prevention of hookworm disease. *Ann. Intern. Med.* **17**, 891–901.

Ashford, B. K., Payne, G. C., and Payne, F. K. (1933a). Acute uncinariasis from massive infestation and its implications. *JAMA* **101**, 843–847.

Ashford, B. K., Payne, G. C., and Payne, F. (1933b). The larval phase of uncinariasis. *P. R. J. Public Health Trop. Med.* **9**, 97–134.

Ball, P. A. J. (1966). The relationship of host to parasite in human hookworm infection. *In* "The Pathology of Parasitic Diseases" (A. E. R. Taylor, ed.), pp. 41–48. Blackwell, Oxford.

Bastidas, G. J. (1969). Effect of ingested garlic on *Necator americanus* and *Ancylostoma caninum*. *Am. J. Trop. Med. Hyg.* **18**, 920–923.

Beaver, P. C. (1961). Control of soil transmitted helminths. *W.H.O. Public Health Pap. No. 10*, 1–44.

Becmeur, A., Lafferre, M. and Lamotte. (1950). L'ankylostomose dans les mines de phosphate marocain. *Gaz. Med. Fr.* **57**, 869–874.

Chandler, A. C. (1925). The epidemiology of hookworm and other helminth infections on Assam tea estates. *Indian J. Med. Res.* **13**, 407–426.

Chandler, A. C. (1926). The prevalence and epidemiology of hookworm and other helminthic infections in India. 3. Central, Western and Northern Bengal. *Indian J. Med. Res.* **14**, 451–480.

Chandler, A. C. (1928). The prevalence and epidemiology of hookworm and other helminthic infections in India. 12. General summary and conclusions. *Indian J. Med. Res.* **15**, 695–743.

Chandler, A. C. (1929). "Hookworm Disease." Macmillan, London.

Chernin, E. (1954a). Problems in tropical public health among workers at a jute mill near Calcutta. II. A study of intestinal parasites in the labor force. *Am. J. Trop. Med. Hyg.* **3**, 94–106.

Chernin, E. (1954b). Problems in tropical public health among workers in a jute mill near Calcutta. 4. Hemoglobin values and their relation to the intensity of hookworm infections in the labor force. *Am. J. Trop. Med. Hyg.* **3**, 338–347.

Chowdhury, A. B., Schad, G. A., and Schiller, E. L. (1968a). The prevalence of intestinal helminths in religious groups of a rural community near Calcutta. *Am. J. Epidemiol.* **87**, 313–317.

Chowdhury, A. B., and Schiller, E. L. (1968b). A survey of parasitic infections in a rural community near Calcutta. *Am. J. Epidemiol.* **87**, 299–312.

Cort, W. W. (1941). The hookworms. *In* "Introduction to Nematology, Sec. II, Part II of Chitwood, B. G., and Chitwood, M. B." (J. R. Christie, ed.), pp. 309–313. Babylon, New York.

Cort, W. W. (1942). Human factors in parasite ecology. *Am. Nat.* **76**, 113–128.

Cort, W. W., Grant, J. B., Stoll, N. R., and Tseng, H. W. (1926a). An epidemiological study of hookworm disease in the mulberry districts of the Yangtze Delta. *Am. J. Hyg.* **7**, 188–252.

Cort, W. W., and Payne, G. C. (1922a). Investigations on the control of hookworm disease. 6. A study of the effect of hookworm control measures on soil pollution and infestation in a sugar estate. *Am. J. Hyg.* **2**, 107–148.

Cort, W. W., and Payne, G. C. (1922b). Investigations on the control of hookworm disease. 7. An epidemiological study of hookworm disease in a cacao estate. *Am. J. Hyg.* **2**, 149–161.

Cort, W. W., Payne, G. C., and Riley, W. A. (1923a). Investigations on the control of hookworm disease. 28. A study of a heavily infested group of people on a sugar and coffee estate in Puerto Rico, before and after treatment. *Am. J. Hyg.* **3**, (Suppl., July), 85–110.

Cort, W. W., Riley, W. A., and Payne, G. C. (1923b). Investigations on the control of hookworm disease. 29. A study of the relation of coffee cultivation to the spread of hookworm disease. *Am. J. Hyg.* **3**, (Suppl., July), 111–127.

Cort, W. W., Grant, J. B., and Stoll, N. R. (1926). "Researches on Hookworm in China." *Am. J. Hyg.*, Monogr. Ser. No. 7.

Ghadirian, E., Croll, N. A., and Gyorkos, T. (1979). Socioagricultural factors and parasitic infections in the Caspian littoral region of Iran. *Trop. Geogr. Med.* **31**, 485–491.

Hairston, N. G. (1962). Population ecology and epidemiological problems. *In* "Bilharziasis" (M. O'Connor, and G. Wolstenholm, eds.), pp. 36–62. Churchill, London.

Henderson, H. E. (1957). Incidence and intensity of hookworm infestation in certain East Texas counties. *Tex. Rep. Biol. Med.* **15,** 283–291.

Heyneman, D. (1977). Parasitic diseases in relation to environment, customs and geography. *In* "Parasites: Their World and Ours" (A. M. Fallis, ed.), pp. 1–23. *Proc. Symp. R. Soc. Can. 19th, Ottawa.*

Hoagland, K. E., and Schad, G. A. (1978). *Necator americanus* and *Ancylostoma duodenale:* Life history parameters and epidemiological implications of the sympatric hookworms of humans. *Exp. Parasitol.* **44,** 36–49.

Hodgman, J. H. (1934). Ankylostomiasis in the gold mines of the Witwatersrand. *Ir. J. Med. Sci.* **6,** Ser. No. 101, 203–222.

Kendrick, J. R. (1934). The length of life and the rate of loss of the hookworms, *Ancylostoma duodenale* and *Necator americanus. Am. J. Trop. Med.* **14,** 363–379.

Kochar, V. K. (1975). Human factors in the ecology and epidemiology of hookworm infections in rural West Bengal. D. Sc. Thesis. Johns Hopkins Univ., Baltimore, Maryland.

Kochar, V. (1977a). Sanitation and culture. I. Social aspects of sanitation and personal hygiene in a rural West Bengal region. *Indian J. Prev. Soc. Med.* **8,** 106–117.

Kochar, V. (1977b). Sanitation and culture. II. Behavioral aspects of disposal of excreta in a rural West Bengal region. *Indian J. Prev. Soc. Med.* **8,** 142–150.

Kochar, V. (1979a). Culture–parasite relationship: sociobehavioral regulation of hookworm transmission in a West Bengal region. *Stud. Med. Soc. Sci.* **1,** 1–84.

Kochar, V. (1979b). Culture and Hygiene in West Bengal. *In* "Sanitation in Developing Countries," (A. Pacey, ed.), pp. 176–185. Wiley, New York.

Kochar, V. K., Schad, G. A., Chowdhury, A. B., Dean, C. G., and Nawalinski, T. (1976). Human factors in the regulation of parasitic infections: Cultural ecology of hookworm populations in West Bengal. *In* "Medical Anthropology" (F. X. Grollig, and H. B. Haley, eds.), pp. 287–312. Mouton, The Hague.

Koshy, A., Raina, V., Sarma, M. P., Mithal, S., and Tandon, B. N. (1978). An unusual outbreak of hookworm disease in north India. *Am. J. Trop. Med. Hyg.* **27,** 42–45.

Martin, L. K., and Beaver, P. C. (1968). Evaluation of Kato thick smear technique for quantitative diagnosis of helminth infections. *Am. J. Trop. Med. Hyg.* **17,** 382–391.

Matsusaki, G. (1966). Hookworm disease and prevention. *In* "Progress of Medical Parasitology in Japan" (K. Morishita, Y. Komiya, and H. Matsubayashi, eds.), pp. 242–244. Meguro Parasitological Museum, Tokyo.

Miller, T. A. (1965). Persistence of immunity following double vaccination of pups with x-irradiated *Ancylostoma caninum* larvae. *J. Parasitol.* **51,** 705–711.

Napier, L. E., and Das Gupta, G. R. (1937). Haematological studies in Indians. 6. Investigations in one hundred cases of marked anemia amongst tea-garden coolies. *Indian J. Med. Res.* **24,** 855–909.

Nawalinski, T. A., Schad, G. A., and Chowdhury, A. B. (1978a). Population biology of hookworms in children in rural West Bengal. I. General parasitological observations. *Am. J. Trop. Med. Hyg.* **27,** 1152–1161.

Nawalinski, T. A., Schad, G. A., and Chowdhury, A. B. (1978b). Population biology of hookworms in children in rural West Bengal. II. Acquisition and loss of hookworms. *Am. J. Trop. Med. Hyg.* **27,** 1162–1173.

Rice, E. M. (1927). Mass treatment for hookworm infection on tea estates in Assam. *Indian Med. Gaz.* **62,** 126–129.

Schad, G. A. (1965). Factors influencing the distribution of hookworm. *Rep. Johns Hopkins Center Med. Res. Training,* 1964–1965, 21–25.

Schad, G. A. (1966). Ecology of hookworms in the soil. *Rep. Johns Hopkins Center Med. Res. Training*, 1965–1966, 42–48.

Schad, G. A. (1979). Effects of leaky sanitation on hookworms and other geohelminths. In "Sanitation in Developing Countries" (A. Pacey, ed.), pp. 31–33. Wiley, New York.

Schad, G. A., Chowdhury, A. B., Dean, C. G., Kochar, V. K., Nawalinski, T. A., Thomas, J., and Tonascia, J. A. (1973). Arrested development in human hookworm infections: an adaptation to a seasonally unfavorable external environment. *Science* **180**, 502–504.

Schad, G. A., Dean, C. G., Kochar, V. K., Nawalinski, T., and Chowdhury, A. B. (1971). Ecology of interacting populations of man and hookworms in West Bengal. *Annu. Meet. Am. Soc. Parasitol. 46th, Los Angeles. Abstr.*, pp. 28–29.

Schad, G. A., Soulsby, E. J. L., Chowdhury, A. B., and Gilles, H. M. (1975). Epidemiology and serology of hookworm infection in endemic areas of India and West Africa. *Nucl. Tech. Helminthol. Res. Proc. Panel*, 41–54. Int. At. Energy Agency.

Schad, G. A., Stewart, T. B., Page, M. R., El Naggar, H. M. S., and Parrish, P. K. (1980). Meatborne ancylostomiasis: a new route for the infection of man with *Ancylostoma duodenale. Annu. Meet. Am. Soc. Parasitol. 54th, Berkeley. Abstr.*, p. 68.

World Health Organization. (1964). WHO Expert Committee on Helminthiasis. Soil-transmitted helminths. *W.H.O. Tech. Rep. Ser.* 277.

9

The Human Environment and Helminth Infections: A Biomedical Study of Four Nigerian Villages

ALPHONSUS B.C. NWOSU

Projects Coordinator
Biomedical Sciences Research Unit
University of Technology
Enugu, Nigeria

Copyright © 1983 by Academic Press, Inc.
All rights of reproduction in any form reserved.
ISBN 0-12-196880-4

I.   Introduction

It is generally accepted that physical and cultural factors have a significant impact on the prevalence of human parasitic infections. Climate is an important limiting factor in the free-living developmental phase of parasites, whereas culture plays a crucial role either in bringing the infective agent and potential host together or in creating barriers that keep them apart. The serious manifestations of helminth infections result, therefore, from the interaction of climate, human ecology, and behavior so much so that different ecocultural zones have their own characteristic helminth diseases. However, the complex matrix of human ecology, culture, and parasitic diseases has not been fully elucidated. In recent times, there has been an upsurge of interest in this concept (Buck *et al.*, 1968, 1970; Hughes and Hunter, 1970; Dunn, 1972, 1976, 1979). Results from our unit and from other investigators in rural areas of Nigeria (Nwosu, 1981; Onubogu, 1978; Hinz, 1966, 1967a, 1967b, 1967c, 1968) indicate that the high prevalence rates are maintained by poverty, illiteracy, and population density. It is obvious that intensity of infection is determined by the extent to which the villager pollutes his environment. It is also clear that there is little hope of reducing the enormous helminth burden of the rural population without drastic changes in human ecology, behavior, and culture. This implies that disease management and control programs should be integrated with socioeconomic development, and to achieve this an understanding human cultural ecology relative to parasitic infections is necessary.

Kochar *et al.* (1970), in their excellent study on rural villages of West Bengal, emphasized the significance of cultural ecology in regulating community hookworm loads (see also Chapter 8, this volume). Their findings have raised hopes of the possibility of controlling parasitic infection through cultural changes. In other words, the rapid improvement of environmental conditions coupled with changes in specific habits of villagers would drastically reduce parasite population densities and consequently enhance the health status of rural communities. This avenue for the control of parasitic diseases needs to be critically evaluated by the developing countries of tropical Africa in view of their limited resources, the high cost of drugs, and the failure of past mass chemotherapy campaigns. Unfortunately, there has been little attempt in rural Africa to analyze (in the manner of Kochar *et al.*, 1970) the various theories on the effect that human cultural ecology has upon helminth diseases. There is therefore little exact information on rural Nigeria, although an environmental study conducted in *Akufo*, a small village in Western Nigeria (Gilles *et al.*, 1964), has yielded valuable information.

Rural villages in Nigeria will probably experience rapid economic advancement in the next decade as a result of deliberate and directed government policy.[1] As the anticipated transformation of the rural environment takes place, changes in culture will follow as the villager adapts to his new milieu, and this will significantly affect the prevalence of helminth diseases. Thus, the intensity of soil-transmitted helminth infections can be expected to decline with improved excreta disposal, although simultaneously irrigation schemes, greater mobility of the rural population, dietary changes, etc., may introduce new parasitic problems. A major objective of this chapter, therefore, is to collate parasitological and ecological data extant in the literature on four village communities that our unit has been studying for the past 4 years. These data together with our results will provide the basis for correlations between environment, habits of the villagers, and helminth infections. Our surveys were part of comprehensive longitudinal field studies of intestinal helminthiases, dracontiasis, and schistosomiasis in rural areas of Anambra State, Nigeria. The basic objectives of the project were to elucidate the epidemiological characteristics of these infections, evaluate the impact of these diseases on the rural economy, and design parasite control programs for the village communities.

II. The Communities

Based on a review of the 1975–1978 health records of hospitals and health centers in local government areas of Anambra State of Nigeria, four zones were delineated with respect to parasitic infections (Nwosu, *in press*). Four villages, *Ovoko* and *Ibagwa* from the northeastern zone, and *Nkalagu* and *Ntezi* from the northwestern zone, were chosen for the studies. The villages were chosen because they were small rural communities with low standards of living. The villagers were in intimate contact with the natural environment, and therefore offered a good setting for the study of community ecology of parasitic diseases. Two of the villages, *Ovoko* and *Ntezi,* were closed-in, isolated communities, whereas *Ibagwa* and *Nkalagu* were more open, with a significant immigrant population. *Ovoko* and *Ibagwa* were served by government health centers, and hospitals in *Enugu-Ezike* and *Nsukka* were less than 15 km away. The hospital at the cement manufacturing company and a health center at *Eha-Amufu* (18 km away) served the *Nkalagu* village community, and there was a government hospital at *Ezzamgbo,* 12 km from *Ntezi.*

---

[1]Federal Republic of Nigeria: Outline of the Fourth National Development Plan 1981–1985. Federal Ministry of Planning, Lagos, Nigeria.

A. General Description, Climate, and Vegetation

The villages lie about 7°E and 6°N of the equator; there is constant and abundant insolation causing high atmospheric temperatures (mean daily temperature is 80 ± 11°F). The mean annual rainfall exceeds 150 cm and shows a marked seasonality in its distribution; there is a long wet season from April to October, followed by a shorter dry season from November to March. The average monthly temperature, precipitation, and relative humidity (RH) data for *Ovoko* and *Isienu* (Nwosu and Anya, 1980) illustrate clearly the hot, humid climate of the area. The high humidity does not permit human perspiration to evaporate freely, thus making it imperative for the villagers to have daily baths, especially after farm work. In villages that are served by ponds, streams, and rivulets (that are also the foci for guinea worm and schistosome infections in the localities), these daily baths are ritualized and have played a role in the maintenance of the infections at high levels. The hot, humid climate also encourages the development and survival of infective stages, intermediate hosts, and vectors of helminth parasites as well as the breeding of houseflies that are significant vehicles for the transmission of intestinal helminthiases.

The topography is rugged and the vegetation is essentially grassland with patches of deciduous forest, constituting what has been called the savanna–forest ecotone. It forms a natural transition zone between the tropical grassland of the northern parts of the country and the rain forests to the south (Igbozurike, 1975).

B. Population, Housing, and Land Use Patterns

The population densities of these villages are low, ranging from 75 to 200/km². The villagers are Ibos, and mostly Christians with some adherents to the traditional religion; a few Hausa Moslems form part of the immigrant element in *Ibagwa*. Except for the few petty traders, most of the villagers lived their entire lives in their respective villages. Although the older members of the population were generally illiterate, most of the younger members (≤ 20 years) were not because all villages were served by schools and Christian churches.

The population structures of the villages as determined from sample surveys are fairly similar except for *Nkalagu* which showed a high male/female ratio, presumably as a result of the cement manufacturing company located at the outskirts of the village which has encouraged male-dominated immigration into the village. *Ovoko* and *Ntezi* show varying degrees of female preponderance. This may be due to the fact that these villages serve as labor reservoirs, losing their adolescent/adult males to the commercial and administrative centers of *Nsukka* and *Abakaliki*. The preponderance of children and the sex ratio of the population are important in correlating defecation behavior and the degree of environmental pollution.

The population is distributed in patrilineal households of 8–24 members dominated by the elder members. Habitation is dispersed, the villages being large collections of scattered households spread across large expanses of arable land. The houses are of two types, the traditional mud-walled houses with thatched roofs, and the cement-walled houses with roofs of corrugated iron sheets. The latter, which are usually better ventilated, indicate the household's improved socioeconomic status. Each household compound may be enclosed either by a wall or more commonly by a fence, and is surrounded by oil-palms, banana/plantain stands, and other economic plants.

The villagers live by farming plots of land (3–8 ha) adjacent to their houses. Food crops are intensively cultivated in these household farms, and a few animals (poultry, sheep, and goats) also are kept. The main cultivated crop is yams, which are planted in large mounds that characterize the farmlands in these localities. Yams may be combined with cocoyam and cassava in a multi-cropping rotational system. Vegetables are also commonly planted in the same farm plots. In addition to the peridomestic farms, there may be larger household farms of 5–15 ha at the periphery or outskirts of the villages where yams (only in *Ntezi*) and more commonly cassava and rice are planted.

Farming activity is seasonal and varies slightly from zone to zone. The typical pattern is for the ground to be tilled with hoes and prepared for the planting of the crops just before and/or after the first rains. This energy-intensive farm work is carried out almost exclusively by the males. There is a lull of 3–4 weeks followed by a peak in farming activities during the rainy season as the farms are "remolded" and weeded repeatedly using hoes. The process of remolding or "rehilling" is also energy-exacting. Taking place after about 2 or 3 months of luxuriant crop growth, it requires the participation of all adolescent and adult members of the household irrespective of sex. It is preceded by manuring of the farms with animal droppings, compost, and extensive human defecation. As a result of the government policy of synchronizing the main school holiday in Nigeria with summers in Europe and North America, schoolchildren have become heavily involved in farmwork during this peak farming season; prior to this, children only helped on the farms after school hours. The implications of this in relation to helminth infections will be discussed later.

The period following remolding is a rest period marked by food scarcity, which is ameliorated by constant harvesting and consumption of vegetables, maize, and various fruits. The harvest period (usually yams are first) is marked by festivities in the villages. The pattern shows both seasonality and sex-linked division of labor of farm work; the men are involved in the more exhausting farm labor such as tillage and making of yam mounds, and the women and children are occupied with household duties and the lighter farm duties such as planting of vegetables and weeding. This farm activity pattern will be correlated later with helminth prevalence rates in different sectors of the community, but it is important to note now that in many respects these villages are self-sufficient stable units, and exist as such.

III. Description of Village Sanitation

Generally, the sanitation level was low in all villages; defecation was indiscriminate in farmlands, refuse disposal was rudimentary, housefly populations were high, and domestic animals freely scavenged refuse and human excreta. The broad similarity in sanitary attributes of the villages notwithstanding, it is essential to quantitatively estimate the sanitary status of each village and isolate local differences in sanitation-lowering behavior so that meaningful correlations and comparisons can be made between the environment and community helminth burdens. To do this, four basic components (i–iv) of environmental sanitation relevant to human helminth infections were used in a scoring system (to be explained later). These were related to human population densities in the villages. Thus the sanitary level of each village was evaluated from (i) the numbers and distribution of pit latrines in the community; (ii) fecal densities in farmlands; (iii) garbage and refuse disposal systems; (iv) housefly population densities; (v) human population densities; and (vi) land availability per household. Of these, the absence of pit latrines and fecal densities in peridomestic farmlands are the most significant factors.

A. Excreta and Refuse Disposal

1. Pit Latrines

Eggs of most helminth parasites exit the host with the excreta and develop to the infective stage in the environment. The absence of pit latrines and sewage disposal systems results in a high level of environmental contamination with infective agents of intestinal helminth parasites and, consequently, in high parasite prevalence rates in the human population. Parasites in this group include the triad of nematodes, hookworms (*Necator americanus*), *Ascaris lumbricoides* and *Trichuris trichiura,* which constitute the principal helminth problem of rural communities in Nigeria.

2. Refuse and Housefly Populations

Houseflies have always been suspected of playing a role in helminth transmission; because of their constant contact with and ingestion of human feces, they

or lesser extent. The groups differed however in literacy levels, nature and sanitary status of households, defecation habits, excreta and refuse disposal practices, and attitudes to chemotherapy. Helminth prevalence rates in the various socioeconomic groups for *Ovoko* showed lower infection levels among the literate population. The illiterate farmers were heavily infected, and it was among this group that neonatal hookworm infections were detected (Nwosu, 1981).

The differences in helminth infection rates in the socioeconomic groups apparently were related to the presence or absence of pit latrines (Nwosu, 1981); this was correlated with literacy, disease awareness, and personal hygiene. Among the literate wage earners and traders in the village, self-medication using anthelmintics such as Mintezol (thiabendazole), Combantrin (pyrantel pamoate), Ketrax (mebendazole), and Antepar (piperazine) was common. The dangers of self-medication apart, this practice in conjunction with reduced "open" defecation results in minimal contamination of peridomestic farmlands.

Schoolchildren present unusual etiological aspects; they have consistently high worm burdens whatever their socioeconomic group. This may be partly because of inadequate latrine hygiene in the schools, resulting in equal exposure of all children (irrespective of their socioeconomic backgrounds) to a highly polluted environment. Most of the village schools are served by only 2–12 pit latrines, and a few schools have none. School populations range from 560 to 1828, and the mean number of children per latrine was 61! In such situations, defecation around school compounds, which is common, contributes to high infection levels among schoolchildren. Perhaps equally important is the change in the primary school year, previously January–December, to a new September–June academic year. This change, despite its other possible advantages, releases schoolchildren to spend more time on the farms during the peak helminth transmission season. This was not so in the previous schedule.

D. Seasonal Aspects of Transmission

Seasonality in helminth infections is a well-known phenomenon. In southern Nigeria, Hinz (1967) and Obiamiwe (1977) observed an increase in total helminth burden at the end of the rainy season and in the first months of dry season. Similar seasonal fluctuations in human hookworm populations have been reported for *Ovoko* and *Isienu,* and the relationship between worm burden and rainfall was investigated in detail (Nwosu and Anya, 1980; Udonsi *et al.,* 1980). The results showed discontinuity in worm transmission during the dry season, when infective agents of soil-transmitted helminth parasites were rarely recovered from contaminated farmlands. In the rainy season, the infective agents are abundant and widely dispersed in the environment; frequent rains help to spread the fecal deposits over wide areas and also provide the required moisture for the development of helminth eggs.

Large seasonal variations in worm burdens are governed by two factors. The first is seasonal fluctuation in populations of infective stages. The second and perhaps more important factor in our analyses implicates the cyclical rhythm of farming activities in the rural village communities, which is dependent on the amount of rainfall. During the rainy season, infective stages of the various helminth parasites are abundant, farming is at peak activity and the (usually barefooted) villagers make frequent contact with hookworm larvae in the topsoil, in pools between yam mounds, and on blades of grass onto which the larvae have been washed by the frequent torrential rainfall. Vegetables are abundant during this season and are consumed in large quantities; some, such as *Solanum* spp., are frequently eaten raw. This relationship between farming activities and infection levels is confirmed by results obtained by Erhadt and Schulze (1961), who found higher hookworm burdens among farmers than in other vocational groups.

Age and sex distribution of worm prevalence rates may also be explained on this basis. Age- and sex-linked division of farm labor, described earlier, showed that men performed the energy-exacting tasks such as preparation of yam mounds, remolding and so on, while the women and children combined household chores with weeding, picking vegetables, and carrying materials to and from the farms. This resulted in a greater exposure of the men to infective hookworm larvae, whereas women and children were more exposed to infective eggs of *A. lumbricoides* and *T. trichiura* as they picked vegetables and frequently consumed some (unwashed) in the process of picking.

Seasonality in dracontiasis and schistosomiasis is related to domestic water supplies. *Dracunculus medinensis* infections are acquired during the dry season exclusively; the reasons for this have been extensively discussed (Onabamiro, 1951; Muller, 1971; Muller, 1979). However, the yearly cycle in domestic water sources in the villages in relation to schistosome and guinea worm infections is rarely discussed. Dracontiasis endemic zones are characterized by serious shortages of drinking water during the dry season when the villagers have consumed all the water collected and stored during the rainy season. In *Ntezi*, the two perennial streams and a well located at the outskirts of the village are 5–8 km from many of the households, and most of the population depends on the artificial pond for their source of drinking water during the dry season. Onabamiro (1951) has calculated that during this season each individual ingests about 75 infected copepods by drinking pond water.

Our records of new schistosomiasis cases in *Nkalagu* during the period 1978–1980 show that the infections were acquired during the later part of the rainy season (August–October). The disease was highly localized in the area, and there were wide fluctuations in prevalence levels between adjacent villages (Nwosu, *in press*). The village under study was served by a small perennial stream that was less than 3 km from the most remote household. The bulinid snail populations in the stream were highest during the rainy season, and cercarial densities reached maximum levels in September and October. Water contact sites, where the villagers bathed, washed clothes, and prepared cassava for their meals, were identified and the number of hours spent by each sex/age-group performing these functions were recorded at bimonthly intervals for the period June–February 1979. The water contact patterns differed between sexes and age-groups, and varied from household to household. The results suggest that schistosome infections were acquired not as a result of villagers seeking drinking water, but from their performance of such chores as peeling and washing fermented cassava for family meals and washing clothes.

E. Polyparasitism

Multiple infections were common in the villages. This phenomenon, that is, an individual infected with several parasites at one time, has been called polyparasitism by Buck *et al.* (1978) and appears to be a feature of helminth infections in rural population in the tropics. The frequency distribution of multiple infections in the four villages shows clearly that the incidence of polyparasitism was highest in the 10–15-year age group, especially in villages with low sanitation scores. Double infections with intestinal nematode parasites were the most common, found in 29–36% of the total population; in Ovoko, the various combinations were hookworm/*Ascaris lumbricoides*, 5.2%; hookworm/*Trichuris trichiura*, 8.9%, and *A. lumbricoides*/*T. trichiura*, 3.6%. Triple infections with hookworm/*A. lumbricoides*/*T. trichiura* were rare (1.3%). The pattern of polyparasitism for the other village communities did not differ markedly except that schistosome and guinea worm infections raised the level of triple helminth infections in *Nkalagu* and *Ntezi* to 18.2 and 21.6%, respectively.

The population at greatest risk to multiple helminth infections is again school-children, which has serious health implications and emphasizes a great and urgent need for intensive school health programs in rural villages.

V. Socioeconomic and Behavioral Factors and Intensity of Infections

One of the major hopes of studies on the interrelationships between environment, culture, and parasitic infections is the attractive alternative of bypassing mass chemotherapy and improving the health status of rural populations through improved sanitation via changes in community habits. The excellent study by Kochar *et al.* (1970) in West Bengal has shown the importance of human factors in the regulation of hookworm populations (also see Chapter 8, this volume). A common feature of the fluctuation patterns of the total helminth burden in the villages under study during 1977–1980 was their tendency to remain stable, indicating the presence of regulatory factors. It is essential to understand the nature of these regulatory factors before a cultural approach can be adopted in the control of helminth infections. For this purpose, a number of mathematical models, used to describe the transmission dynamics of parasitic infections, stable states, and breakpoints in host–parasite relationships (Anderson, 1976; Anderson and May, 1979; May and Anderson, 1979) have been useful. This work does not seek to explore these mathematical models in detail but to derive from them a simple method for estimating transmission rates for the various helminths and to isolate those factors in the living habits of the villagers that expose them to infections. It is only when such "risk factors" are known that definite community health-promoting behavior may be initiated in the villages.

A. Man–Infective Agent Contact: Risk Factors

The number and dispersion of infective agents in the environment determine the transmission level of helminth parasites. This means that the worm load of an individual in a community is a function of the frequency of contact between that individual and infective agents. For each village, the infective agent population is related to the village's sanitary status and fluctuates seasonally in consonance with humidity cycles. Both factors are constants within small, closed village communities so that the level of infection becomes a function of the degree of exposure to infective agents. Correlations of helminth prevalence rates in different ages, sexes, and occupational groups with group-specific activities and behavior indicate aspects of community life that regulate exposure to infective agents of helminth parasites. Simple calculations and correlations of this nature for the villages emphasize the role of farming activities in hookworm infections and the effect of consumption of raw unwashed vegetables on maintenance of *A. lumbricoides* and *T. trichiura* infections.

The results are especially interesting in the case of schistosome infections. The risk factor is a function of the duration of water contact during the transmission season, and this in turn is determined by the distance of the household from the stream. As was pointed out earlier, schistosome infections are acquired by the villagers in *Nkalagu* as they use the streams for domestic purposes other than drinking water. The provision of clean piped water to the village for drinking purposes only would therefore not solve the problem. Indeed, piped drinking water has been supplied to *Nkalagu* for the past 15 years without affecting the schistosome infection level. For an appreciable drop in infection level to occur, the piped water supply must be easily available to all households in sufficient quantities for all domestic uses.

There was excellent correlation between dracontiasis and drinking pond water; the risk factor is sharply defined and points to the provision of piped drinking water to the *Ntezi* community as the solution to the problem. The reasons that this may not be feasible in the immediate future in this village are discussed by Nwosu *et al.* (1982).

B. Defecation Behavior

It has been established that the decisive factors in the transmission of hookworms, *A. lumbricoides,* and *T. trichiura,* which constitute the bulk of the helminth burdens of these villages, are poor latrine hygiene and indiscriminate defecation. The infective agents of these parasites have poor lateral migratory capacities and therefore aggregate around defecation sites. The sites are determined by defecation behavior, an integral part of village culture which cannot be divorced from community ethnography. Ethnic differences are not pronounced among the villages under study and defecation patterns are similar, showing higher fecal densities in peridomestic household farms. The topographical distribution of feces on the farmlands as described by Udonsi *et al.* (1980) showed some degree of overdispersion that suggested repeated use of defecation sites. Fecal samples taken from the defecation sites during the transmission (rainy) season (July–September) revealed worm-egg counts of 4082 ± 182 epg (eggs per gram feces) in the peridomestic farmlands, and 2051 ± 483 epg in the tree/shrub groves at the outskirts of the villages. These data when combined with observations of age distribution of epg counts and defecation practices suggest that children are largely responsible for pollution of the periodomestic farms. On questioning, villagers 20 years and older stated that they usually defecated in the groves although 10–15% of this age group admitted to occasional defecation in peridomestic farmlands in the very early mornings and late evenings. It is therefore clear that the high levels of infective stages in the environment are largely caused by the promiscuous defecation behavior of the younger elements of the population, who incidentally also carry the highest worm loads in the community.

Cocoyam plots were more heavily polluted than yam and cassava plots (presumably because the large broad cocoyam leaves provided shade and privacy), but the degree of difference does not permit these plots to be designated ''defecation grounds'' as identified by Kochar *et al.* (1970). Kochar *et al.* had clearly shown that in West Bengal fecal pollution of the environment was highly localized and restricted to about 1.0–2.6% of the total community area (see Chapter 8). Our findings and observations do not agree, but we believe that the mild degree of overdispersion in fecal distribution in the villages under study is caused not by defecation behavior but by microclimatic heterogeneities. The implications of differences in defecation behavior between rural villages in West Bengal and southern Nigeria with regard to prevalence and intensity of intestinal worm infections are obvious. It would have been interesting to compare data on worm populations in the two geographical areas, but figures on infection levels in West Bengal were not given.

The various aspects of defecation behavior described above show that promiscuous defecation by children near households is largely responsible for the high prevalence rates of intestinal worm infections in the villages. As has been repeatedly pointed out, these children constitute the wormy persons whose egg output contributes over 70% of the total egg input to the environment. It is therefore essential that improvement of the health status of rural populations in southern Nigeria through better sanitation and excreta disposal methods start with the younger age groups. There is a high incidence of nonuse of latrines (when these are available) in this subpopulation, but it was observed that this was because the latrines, as they were constructed, were unsafe for children. In such cases the children defecated on banana leaves or waste paper inside the household. The feces were wrapped up and thrown into the latrines later. Pit latrines appropriately designed to incorporate safety measures for children would ensure wider usage, leading to minimal environmental pollution and, consequently, reduced worm burdens.

An important fallout from analysis of defecation behavior is the possibility that the land use patterns, especially the multicropping system in which cocoyam plots are not prominent, may play a positive role in reducing the overall level of fecal pollution. This would be a factor in regulating community worm loads, maintaining them at the observed steady states. The ways in which land use patterns and cropping systems (especially cocoyam hectarage) affect defecation behavior and level of pollution of farmlands are currently under investigation.

Indiscriminate urination, especially into streams, does not qualify as defecation behavior, but it is important in considering schistosome infections in *Nkalagu*. In this village the practice of urinating into the streams was exclusive, and widespread, among the children. Of the schoolchildren questioned, 86.2% admitted to urinating frequently into the water as they bathed, swam, and played. When the schistosome egg counts of this age group are considered, the implications of this unhygienic practice for the prevalence of urinary schistosomiasis are obvious.

C. Diet, Malnutrition, and Helminthiases

Dietary surveys of selected households which cut across socioeconomic strata showed a considerable dependence on starchy staples such as cassava, yams, and cocoyams. Animal protein was scarce and was denied to the children who supplemented their starch diets with wild rodents and freshwater crabs and snails

(*Nkalagu*). Roasted in open fires before consumption, these resulted in a high incidence of paragonimiasis among children in the *Okigwe* area (Nwokolo, 1974). In our study villages, the scarcity of meat in the diet explains the absence of common meat-transmitted helminth infections, notably *Taenia* spp. The only exception is *Ibagwa*, which has a cattle market and an appreciable immigrant Hausa population. A type of barbecued beef (called *suya* throughout Nigeria) which originated in the northern (Hausa) parts of the country is widely consumed. The eating of *suya* has been associated with tapeworm disease (Dada, 1978; 1979), and it is therefore not surprising that *T. saginata* infections are restricted to the *Ibagwa* community.

The dietary composition in the villages is similar to that in *Ilesha* and *Akufo*, western Nigeria (Collis *et al.*, 1962a; Gilles *et al.*, 1964), and typifies the dietary situation among rural populations of southern Nigeria in its lack of protein-rich staples. In the northern parts of the country, the traditional diets provide a well-rounded nutritional regimen; the differences in the nutritional values of diets in these communities are reflected in the growth curves of the children (Collis *et al.*, 1962b). Protein-calorie malnutrition (PCM) is common in the villages under study, and growth curves of children show these to be below the optimum for Nigerian children.

The susceptibility of the two populations to helminth infections and the manifestations of disease are different because of the intimate relationship between the nutritional status of the host and the pathogenicity of helminth parasites. Data for this comparison again are not available but some deductions may be made from observations on worm burdens/disease levels of the study communities.

The worm burden per individual, even in the most intensely infected groups, were generally below the intensity associated with clinically recognizable symptoms. Hospital cases were few (Nwosu and Anya, 1980); but the morbidity effects of the infections on children were obvious, although there was no clearcut relationship between morbidity and worm burden. In many cases high worm burdens ($\geq 10,000$ epg) were well tolerated by some children, and in our experience morbidity effects were closely linked to malnutrition. It may well be that the level of worm disease in a rural community is not purely a function of high prevalence and intensity of infection but is induced by malnutrition. For this reason, because PCM was common among children in the villages, the low number of hospital cases was surprising. Perhaps this is not an accurate representation but merely a result of the apathetic attitude of villagers to chronic but nonfatal diseases, which leads to low hospital attendance rates. This attitude is best illustrated from our experience in *Ntezi* where we recorded a hospital attendance rate of 0.05% among the diseased (dracontiasis) population for a variety of related reasons ranging from ignorance, apathy, and resignation to disease (36.41%), preference for local therapy (23.80%), and a grossly inadequate health care system (21.09%), to the high cost and doubtful efficacy of available drugs (5.61%).

Nutritional status in rural villages is not consistent but fluctuates with food supply, which in turn depends on the seasonal cycles of planting and harvesting of food crops. The dietary composition of selected households in *Ovoko* and *Ntezi* during the postplanting season (June–August) and the harvest season (October–December) clearly illustrates this fluctuation pattern. This seasonal cycle of food availability has nutritional implications that may affect susceptibility to infections, but this has never been studied. The only deduction that is permissible from the data in the literature and from our observations is that the postplanting period, when food is insufficient in both protein and calories, corresponds to the worm transmission season. It is therefore not surprising that the few recorded cases of helminthiases in these localities occurred during this period.

D. Social Habits and Helminth Infections

Certain social and recreational habits lead to greater exposure of some individuals to helminth infections, for example, the relationship between palm wine drinking and guinea worm infections. Palm wine is fermented palm sap which, diluted with water, is widely drunk throughout southern Nigeria. The alcohol content is low (0.5–7.1%) so that contaminants remain viable even after long periods. In *Ntezi,* palm wine is diluted with pond water infested with copepod intermediate hosts of *Dracunculus medinensis*. In the *Abakaliki* urban area 20 km from *Ntezi,* appreciable numbers of infected copepods were recovered from palm wine sold in bars, and we established that *Ntezi* was the source of the wine. A significant percentage of the *Abakaliki* urban population, although they did not ordinarily drink pond water, constituted the "regulars" of local palm wine bars and were infected with guinea worms (Nwosu and Chime, *in press*). Other social habits of the villagers are not relevant to helminth transmission except, perhaps, the water contact pattern in *Nkalagu* which has acquired a social dimension. The women get out of hearing range of the menfolk to exchange local gossip by going to the stream while the children frolic in the water. Higher schistosome infections result from the prolonged exposure to cercariae-contaminated water. Theoretically, these social habits will become less hazardous with improved domestic water supplies and environmental sanitation. It augurs well for the health of the rural population in Nigeria that the provision of clean and adequate piped water to villages has a high priority rating in the country's development plan.

VI. Strategies for Control of Helminthiases in Rural Nigeria

A major aim of our study of community ecology of helminth infections in the villages was to gain insight into the complex interrelationships between environment and disease in order to formulate effective control programs for each locality. The failure of past control programs, some of which were massive and internationally backed (such as the malaria and schistosome control programs), has emphasized the need for a new framework that takes into account the total environment, physical, biological, and cultural, for the formulation of future programs. The simple fact that we have emphasized is that human ecology and behavior are important factors determining parasite infection levels. A theoretical framework for parasite control must therefore aim at improving the sanitary status of the environment and simultaneously at changing the habits and culture of the villager within his socioeconomic matrix. Results from Southeast Asia (May, 1973) and the Ryukyu Islands (Marshall, 1973) point to the crucial role that rapid improvement of the environment, coupled with definite health-promoting changes in human habits, could play in minimizing parasitic infections and consequently in improving community health. Vector control programs and mass chemotherapy campaigns which formed the basis of the old approach should therefore be seen as part of improvements in the environment and health habits of rural communities. From this new perspective, an integrated approach is needed that takes into account the local conditions of the general problems of helminth infections in village communities: latrine hygiene, water supplies, farming activities, literacy level, health education, and mass chemotherapy.

A. Socioeconomic and Technical Aspects of Control Programs

The widespread prevalence and high intensity of helminth infections form part of the vicious cycle between disease and poverty so noticeable in these villages. The helminth problem is an insidious one, not dramatic in its morbidity as is malaria, but one which slowly and quietly saps the strength of the afflicted population to a state of debility that renders them incapable of sustaining economic activities at the level necessary to foster development of the villages. Thus, the villager remains economically poor, partly because of his poor health status, and in this state of poverty and ignorance he is not able to do much to improve his health.

The crucial question is how to break this cycle by incorporating not only parasite control programs but the total concept of primary health care into rural development plans. In developing countries where over 70% of the population is rural, this question has become political, and in Nigeria the term "integrated rural development" has become a slogan used to highlight the need for economic development programs of villages to have a total, ecological base.

The current attitude is that improving the economic growth of villages will bring in its wake better health for the villages. This approach is idealistic because it aims at improving the standards of living of the villagers, rather than merely freeing them from the onslaught of parasitic infections. Using this approach, developing countries should focus their scarce resources not only on snail control programs (for example) but on the provision of adequate piped water supplies for domestic use. Such water supplies should be located within 100–200 m of the households and designed for the total needs of the families by providing facilities for washing clothes, preparing cassava, etc. and not only for drinking water. When this is done, it will release the villager from the enormous pressure of organizing his daily routine around obtaining his domestic water supplies, as well as minimize the incidence of the whole spectrum of water-borne diseases.

We also believe that if improved farming practices are introduced and agro-based industries sited in the villages (with the necessary educational and administrative support) to improve the earning capacity and literacy level of the villager, improved housing and latrine hygiene will follow with the resultant elimination of soil-transmitted nematode infections.

The elimination of parasitic infections through economic growth should therefore be the ultimate aim of control programs. A major constraint to this approach is that it will have to take place over a very long period in view of the limited resources of developing countries and the multivarious facets of development.

Specific sanitation improvements and vector control programs, albeit with limited objectives, must be undertaken in localities where infections are widely prevalent. In *Ntezi* we are currently attempting a dracontiasis control program based on eliminating pond copepod populations during the transmission season by using insecticides. Our experience shows that for such control programs to be effective the cooperation of all sectors of the community is essential. The program must be simple and must not require technical expertise for its execution. More importantly, the program should be generated or maintained from within the community itself.

The various steps involved in our program will be stated briefly. Preliminary laboratory investigations on dose-mortality rates of copepods were conducted and the results tested in 10 artificial ponds located at the farms. During this period, the ponds were not used and the buildup rates of copepod populations were monitored; this required the cooperation of the chiefs, councillors, and elders of the village. Based on the copepod population buildup rates, the number of ponds in the village, and their rates of use, dates for treating the various ponds were scheduled. Literate villagers (usually teachers) were recruited and instructed in the insecticide dose rates for the ponds in their localities. Weekly supervision routines involving copepod sampling of treated ponds ensured compliance.

B.   A New Approach to Mass Chemotherapy Campaigns

Mass chemotherapy has always featured prominently in parasite control programs because it is the best way of drastically reducing the numbers of diseased individuals in the community. Its importance in rural health improvement will increase in the next decade throughout the developing world as populations increase rapidly (because of high birth rates), leading to overcrowding and increased poverty. The basic issue becomes maximization of the possible benefits derivable from communitywide chemotherapeutic campaigns. A solution was suggested by Nwosu (1980, 1981), who showed how mass chemotherapy directed at the most intensely infected subpopulation in the community and timed at the season unfavorable for transmission would reduce infection rates with minimal costs.

The initial results (1978–1979) showed that such strategic mass chemotherapy campaigns initially achieve a tremendous success in reducing infection levels, but data (Nwosu, 1980) on infection levels and infective larval populations in these communities show that in the long run this success may be limited. The reasons for this are environmental and underline the need to view mass chemotherapy as part of health-promoting behavior that must be combined with improved environmental sanitation. In other words, for the success of strategic mass chemotherapy to be sustained and made permanent, it must be backed by local environmental sanitation campaigns. However, our mass chemotherapy campaign against intestinal helminthiases in *Abbi*, which is a closed village community at the outskirts of *Nsukka*, is yielding very encouraging results in the absence of an environmental sanitation program. Similarly, the results of our mass chemotherapy campaigns against schistosomiasis in *Nkalagu* are very encouraging, showing promise of successful local control of the disease.

The quintessence of strategic mass chemotherapy is identifying and treating the subpopulation in the community that carries the bulk of the worm burden. This subpopulation of wormy persons is easily determined from the frequency distribution of infections (percentage infection $\times$ egg output) in the various age, sex, and occupational groups. Because of overdispersion, this subpopulation is usually less than 25% of the total population. If these persons are successfully treated within a short time during the nontransmission period when there is no danger of reinfection, the reduction of environmental contamination with infective agents will exceed 70% so that very few individuals will acquire the infections during the next transmission season.

By continuously identifying and treating the diminishing populations of wormy persons over a period of 3 to 4 years, it should be possible to reduce the level of infective agents in the environment to a level below the transmission threshold even without improved latrine hygiene.

The choice of drug is also important and must be based on data obtained from preliminary investigations for the locality. The following attributes are necessary: broad-spectrum anthelmintic (since polyparasitism is common) with high worm egg reduction rates, minimal side effects, uncomplicated treatment regimes (single-dose treatments are ideal), availability, cost and acceptability to local population, and so on. Based on these parameters, Mintezol (Merck) for intestinal nematode infections, and a single dose Ambilhar/Metrifonate (CIBA/Bayer) for urinary schistosomiasis, were used. Treatment regimes using these drugs produced over 80% worm egg reduction rates, and the campaign periods were usually the dry season months (November–March). Zentel (albendazole) is currently the anthelmintic of choice in mass chemotherapy campaigns because of its broad spectrum efficacy and high (95%) worm egg reduction rates. Dracontiasis therapy campaigns were not undertaken because of the unsuitability of available drugs.

C. Vector Control

Vector-borne helminth diseases *strictu sensu* such as filariases were not common in the villages, but the widespread distribution of mosquitoes in the villages and movements of the population into adjoining filariasis-endemic zones in northern and southeastern zones of the country render these villages potentially hazardous. Because of these factors, and the ubiquity of malaria, vector control cannot therefore be eliminated from control programs. The control of insect vectors of disease constitutes a distinct area in itself that cannot be meaningfully reviewed within this chapter. However, it has become apparent that attempts to control vectors without changing the environment produce only palliative effects as the environment sooner or later will be recolonized. Therefore, it is essential to consolidate the effects of insecticides in reducing vector populations with cultural practices that alter permanently the breeding and resting sites of the vector. This will also have the added advantage of minimizing environmental pollution caused by excessive insecticide use.

It is debatable whether bulinid snails are vectors or intermediate hosts of *Schistosoma haematobium*. It is also doubtful whether the application of molluscicides on a large scale to control these snails will lead to a reduction in schistosome infections commensurate with the costs of such programs. The highly localized nature of schistosome infections suggests that limited molluscicide application during the transmission season, and reduced water contact through behavioral changes, would suffice.

VII. Conclusion

This chapter has focused on the tremendous helminth burden carried by villagers in developing countries of the tropics such as Nigeria and has emphasized the importance of helminth infections in rural communities (Wyatt and Wyatt, 1967; Duke, 1978; Ejezie, 1979). The infection levels that have been reported for the villages studied are high, paralleling those found in villages in similar bio-geographical zones of the country more than a decade ago (Hinz, 1967; 1968). If a marked drop in helminth infections is to occur, a fundamental change in the complex matrix of interrelated components that permits parasite transmission is required. Unless this fundamental change is made, the problem will increase with the high rate of increase of rural populations, posing a significant task for rural health services. It is unfortunate that government programs to improve the health and living standards of the people have previously been restricted to urban areas, but recently there has been increased awareness that economic development of the country will have to be agriculturally and rurally based. It is imperative to restate at this time the parasite (helminth) problems of rural populations and to point out the relationship between carelessly planned development programs and disease (Hughes and Hunter, 1970; Waddy, 1974; Farvar and Milton, 1973).

The spectrum of helminths varied slightly between villages but the general pattern was the triad of hookworm/*Ascaris lumbricoides*/*Trichuris trichiura*, common to all villages, over which were superimposed schistosome infections (in *Nkalagu*) and guinea worm infections (in *Ntezi*). The basic factors in the endemicity of these helminths were poor sanitation and unhygienic domestic water supplies; high intensity of infections resulted from ecocultural factors that brought the villagers into constant contact with infective agents of the parasites. A new framework for the control of helminth infections is advocated, based on these factors and aimed at improvements in rural sanitation and health-promoting behavior. The overall objective should be to regulate parasite populations in the community by greatly reducing the transmission potential (Bradley, 1972). It is our belief that these improvements should result from economic growth of the villages.

The role of improved sanitation in reducing helminth infections is well known (Weir, 1952; Sahba and Arfas, 1967; Barclay, 1966) but the possibility of altering human behavior to minimize contact with infective agents and thereby reduce infection levels has been received with some cynicism (Nelson, 1972). However, the study by Ghadiran *et al.* (1979) in Iran shows the crucial role of ecological-cultural factors in helminth infections. This approach presents us with an attractive alternative method of controlling helminth infections by discouraging those individual and community living habits that enhance infections. It should be the aim of epidemiology, given the failure of previous parasite control programs, to try out this alternative by identifying aspects of human ecology and behavior that are related to parasitic diseases.

Mass chemotherapy would be required to accelerate the pace at which definitive health-promoting behavior reduces the helminth burden of a community.

Stürchler *et al.* (1980), in a recent study on eight Liberian villages, stated the need for mass treatment, health education, and improvement in environmental hygiene to control helminth infections. These investigators also pointed out the high cost of mass chemotherapy campaigns, calculated as US $4.00 per person. To reduce costs and ensure maximum benefits a new approach to mass chemotherapy is suggested which takes account of overdispersion of parasite populations in the community and discontinuity in transmission, and emphasizes the treatment of the most intensely infected subpopulation (wormy persons) during the season unfavorable (dry) for transmission so as to minimize reinfection and decrease the frequency of treatment schedules. In *Ovoko* (and *Isienu*) where this program is under trial, the cost of treatment per person using Mintezol is US $2.84 ($1.78 for Zentel); the total cost of treating the 1924 wormy persons in a population of 6892 is about US $5,500, one-third of the cost of treating the entire population. Infection levels at the end of the first year diminished by 70.2%.

Frequency distribution analyses of helminth infections showed that wormy persons are usually preschool and schoolchildren in the community. It is among this age group that pathological effects of helminthiases are most pronounced. The high worm populations among children also ensure that the average female parasite is mated, so that fertile ova are passed out with feces, whereas in the less heavily parasitized sectors of the population a higher proportion of nonfertile ova are passed. It is therefore necessary that rural health improvement programs, in Nigeria and throughout the developing world, take account of this vulnerability of children to parasitic infections. Their low resistance to diseases due to these infections results from their poor nutritional states. Results from Guatemala and Chile (Ascoli *et al.*, 1967; Scrimshaw *et al.*, 1968; McCormick *et al.*, 1977) justify this orientation and stress the need for a complete integrated approach to rural development, which must have a sound ecological base.

In Nigeria, for example, billions of dollars will be spent in the next 5 years to develop the various river basins to provide irrigation for rural agriculture. As the irrigation schemes begin to increase rice production in the Northeastern zone of Anambra State (where *Nkalagu* and *Ntezi* are located), increased dispersion of bulinid snails will occur. More villages will become potentially hazardous as a consequence, and with the increased population movements attendant on agrobased development the prevalence of urinary schistosomiasis will be accentuated, creating a new problem for the area. Increase in helminth infections would therefore be expected in rural villages of Nigeria with improperly planned rural development programs. The hope has been expressed in this chapter that the public health component of development especially with regard to helminth infections will be built into the various developmental activities planned for rural villages in developing countries.

Acknowledgments

I am indebted to Professor A. O. Anya for his encouragement and support, which have made it possible for me to embark upon this study. Generous research grants from the University of Nigeria and the Anambra State Ministry of Health, and liberal free supplies of drugs from Merck, Sharpe & Dohme (Nig.) Limited, May & Baker (Nig.) Ltd., and CIBA-GEIGY (Nig.) Ltd., are hereby gratefully acknowledged. I also thank the chiefs, village heads, teachers, and field assistants (too numerous to mention individually) who assisted in these studies, and Mrs. E. Ihekweazu for English translations of the papers by Hinz.

Finally, I needed and obtained the kind understanding of my wife and family to stay away from home frequently as I lived with the villagers. This work would not have been possible without this understanding.

References

Adi, F. C. (1980). "Health Education for the Community." Nwamife Publ., Enugu, Nigeria.

Anderson, R. M. (1976). Dynamic aspects of parasite population ecology. *In* "Ecological Aspects of Parasitology" (C. R. Kennedy, ed.). North-Holland Publ., Amsterdam.

Anderson, R. M., and May, R. M. (1979). Population biology of infectious diseases—Part I. *Nature (London)* **280**, 361–367.

Barclay, R. (1966). A Rural Sanitation Project in Sabah (North Borneo).

Ascoli, W., Guzman, M. A., Scrimshaw, N. S., Flores, M., and Gordon, J. E. (1968). Nutrition and infection field study in Guatemalan villages, 1959–1964. V. Disease incidence among preschool children under natural conditions, with improved diet and with medical and public health services. *Arch. Environ. Health* **15**, 439–449.

Bradley, D. J. (1972). Regulation of parasite populations: A general theory of the epidemiology and control of parasitic infections. *Trans. R. Soc. Trop. Med. Hyg.* **66**, 667–707.

Buck, A. A., Sasaki, T. T., and Anderson, R. I. (1968). "Health and Disease in Four Peruvian Villages." Johns Hopkins Univ. Press, Baltimore, Maryland.

Buck, A. A., Anderson, R. L., Sasaki, T. T., and Kawata, K. (1970). "Health and Disease in Chad." Johns Hopkins Univ. Press, Baltimore, Maryland.

Buck, A. A., Anderson, R. I., and Macrae, A. A. (1978). Epidemiology of Polyparasitism. I: Occurrence, frequency distribution of multiple infections in rural communities in Chad, Peru, Afghanistan and Zaire. *Tropenmed. Parasitol.* **29**, 61–70.

Collis, W. R. F., Dema, I., and Lesi, F. E. A. (1962a). Transverse survey of health and nutrition, Pankshin division, northern Nigeria. *West Afr. Med. J.* **10**, 131–154.

Collis, W. R. F., Dema, I., and Omololu, A. (1962b). On the ecology of child nutrition and health in Nigerian villages. *Trop. Geogr. Med.* **14**, 201–229.

Croll, N. A., and Ghadirian, E. (1981). Wormy persons: Contributions to the nature and patterns of overdispersion in persons with *Ascaris lumbricoides, Ancylostoma duodenale, Necator americanus* and *Trichuris trichuria. Trop. Geogr. Med.* **33**, 241–248.

Dada, B. J. O., and Belino, E. D. (1978). Prevalence of hydatidosis and cysticercosis in slaughtered livestock in Nigeria. *Vet. Rec.* **103**, 14.

Dada, B. J. O., Adegboye, D. S., and Mohammed, A. N. (1979). The epidemiology of *Echinococcus* infection in Kaduna State, Nigeria. *Vet. Rec.* **104**, 321–323.

Dipeolu, O. O. (1977). Field and laboratory investigations into the role of *Musca* spp. in the transmission of intestinal parasitic cysts and eggs in Nigeria. *J. Hyg. Epidemiol. Microbiol. Immunol.* **21**, 209–214.

Dipeolu, O. O. (1980). The role of *Musca* in the contamination of food. *Proc. Int. Congr. Trop. Med. Malariol., 10th.*

Duke, B. O. L. (1978). ''The relevance of parasitology to human welfare today: Medical aspects.'' *Symp. Br. Soc. Parasitol.* **16**, 1–40.

Dunn, F. L. (1972). Intestinal parasitism in Malayan aborigines (Orang Asli). *Bull. W.H.O.* **46**, 99–113.

Dunn, F. L. (1976). Human behavioural factors in the epidemiology and control of *Wuchereria* and *Brugia* infections. *Bull. Public Health Soc. Malays.* **10**, 34–44.

Dunn, F. L. (1979). Behavioural aspects of the control of parasitic diseases. *Bull. W.H.O.* **57**, 499–512.

Ejezie, G. C. (1979). The pattern of parasitic infection in villages of Lagos State, Nigeria. *Trop. Geogr. Med.* **31**, 503–508.

Erhadt, E., and Schulze, W. (1961). Die verbreitung der ankylostomiasis des menschen in Asien unter besonderer berucksichtigung der angaben seit 1939. *In* ''Welt-Seuchen Atlas III''.

Farvar, M. T., and Milton, J. P. (1973). ''The Careless Technology: Ecology and International Development.'' Tom Stacey Publ., London.

Ghadirian, E., Croll, N. A., and Gyorkos, T. W. (1979). Socio-agricultural factors and parasitic infections in the Caspian Littoral region of Iran. *Trop. Geogr. Med.* **31**, 485–491.

Gilles, H. M., (1965). ''Akufo: An Environmental Study of a Nigerian Village Community''. Ibadan Univ. Press, Nigeria.

Hinz, E. (1966). Einfach und mehrfachbefall mit darmhelminthen in der bevolkerung der west-afrikanischen regentropen. *Tropenmed. Parasitol.* **17**, 427–442.

Hinz, E. (1967a). Vergleichende untersuchungen uber den darmhelminthenbefall bei der bevol-kerung sundnigerias in verschiedenen jahren. *Tropenmed. Parasitol.* **18**, 162–171.

Hinz, E. (1967b). Der jahreszeitliche verlauf von darmhelmintheninfektionen bei der bevolkerung der westafrikanischen regentropen. *Tropenmed. Parasitol.* **18**, 172–179.

Hinz, E. (1967c). Geschlechts und altersunterschiede im darmhelminthenbefall bei der bevolkerung sudnigerias. *Tropenmed. Parasitol.* **18**, 335–342.

Hinz, E. (1968). Regionale unterschiede im vorkommen von helminthosen beim menschen in sud-nigeria. *Tropenmed. Parasitol.* **19**, 227–244.

Hughes, C. C., and Hunter, J. M. (1970). Disease and Development in Africa. *Soc. Sci. & Med.* **3**, 443–493.

Igbozurike, U. M. (1975). Vegetation Types. *In* ''Nigeria in Maps: Eastern States'' (G. E. K. Ofomata, ed.). Ethiope Publ., Benin, Nigeria.

Ikeme, M. M. (1976). Human hookworm infections: a diagnostic dilemma? *J. Med. Pharm. Mark.* **4**, 295–298.

Jusatz, H. J. (1966). Biometereological and geomedical aspects of human ecology. *Int. J. Bio-metereol.* **10**, 323–334.

Kochar, V. K., Schad, G. A., Chowdhury, A. B., Dean, C. G., and Nawalinski, T. (1970). Human factors in the regulation of parasitic infections: Cultural ecology of hookworm populations in rural West Bengal. *In* ''Medical Anthropology'' (F. X. Grollig, and H. B. Haley, eds.). Mouton.

Marshall, C. L. (1973). Some exercises in social ecology: Health, disease and modernisation in the Ryukyu Islands. *In* ''The Careless Technology.'' Tom Stacey Publ., London.

May, J. M. (1973). Influence of environmental transformation in changing the map of disease. *In* ''The Careless Technology.'' Tom Stacey, Publ., London.

May, R. M., and Anderson, R. M. (1979). Population biology of infectious diseases: Part II. *Nature (London)* **280**, 455–461.

McCormick, M. C., Shapiro, S., and Horn, S. D. (1977). The relationship between infant mortality rates, medical care and socio-economic variables, Chile 1960–1970. *Proc. Int. Meet. Int. Epidemiol. Assoc., 8th,* San Juan, Puerto Rico.

Muller, R. (1971). *Dracunculus* and dracunculiasis. *Adv. Parasitol.* **9**, 73–151.

Muller, R. (1979). Guinea worm disease: epidemiology, control and treatment. *Bull. W.H.O.* **57**, 683–689.

Nelson, G. S. (1972). Human behaviour in the transmission of parasitic diseases. *In* "Behavioural Aspects of Parasite Transmission" (E. U. Canning, and C. A. Wright, eds.). Academic Press, London.

Nnochiri, E. (1968). "Parasitic disease and urbanization in a developing community." Oxford Univ. Press, London.

Nwokolo, C. (1974). Endemic paragonimiasis in Africa. *Bull. W.H.O.* **50**, 569–571.

Nwosu, A. B. C. (1980). Strategic mass-chemotherapy for the control of common protozoal and helminth infections of humans in Nigeria—trial results. *Proc. Int. Congr. Trop. Med. Malariol., 10th.*

Nwosu, A. B. C. (1981). The community ecology of soil-transmitted helminth infections of humans in a hyperendemic area of southern Nigeria. *Ann. Trop. Med. Parasitol.* **75**, 197–203.

Nwosu, A. B. C. (1981). Human neonatal infections with hookworms in an endemic area of southern Nigeria—a possible transmammary route. *Trop. Geogr. Med.* **33**, 105–112.

Nwosu, A. B. C. (in press). Parasitic Diseases in Igboland: a study in medical geography. *In* "A Survey of Igboland" (G. E. K. Ofomata, ed.). Fourth Dimension Publ.

Nwosu, A. B. C. (in press). Ecology of schistosome transmission in Anambra State of Nigeria. *Tropenmed. Parasitol.*

Nwosu, A. B. C., and Anya, A. O. (1980). Seasonality in human hookworm infection in an endemic area of Nigeria, and its relationship to rainfall. Tropenmed. Parasitol. 31, 201–208.

Nwosu, A. B. C., and Chime, A. B. (*in press*). Palm-wine as a significant vehicle for the transmission of guinea-worm and common protozoal and helminth infections in endemic areas of Anambra State of Nigeria. *Trans. R. Soc. Trop. Med. Hyg.*

Nwosu, A. B. C., Ifezulike, E. O., and Anya, A. O. (1981). Endemic dracontiasis in Anambra State of Nigeria: geographical distribution, epidemiology, clinical features and socio-economic impact. *Ann. Trop. Med. Parasitol.* **75**.

Obiamiwe, B. A. (1977). The pattern of parasitic infection in human gut at the specialist hospital, Benin City, Nigeria. *Ann. Trop. Med. Parasitol.* **71**, 35–43.

Onabamiro, S. D. (1951). The transmission of *Dracunculus medinensis* by *Thermocyclops nigerianus* as observed in a village in south-west Nigeria. *Ann. Trop. Med. Parasitol.* **45**, 1–10.

Onabamiro, S. D. (1952). The geographical distribution and clincial features of *Dracunculus medinensis* in south-west Nigeria. *West Afr. Med. J.* **1**, 159–165.

Onubogu, U. V. (1978). Intestinal parasites of school children in urban and rural areas of Eastern Nigeria. *Zentralbl. Bakt. Parasitenk. Infektionskr. Hyg.* **242**, 121–131.

Sahba, G. H., and Arfaa, F. (1967). The effect of sanitation on ascariasis in an Iranian village. *Trop. Geogr. Med.* **19**.

Sahba, G. H., Arfaa, F., and Bijan, H. (1967). Intestinal helminthiasis in the rural area of Khuzestan, South-west Iran. *Trop. Geogr. Med.* **19**.

Scrimshaw, N. S., Taylor, C. E., and Gordon, J. E. (1968). "Interactions of Nutrition and Infection." *W.H.O. Monogr. Ser.,* No. 57.

Sturchler, D., Stahel, E., Saladin, K., and Saladin, B. (1980). Intestinal parasitoses in eight Liberian settlements: prevalences and community antihelminthic chemotherapy. *Tropenmed. Parasitol.* **31**, 87–93.

Udonsi, J. K., Nwosu, A. B. C., and Anya, A. O. (1980). *Necator americanus:* population structure, distribution, and fluctuations in population densities of infective larvae in contaminated
farmlands. *Z. Parasitenk.* **63,** 251–259.

Waddy, B. B. (1974). Tropical medicine and industrial development. *J. Trop. Med. Hyg.* **77,**
19–21.

Weir, J. M., Wasif, I. M., Hassan, F. R., Attia, S., and Kader, M. A. (1952). An evaluation of
health and sanitation in Egyptian villages. *J. Egypt. Public Health Assoc.* **27,** 61–114.

Wyatt, J. L., and Wyatt, G. B. (1967). An analysis of the patients seen at Igbo Ora rural health
centre, western Nigeria, during the year July 1964 to June 1965.

10

The Transmission of *Trypanosoma cruzi* Infection to Man and Its Control

P. D. MARSDEN

Department of Medicine
University of Brasilia
Brasilia, Brasil

I. Introduction

One of the most important subjects of current research on Chagas' disease relates to human ecology. Two aspects can be defined: one is the attitude of people who live in areas of active transmission and their willingness to help, and the other relates to technical personnel involved in control. These aspects, which are discussed in this section, require insight into the epidemiology of transmission. It is therefore necessary to give some background details before their importance can be appreciated.

To prevent human infections with *Trypanosoma cruzi*, it is most important to reduce domestic triatomid bug populations so that the risk of transmission becomes negligible. The major advance that made this feasible was Müller's discovery that chlorinated hydrocarbon compounds (Kean *et al.*, 1978) had excellent residual insecticide activity. Domiciliated reduviid (Reduviidae) bugs, because they are largely confined to the house environment, are more accessible to this method of control than winged Diptera such as *Anopheles* which only visit human tenants. Initial trials in the late 1940s and early 1950s confirmed expectations with large bug mortalities. Indeed, there is a famous telegram sent to the Brasilian Ministry of Health in 1947 declaring that the problem of Chagas' disease would be solved using this method (De Brito, 1968).

However, subsequent observations showed that the degree of success depended on the type of insecticide used, its frequency of application, and the species of bug against which the control measure was directed. When insecticide activity had disappeared, the possibility of reinvasion of the house after a few months was very real in certain situations, that is, those in which the vector had a wide ecological valence or another effective vector species had invaded the domestic habitats from sylvatic foci. It is often difficult to gain access to the most severely affected families because they are scattered in remote rural areas lacking roads or other means of communication. Economic inflation is now making house spraying an expensive operation, particularly because insecticides and gasoline are often imported.

In spite of these difficulties, the ministries of health of countries such as Venezuela, Brasil, and Argentina have made progress in removing the threat of transmission from large areas of their countries. A large part of the known endemic area in Brasil has been subjected to a spraying program (Marques, 1979).[1]

Detailed information regarding the responsible bug vectors and other transmission cycles present in rural and periodomestic environments is essential before a control program can be planned. Other factors influencing priorities of the areas to be sprayed will be available lines of communication (roads), the importance of the area relative to the economic development of the country as a whole, and the prevalence of human disease in the area.

II. Transmission to Man without the Insect Vector

Although most patients with *Trypanosoma cruzi* infections are infected by contaminated bug feces, there are other methods of transmission. Infection by blood transfusion was first reported in 1936; this method of transmission and others have been reviewed by Dias (1979a). He presents an extensive list of investigations of the prevalence of blood donors with positive serology often reaching 10–20%. Amato Neto (1979) has suggested that 20,000 infections per year might occur in Brasil. With increasing awareness of this risk accidents of this

---

[1]Since this review was written, the Brasilian Ministry of Health has been voted sufficient money to mount control programs in all unsprayed affected areas.

type will diminish; however, more than 100 have been reported. Since living *T. cruzi* are introduced directly into the blood stream, such cases are usually particularly acute. The trypomastigote survives well in stored blood; Sullivan (1944) recovered live flagellates from a blood specimen drawn 250 days previously. The discovery by Nussenweig *et al.* (1953) that stored blood can be sterilized with 1 : 4000 gentian violet added 24 hr before transfusion has enabled blood banks to use sero-positive blood when there is a shortage. At the University of Brasilia, we have used this technique for many years without mishap; unfortunately, blue blood is not very acceptable to patients and gentian (or crystal) violet is rather variable in composition. It has recently been suggested that Amphotericin B may sterilize blood effectively (Cruz *et al.*, 1980). In highly endemic areas where serology is occasionally unreliable, addition of gentian violet to all blood before transfusion has been recommended (Rassi and Rezende, 1976). Kidney transplants can also be a source of *T. cruzi* infection (Chocair *et al.*, 1981).

Dias (1979a) has also reviewed the problem of congenital Chagas' disease. Usually, mothers are in the indeterminate phase of the disease in which parasitemia can be demonstrated by suitable xenodiagnosis in only about 50% of patients. Bittencourt (1976) found placental lesions in the cases that she studied, and *T. cruzi* infection in the mother has been suggested as a cause of abortion (Tervel and Nogueira, 1970). Bittencourt *et al.* (1972) estimated that 2% of premature babies in a maternity hospital in Salvador had congenital Chagas' disease, and a similar incidence has been noted in experimental animals (Mello and Borges, 1981). In Chile, Howard (1962) encountered 1 case of transplacental transmission for every 20 premature babies under 2 kg, a frequency greater than is caused by toxoplasmosis and, in his experience, equalling the frequency attributable to syphilis. Although more work is needed, the review by Dias (1979a) of field studies suggests that in the general community the prevalence is not very significant.

Infection in the neonate is also possible by transmission in the mother's milk, as was shown in man by Mazza *et al.* (1936) and in experimental animals by Miles (1972). More than 100 cases of congenital Chagas' disease have been described in the literature; many were severe, with cardiac or meningeal involvement. However, the disease may be mild, with fever or hepatosplenomegaly the only sign. Normally, parasites can be easily detected in the peripheral blood. *T. cruzi*-specific IgM antibodies present in neonatal sera are also diagnostic (Amato Neto *et al.*, 1977).

Accidental transmission to man is also possible either as the result of a laboratory accident or by ingestion. It is not surprising that more than 50 laboratory infections have occurred, because *T. cruzi* is the most infectious of the human blood protozoa, and protozoologists are not accustomed to handling high-risk organisms (Marsden, 1976). Meningoencephalitis and megasyndromes have subsequently occurred in infected medical workers. It is unfortunate that these occurrences have not been better documented because often a great deal is known about the inoculum and manner of infection. Common accidents occur by inoculation with infected syringes or while pipetting cultures. Some laboratory infections are mysterious, but the aerosol infections of raccoons that were induced in Washington (Winslow, 1964) should be remembered, and habits such as blowing over jars of infected bugs to drive them away from the top should be discouraged. On two occasions in the author's experience, technicians who had worked with bugs for a long time suffered from impaired judgment and allowed insects (in one case infected insects) to feed on their arms. Attempts should be made to provide variety in the work of personnel in a Chagas' experimental laboratory. (I sent my people to the cinema when I thought concentration was poor.) The drug nifurtimox (Lampit) should always be available and in the event of a genuine risk of infection treatment at a daily dose of 8 mg/kg body weight should be started immediately pending serology at 30 and 60 days.

Apart from pipetting accidents, oral transmission to man is not well documented although it is easy to infect animals by this route (Marsden, 1967). Indeed in nature insectivores are most often infected by eating bugs. There have been two microepidemics in Brasil in which oral transmission was suggested as the route of infection in man. In Belem, Para, on the mouth of the Amazon, human Chagas' disease is almost unknown and positive serology is rare (Lainson *et al.*, 1979), yet three acute cases occurred in children of a single family who had never left the locality (Shaw *et al.*, 1969). No bugs were found in the house but seven sylvatic species in the area are known to be infected, and the *T. cruzi* zymodemes common to these bugs and man have been identified (Miles *et al.*, 1978). It is possible that an infected bug entered the house and fell into the cold soup people customarily prepare (Lainson *et al.*, 1980). In an agricultural school in Rio Grande do Sul, 17 people were infected and 6 died; contamination of food with infected opposum urine has been suggested as the cause of the epidemic. Treatment with steroids as a result of initial misdiagnosis may have modified the diaease (Di Primio, 1971). In animals with high parasitemias, trypanosomes which may be present in the saliva and urine (Marsden and Hagstrom, 1968) could constitute an infective risk for man.

III. Transmission to Man by the Insect Vector

It is possible that blood-sucking Triatominae and *Trypanosoma cruzi* evolved together from more primitive ancestors and that theirs is an association of great antiquity. This might explain why Triatominae are usually so readily infected with *T. cruzi* and why they incubate the infection better than other insect vectors of medically important protozoa. The majority of Hemiptera (bugs) have piercing mouthparts to suck plants to which they frequently transmit flagellates of the *Phytomonas* group (Sherlock, 1979a; Wallace, 1979). From these Hemiptera may have evolved the large group of the family Reduviidae which suck arthropod haemolymph and are predatory on other arthropods. Their powerful piercing mouthparts inject toxic proteolytic saliva which is extremely painful to man, and they are infected with the *Crithidia* group of flagellates. Indeed members of this group can infect blood-sucking Triatominae as was illustrated by the discovery of a colony of *Triatoma infestans* infected with *Blastocrithida triatominae* (Del Prado, 1972). This group of insects and their flagellates may have adopted a warmblooded host into their cycles giving rise to the Triatominae-*Trypanosoma cruzi* complex as we know it today. Why this process should have occurred mainly in the New World is not clear.

Since the early experiments of Brumpt, we have known that a variety of arthropods other than Triatominae, including ticks, bedbugs, and mosquitoes, can incubate *T. cruzi* in the laboratory (Brumpt, 1912a). At least eight other families of arthropods can be infected (Pipkin, 1969); however, their role in transmission to man is likely to be negligible. The roles of fleas and bedbugs need to be further defined. They are common in poor housing in endemic areas, and bedbugs may proliferate after insecticide application; transmission might be possible if such infected insects were crushed on the skin. Certainly, *T. cruzi* remains infective in dead triatomids for months in the refrigerator (Soares and Marsden, 1979).

The posterior station transmission of *T. cruzi* by reduviid bugs was first demonstrated by Brumpt (1912b). Most human infections occur in this manner: during or after feeding, the bug defecates on the skin, the metacyclic trypanosomes present in this dejecta multiply on gaining entry to man's tissues, and the infection persists indefinitely. No spontaneous cures in terms of sterilization of infection are known, and indeed very few are adequately documented after specific treatment. These events determine whether a patient will carry the label "chagasic" for the rest of his life with all that implies in terms of developing heart or gut disease, getting a job, and raising a family (Macedo, 1979). They are, therefore, worth examining in some detail.

The recent monograph by Lent and Wygodzinsky (1979) describes over 100 Triatominae. Although more than 50 are known to be infected with *T. cruzi* and no resistant species are known in nature, relatively few are important in human transmission because triatomid ecological niches rarely include contact with man. Given that the bug species in question has close contact with man, many factors will influence the success of transmission.

There is evidence from field observations in a highly endemic area that some subjects escape infection for many years while living in a high-risk environment.

Uninfected 9-year-old children who have lived all their lives in houses with high densities of infected bugs and with younger infected siblings have been observed to develop acute Chagas' disease while under study (Minter, 1978). An attempt to assess the risk of infection based on a calculation of the density of infected domestic vectors has been reported (Minter *et al.*, 1973); however, on reviewing the evidence this is seen to be an oversimplification.

The feeding activities of domestic vectors under natural conditions are unknown, but Rabinovitch *et al.* (1979) have calculated the average feeding frequency of *Rhodnius prolixus* in the natural domestic environment. In houses with typical insect population densities this frequency, estimated at 9 bites/person/day, could rise to 58 in exceptional circumstances. This species is quite voracious; the feeding frequency will be lower for *Triatoma infestans* and much lower for *Panstrongylus megistus,* a very sluggish bug. In Mambai, Goias, fewer than 2 bites/person/day were estimated in two houses for adult *T. infestans* (Schofield, 1980a). In Sao Felipe, Bahia, the author sat for two nights in a house with many *P. megistus* present on the walls and was not approached by a single bug; observation of marked bugs showed that in fact many remained in the same spot for as long as 48 hr.

The nocturnal activity of these important domestic vectors is of the greatest importance to human transmission, determining not only the contamination of the skin but also the exact timing with which it occurs. Obviously, even if only a small proportion of bugs contaminate the human subject before he wakes, then the chances of infective trypanosomes being rubbed into the skin or conjunctiva upon waking are much greater. Laboratory observation in an artificial arena by Schofield (1975) suggests that the majority of species examined showed activity immediately after lights were turned off. The time of defecation after feeding varies with the bug species but all the three important vectors mentioned above defecate during or shortly after engorgement. This is in contrast to other species such as *Triatoma protracta* which, as its name suggests, often defecates after a protracted time away from the host. The time before defecation has been the subject of several studies because of its relevance to transmission (Zeledon *et al.*, 1977a; Rocha e Silva *et al.*, 1979a). After the rectal contents are voided the blood meal is concentrated in the stomach by the passage of drops of clear urine through the rectum; in infected bugs this urine is rich in metacyclic forms (Zeledon *et al.*, 1977b). Usually by the time this process occurs the insect has left the host skin.

The efficiency of the bug in ejecting a large number of tryptomastigotes at the time of defecation is also important. Although triatomid bugs are generally most efficient incubators of *T. cruzi*, refractoriness is well documented in laboratory experiments and does not depend on the quantity of trypomastigotes ingested (Miles *et al.*, 1975; Torno *et al.*, 1981). This refractoriness, which occurs in individuals in a susceptible colony, has a genetic basis (Maudlin, 1976). The concentration of flagellates within the rectum of individual bugs studied sequentially over 503 days varied greatly although they were always detectable (Marsden and Alverenga, 1975). In other experiments, spontaneous loss of infection has been noted (D'Alessandro and Mandel, 1969).

Another nearly unknown factor is the relationship between the strain of *T. cruzi* and the bug species involved. Many authors have suggested that the local bug species better incubates the local strains of *T. cruzi* and should be used as the xenodiagnostic agent. Certainly in Sao Felipe, Bahia, infected *P. megistus* contains rectal concentrations of flagellates rarely achieved in the laboratory. In contrast, in Mambai, Goias, rectal flagellates in *T. infestans* are frequently sparse. There is some evidence that in this area *T. infestans* has replaced *P. megistus* as the domestic vector. Recent work with *Dipetalogaster maximus* has shown that this Mexican bug incubates Brasilian strains of *T. cruzi* equally as well as does the local vector (Marsden *et al.*, 1979a), but this question requires further investigation.

Other considerations in addition to the strain of *T. cruzi* constitute the second group of factors influencing transmission. The number of trypomastigotes necessary to initiate an infection in man is not known. This obviously will depend on the transmission route, and it is possible that the introduction of one trypomastigote directly into the blood stream (as in transfusion) would be sufficient. However, there is no ethical way of determining this because complete cure of human *T. cruzi* infection is still rare even after chemotherapy. Experiments such as those that established that a minimum of 300 to 450 African trypanosomes were necessary to initiate an infection in man cannot be performed (Omerod, 1970).

When studying perconjunctival penetration, Marsden (1969) found bug-derived metacyclic trypomastigotes to be more infective than bloodstream-derived trypomastigotes of the same strain. In another assessment of a different strain by syringe inoculation, the reverse was true (Neal and McHardy, 1977). Although trypanosome penetration of cells has been observed *in vitro* (Dvorak, 1976), the precise mechanism is not known.

Many experiments have shown that the number of trypanosomes in the inoculum modifies the course of infection in the mammalian host (Marsden and Hagstrom, 1968). In the artificial situation of an inbred mouse model, single trypanosomes can initiate a fatal infection (Marsden *et al.*, 1977). Several strains were cloned in animals in our laboratory, but it should be noted that these strains had been laboratory-maintained for years; with new field isolates, it is frequently difficult to raise patent infections in mice.

A third group of factors relating to the microclimate of the skin or mucous membrane comes into play when the feces containing the metacyclic trypomastigotes are deposited on the host integument. Conjunctival penetration is easily induced in mice, probably because the membrane is thin and moist from lubrication with an isotonic liquid. Skin penetration is more difficult; many workers have failed to induce infections through "unbroken" skin (Pipkin,

1969). The term unbroken skin must be interpreted with caution; ectoparasites that may not be macroscopically evident, gland orifices, and other factors may have an effect on skin integrity. Experiments showing the decline in the number of infections acquired from a standard skin-contaminating drop related to the time after shaving the skin emphasize the importance of skin integrity in denying entry (Marsden, 1967). If the patient has an immediate skin reaction to the bug bite, he may scratch the site of the bite, breaking the skin surface (Costa et al., 1981).

The microclimate at the skin-air interface is also significant because the temperature–humidity ratio determines the dessication of the liquid feces. Chagas (1921) insisted that trypomastigotes are very sensitive to drying. In our laboratory at ambient temperatures (22–26°C) infectivity is lost in 30 min (Soares and Marsden, 1981. At 100% humidity, a rise in temperature within the tropical temperature range causes a very significant drop in infectivity (Alvarenga and Marsden, 1975). Contrary to a previous report, human sweat does not have trypanocidal properties (Soares and Marsden, 1980).

The fourth and final group of factors that could influence successful transmission to man are related to the human host and are still poorly understood. The majority of cases of acute Chagas' disease occur in the first decade of life; and, as can be shown in animal models, age may be a factor determining susceptibility. Any form of immunosuppression as a result of malnutrition, drugs, or primary failure of a component of the immune response could increase host susceptibility. There is no evidence to suggest that any human subjects demonstrate innate resistance such as can be shown in inbred mouse systems (Treischmann et al., 1978). There is some evidence to suggest that superinfection can occur and will influence the development of Chagas' disease (Macedo, 1973; Deane et al., 1981).

In conclusion, although a single night's exposure to these bugs in a house could effect transmission as was suggested in the case of Charles Darwin, the chance is remote since certain conditions have to be fulfilled. The high concentration of infected vectors in close proximity to man is in marked contrast to the conditions of transmission of human African trypanosomiasis.

IV. Transmission Cycles Involving Bugs and Animals and Their Relevance to Man

Carlos Chagas himself discovered the main elements of the transmission cycles after initially finding Trypanosome cruzi in house-dwelling Panstrongylus megistus. He later identified two important mammalian hosts in the domestic environment, man and the domestic cat (Chagas, 1909). He discovered infection in armadillos, and recognized *Panstrongylus geniculatus* as the vector in this purely sylvatic cycle in armadillo burrows (Chagas, 1912).

Subsequently, transmission cycles involving a wide range of hosts have been reported from almost every country where *T. cruzi* infections are endemic. Numerous species from at least 24 families of mammals have been identified as definite hosts of *T. cruzi* under natural conditions (Barretto, 1979). Birds are not infected, possibly due to innate immune factors and high body temperature, nor have infected reptiles been found in nature. Several authors have attempted a classification of such cycles based on their importance relative to human transmission (Zeledon, 1974; Barretto, 1976; Miles, 1979). It is useful to consider mammals and their triatomid vectors together in this context since in nature they occupy the same habitat.

Occasionally, sylvatic Triatominae invade houses. For example, the species *P. geniculatus,* although breeding in animal hiding places, often appears in houses. In urban São Paulo, *P. megistus* were uninvited guests at several dinner parties in the center of town. They originate in small, residual, woodland park areas and probably live in opossum or rodent nests. *Triatoma protracta* commonly invades houses in California. In all three species, winged adults can be found flying into the houses at night, probably attracted by light (Sjogren and Ryckman, 1966). Because some of these bugs are infected, the possibility of transmission to man exists, and because all flying females are inseminated, house colonization can occur.

Many more triatomid bugs never invade houses, remaining in a sylvatic habitat. Transmission of *Trypanosoma cruzi* to man by these species can occur only if man invades their habitats. For example, *Dipetalogaster maximus,* the largest known triatomid bug, is restricted to the tip of the Baja California peninsula in Mexico where it is found on hilltops at the base of rock piles. It is unusual to capture a specimen with a blood meal because blood sources are scarce, but a human feed has been reported, and wild bugs may harbor *T. cruzi* (Marsden *et al.,* 1979b). This species attacks man in daylight when he is seated on the rocks. In Argentina, *Triatoma patagonia* has been observed to attack campers at night.

Wild animals invading houses could increase the risk of transmission of infection, although their role has been difficult to assess. Several genera of bats have been found to cohabit with man and to incubate *Trypanosoma cruzi* infections. Infected opossums have been captured from the United States to Argentina; they tolerate *T. cruzi* infections well and parasitemia is easily detectable. Some species (*Didelphis azarae*) invade houses and nest in roof materials, etc. Rats may share both sylvatic and domestic habitats, moving between one and the other (Rocha e Silva *et al.,* 1975). In a recent epidemic of acute Chagas' disease, the prevalent *Rattus* species was noted to harbor *T. cruzi* of the same zymodeme as that which causes disease in man (Barrett *et al.,* 1979; Barrett *et al.,* 1980).

Both dogs and cats have been recorded as having high rates of infection, and in some areas they are important domestic infection reservoirs. Dogs also may live outside the house and establish links with sylvatic cycles. Dogs, especially when living in the house with suckling litters, may provide an important blood meal source for domestic bugs. Cats are less important since they invariably hunt at night when the bugs are active. There is evidence of a closed cycle of infection by rodents eating bugs in the house and in turn being eaten by the cats (Minter, 1976a). Pigs and larger domestic animals have little importance in transmission cycles, and although they can be infected experimentally show very low parasitemia (Marsden et al., 1970). In Bolivia and Peru guinea pigs are reared for food, often in the house, and are frequently infected with T. cruzi. A bug colony may be maintained along with the guinea pigs (Herrer, 1964).

Some of the wild Triatominae living in sylvatic habitats show signs of domiciliation with a varying capacity to colonize houses. Rhodnius neglectus, for example, is usually found in the crowns of palm trees, but occasionally adults and immature stages are found in houses. Palm trees are particularly important and many species have been listed as occurring in these (Zeledon and Rabinovich, 1981). Also, because these trees frequently yield useful products for roofing, soap, etc., they are left standing when the forest is cleared for farming.

Some species such as Triatoma dimidiata, T. sordida, and T. brasiliensis are frequently found in houses but also occupy many natural habitats. For example, it is common to capture as many T. dimidiata or T. brasiliensis around a house as inside the infested dwelling (Zeledon et al., 1975). In Sao Paulo State, when T. infestans was eradicated by a spraying program T. sordida was observed to enter houses and occupy its vacated domestic habitat (Forattini et al., 1973). In Venezuela, T. maculata may similarly replace R. prolixus (Ferrer, 1976).

The final group of bugs includes those that are more common in the domestic environment and rarely occur outside the house. The best example is T. infestans, but P. megistus in northern Brasil is another good one. P. megistus exists as a sylvatic species in southern Brasil, but in the northeast it becomes an exclusive house dweller. Genetic variation has been suggested as an explanation (Pessoa, 1962); humidity dependence has also been suggested (Forattini, 1972). The geographical distribution of certain bugs does seem related to climatic factors (Bustamante, 1957). Comments are frequently made about the danger of invasion of the Amazon basin by important domiciliary vectors; however, T. infestans must have already been introduced many times by man but has failed to adapt. T. sordida or R. prolixus arriving in the feathers of migrating birds have also failed to establish infections in houses in this area.

V.   Behavior of Domestic Bug Populations

Sherlock (1979a) has prepared a useful map showing the general geographical distribution of important vectors (Fig. 1). The best example of a bug vector

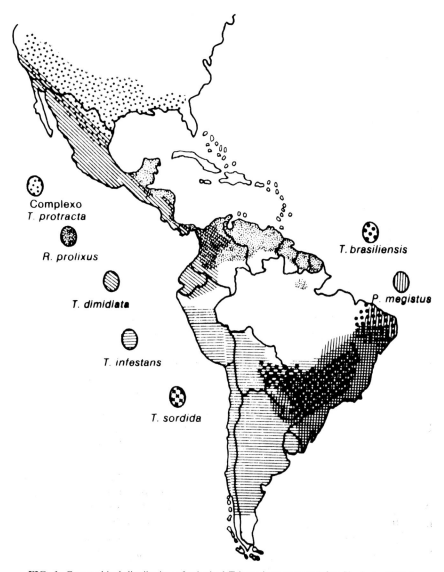

FIG. 1. Geographical distribution of principal Triatominae vectors (after Sherlock, 1979a).

dependent on the homes of man for its survival is *Triatoma infestans*. It has been suggested that the adaptation of this bug to man's domiciles occurred in the Andean region of Bolivia where they were first noted in the sixteenth century (Martins, 1968). The preColumbian cave homes of early man were probably little different from the animal burrows the insect originally frequented (Da Silva *et al.*, 1979). Today this species, rarely encountered in a sylvatic habitat, is the principal vector of Chagas' disease in Chile, Argentina, Bolivia, Peru, Uruguay, Paraguay, and Southern and Central Brasil, extending as far north as the State of Pernambuco. As its name suggests, domestic infestations are heavy and several thousand bugs have been captured in one house (Dias and Zeledon, 1955). Yet, although a most effective *Trypanosoma cruzi* vector, its dependence on the domestic environment means that it is particularly vulnerable to house spraying.

Panstrongylus megistus is an important domiciliary vector in northeast Brasil, and in southcentral Brasil it has been supplanted by *Triatoma infestans*. In São Felipe, Bahia, where Miles (1975) carried out a very thorough assessment of sylvatic cycles, this species was never encountered outside homes or chicken houses. In the author's experience, demolition of houses reveals much lower population densities of *P. megistus* than of *T. infestans* (about 500 *P. megistus* in a heavily infected house in Sao Felipe, compared with over 1000 *T. infestans* in a similar house in Mambai). Another difference is that in Brasil *T. infestans* is found in the upper part of the walls and sometimes in the roof, but *P. megistus* inhabits the lower wall segments (De Belder *et al.*, 1978; Marsden, 1980). Schofield (1979) suggests that a difference in ambient temperature between these wall zones could be responsible for this behavior, which has not been observed in laboratory colonies.

Rhodnius prolixus is the main vector of *Trypanosoma cruzi* in Venezuela, Columbia, and in parts of eastern Central America. The highest domestic densities have been recorded with this species which reproduces rapidly. Because *R. prolixus* also inhabits palm trees, the fronds of which are used for roofing, reinfection of the house by adding such material is common (Pifano, 1973). Small instars and eggs can be carried by migratory birds (Gamboa, 1973). Sherlock (1979a) suggests that scattered reports of captures of *R. prolixus* in Brasil as far south as Sao Paulo could be due to bugs excaping from laboratories where they are used for xenodiagnosis; it is more likely that *R. neglectus* has been misidentified.

Bugs enter houses in two ways, either actively by flying or walking or by passive transfer as was mentioned in the case of *R. prolixus* in palm roofing. Although adult bugs can be stimulated to fly in the laboratory, it is not known how often they do so in nature (Lehane and Schofield, 1978). The author has rarely observed the flight of *P. megistus* and *Triatoma infestans* although people living in endemic areas report that bugs fly into houses when it is hot and humid (e.g., before a thunderstorm); flight may be stimulated by starvation as well as by ambient temperature. Of the three species mentioned above only *R. prolixus* can be captured with any frequency in light traps.

Passive transfer in peoples' clothing and baggage is well documented for *T. infestans* (Soler *et al.*, 1969; Prata, 1980) and the upholstery of railway carriages may also be infested (Neghme *et al.*, 1960). Some bugs travel great distances and can survive for months without food. Dias (1979a) cites the example of an acute case of Chagas' disease occurring in a man who had never left his apartment in Rio de Janeiro. The origin of the infection remained obscure until the maid discovered a recently engorged infected *T. infestans* in a sack of rice sent as a gift from an endemic area of Goias.

It is not known how long it takes for a population of bugs to develop to a number that poses a transmission threat once a gravid female bug has gained access to a house. Much is known about the growth of populations in the laboratory (Szumlewiecz, 1976), but this is not the same situation because blood meals are provided on a regular basis and no enemies are present. Thus, although several cycles are possible in the course of a year in the laboratory, it is thought that in houses only one annual cycle occurs in *T. infestans* and *P. megistus,* and two in *R. prolixus* (Sherlock, 1979a). Based on field observations, Schofield (1980a) suggested two cycles may be possible with *T. infestans.* Data from monthly house captures showed that bug populations of adults appear to peak during the rains, the time when people are more restricted to the house.

Bugs in the house wall habitat are exposed to many hazards and have a notable capacity to hide during the day. They prefer dark, rough, dry surfaces and possess several sense organs to detect such conditions (Schofield, 1979). They are frequently covered with dust, making them difficult to detect. In demolition work, bugs will not be found where termites or ants are discovered in the wall cracks. Ants and parasitic hymenoptera cause significant egg mortality. Laboratory colonies have to be protected against ants which can kill even adult bugs; how tiny pharaoh's ants can kill the giant *Dipetalogaster maximus* is not clear to the author. Barrett (1976) has reviewed the insects and spiders which prey on bugs. Insecticide spraying will usually kill their natural enemies which are often more sensitive than the bugs.

Schofield (1980b) has calculated that only a small proportion of bugs reach maturity; a considerable part of this mortality must be due to predators. Chickens and man, and to some extent lizards and mice, depend on sight to locate and kill bugs (Gomez Nunez, 1969). Overcrowding of bugs because of shortages of domestic habitats in suitable houses does not seem to occur. Laboratory experiments with *R. prolixus* suggested that density is not a limiting factor in nature (Rodrigues and Rabinovitch, 1980). Indeed, a fecal aggregating pheromone has been demonstrated that is unfortunately ephemeral and cannot be used to seed traps. In a house where half the wall cracks were eliminated by plastering, *T. infestans* simply doubled up in the other half of the house (Schofield and Marsden, 1982).

Bugs are obligatory blood feeders, but the type of blood appears to be determined by availability rather than by preference. Thus, a wall population of *T. infestans* was observed to feed successively on chickens, pigs, and man as the opportunity arose (Marsden *et al.,* 1979c). Minter (1976b) has reviewed information regarding blood meals identified in various species and concluded that most domestic bugs are adventitious feeders. Certain bug species show a pre-dominant type of blood meal, but this may be a result of opportunity; examples include *T. sordida* and avian meals and rodent meals in *T. rubrofasciata*. Often more than one bug species is present in the same house, but when *T. infestans* is present it is dominant. A good example is cited by Leal Costa (1955); not long ago it was common in the city of Salvador to find *Triatoma rubofasciata* trans-mitting *Trypanosoma conorhini* among rats in the roof of the same house in which *T. cruzi* transmission was being effected by *P. megistus*. An adequate blood meal is necessary for growth and development of each of the five immature stages and for oviposition by the adult females. All stages take many times their own weight in blood, and mean blood meals have been estimated for instars of many species (Fig. 2). The molt from a fifth-stage larva to an adult is particularly dependent on ingestion of a relatively large meal. Adult bugs may live many months, and the life cycle may extend over 2 years from the hatching of the egg to the death of the individual adult. The egg production and longevity of tri-atomine adults has recently been reviewed; *Triatoma infestans* adults live from 8 to 16 months and lay a mean of 240 eggs (Zeledon and Rabinovich, 1981). Bugs that ingest *Trypanosoma cruzi* with their first blood meals as first instar larvae usually remain infected for life. In collections from households the proportion of infected bugs rises with age, and the adult infection rate can be used as a convenient measure of transmission risk in the field (Minter, 1978; Marsden *et al.*, 1982). Females are inseminated shortly after molting, and there is evidence that they can produce viable eggs for 1 year after separation from the males (Szumlewiecz, 1969).

In the household, bugs are usually concentrated in walls near blood meal sites such as the bedroom wall along the bed, or behind nesting chickens. When feeding on sleeping people they are easily disturbed by torchlight or movement

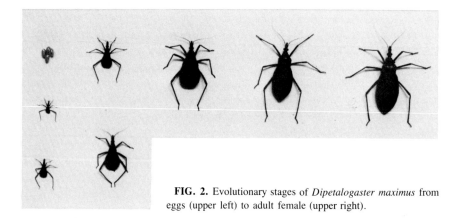

FIG. 2. Evolutionary stages of *Dipetalogaster maximus* from eggs (upper left) to adult female (upper right).

and will withdraw the proboscis and move away from the feeding site. After engorgement they rest in the bed clothes, under the bed frame, or in wall cracks to digest their meal; they will not be ready to feed again for several weeks. Contrary to what is written, the bite can often be felt as a needling sensation, but it is not sufficiently painful to wake a sleeping man. Schofield (1979) suggests that location of a host (prey) is governed by air temperature gradients and influenced by carbon dioxide and other factors. The concept that the concentration of trypanosomes ingested influences the eventual density of infection has little experimental support (Miles *et al.,* 1975), and the type of blood meal (chicken versus mammalian) has no effect on the maintenance of rectal flagellate infections (Miles, 1973).

In Mambai, two cross-sectional surveys for bug distribution and density showed that in spite of combative measures by the householders house infestations by *T. infestans* rose significantly over a period of a few years although densities remained much the same (Marsden *et al.,* 1982). The author has seen isolated hamlets in which living conditions were poor and almost all houses were infested. The success of this species is notable in terms of its cohabitation with man; because of this, it is the target for urgent measures. One-third of the inhabitants of Mambai have positive serology for *T. cruzi;* in areas where *T. infestans* has been present for a relatively short time the rate of seropositivity will be lower (Dias, 1976).

VI. Human Ecology and *Trypanosoma cruzi* Transmission

There still exist many uninhabited areas in the Americas where sylvatic animals and bugs peacefully coexist without human intervention. Mello (1980) has described such a locality in Goias State, Brasil. She noted the ingress of infected *Triatoma infestans* into the area in a recently constructed house. The entry of man may introduce such important vectors; his modification of the environment by cutting down the forest and creating farm land must have a profound effect on sylvatic bug populations when animal hosts flee or are killed (Da Silva *et al.,* 1979). Some bugs such as *T. sordida* adapt to the changed surroundings and come to live in close proximity to man. However, for reasons that are unclear many other species cannot make this adaptation.

There can be no doubt that poor socioeconomic conditions are associated with bug infestation of houses and the presence of Chagas' disease. The modern city of Brasilia was constructed in the center of one of the most highly endemic areas in the world, but concrete apartment blocks have replaced the earlier mud and straw huts. However, active transmission occurs in some localities only a few hours' journey away. Access to such localities is usually made difficult by roads that become impassable in the rains, and they are backward in terms of education and economic development.

Illiterate subsistence farmers frequently move from one area to another. In Mambai (Marsden *et al.*, 1982) more than 50% of the population moved to another region in 29% of the farming communities present in the rural area. With small family economies, houses are sometimes built within a week or two using locally available materials such as mud, stick, straw, and palm. That such houses are suitable for bugs and show higher infestation rates than more permanent dwellings has been known for a long time (Miranda, 1952; Lucena, 1962); in fact, such houses are known by a variety of names in Brasil. A higher seropositivity rate for *Trypanosoma cruzi* can be shown in children dwelling in such houses (Mott *et al.*, 1978).

The construction of such houses, in terms of the technique and materials used, varies greatly from place to place. In a cold Andean climate the house has to be more substantial (Schenone *et al.*, 1978) and stone walls often mean that the bugs are principally in the roof. In tropical Brasil a common house construction method is as follows. A framework for the roof and walls is erected of wooden uprights cut from the surrounding brush, and a latticework of split canes or bamboo is woven between the uprights to form the walls. To these are applied a moist mud, sand, and lime adobe mix which is forced between the lattice and smoothed with the hand. The formulation of this adobe is important, because cracking is delayed or prevented with certain mixes. The incorporation of cow-dung, if available, helps by acting as a binding agent. Other binding agents used have been as diverse as horse or human hair, straw, whale oil, and molasses. Between the tie beams of the roof, wooden poles support either Portuguese tiles or split palm fronds. Many houses, while showing one dominant type of con-struction, may be mixtures of various types of materials. Also later additions may be of different construction (Figs. 3 and 4).

One cannot help admiring the speed and skill with which rural Brasilians provide houses for their families. Single handed, they build cool, pleasant homes in a matter of weeks. If a little capital is available better materials can be used, such as mud bricks for the walls and oven-fired (rather than sun-dried) tiles for the roof. A coat of plaster applied later over the bricks and whitewash provides a wall that may last for many years. In fact, many historic buildings surviving from imperial times in towns in Brasil were constructed in the same manner. (Similar wattle-and-daub houses were used in England for centuries).

The design of most houses in rural Brasil, while having infinite minor varia-tions, is basically the same. By the front door you enter a living room provided with benches on which the family and visitors sit. Frequently, a small religious shrine is present and a few photographs from magazines are tacked to the wall (a

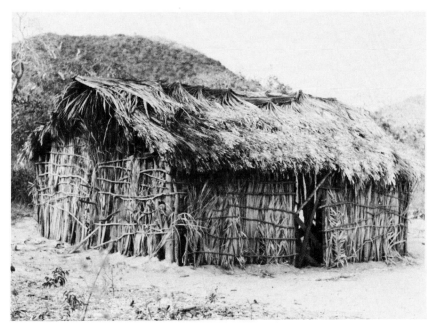

FIG. 3. At demolition, 1103 *Triatoma infestans*, 81% of which were in the roof, were captured in this house which is constructed entirely of palm.

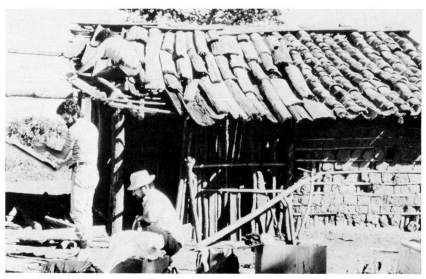

FIG. 4. Illustrating a house composed of several materials. The left side of the roof is tree bark and the right side Portuguese tiles; the left side of wall is upright wooden piles and the right side adobe and bamboo.

common site behind which to find bugs). Behind this reception room there is a varying number of bedrooms which are linked by a corridor leading from the front room to the kitchen at the back. Bugs are rare in the kitchen which has walls smoke blackened from the constantly burning wood stove.

The most frequent sites to encounter bugs are the bedrooms, especially in those walls adjacent to beds, because it is in these beds that their blood meal sources will repose. Apart from the beds there is little furniture in the bedrooms, merely a few hooks to hang clothes and an occasional shelf. Shelves are not common, probably because the wall constructions would not support the weight. Clothes are frequently kept in boxes under the bed; the habit of keeping one's personal belongings under the bed is common even among quite wealthy Brasilians, and money is frequently found under the pillow when examining beds for bugs. If windows exist in the bedrooms, they are usually kept shut to guard valuables and the low light intensities in such rooms must favor bug activity (Latham et al., 1980). Hammocks offer less chance of bug contact, but in Ceara State, where hammocks are used, Triatoma brasiliensis has been found to congregate in the wall near the points of attachment (Sherlock, 1981).

The progression of newly constructed houses to their eventual decay should be accurately documented. The combination of fierce tropical sun and torrential rain has a rapid effect, and the mud walls quickly develop hairline cracks which widen to form ideal hiding places for the bugs. Rain dropping from the eaves forms little streams running parallel to the wall which eventually expose and undermine the uprights. When walls start to lean outward they are often propped up by stout timbers to last for another season. In old houses of fragile construction the presence of the family ensures maintenance; as was recently shown in Sao Felipe, when the family moves out deterioration is rapid; rain begins to come through the roof and the walls start to fall down. Often a house will have a series of owners and the last may be an old relative or single person looking for any sort of roof who is content to inhabit a deteriorating structure. In one instance well known to the author, the family head moved into a small, new, well-constructed house nearby, leaving his numerous children and wife in a bug-ridden, decaying structure. Because of a shortage of land a new house is frequently built near the old one. Adequate drainage and wind direction are important considerations in the siting of the kitchen, and a house constructed upwind might have less chance of receiving flying insects from the old house. People move because of deterioration in the old house structure, rarely because of the bug nuisance (Marsden et al., 1982). Frequently, bugs are introduced from the old house via the furniture and bedding; timbers, doors, and windows also are removed and incorporated into the new house. This is the time to use the insecticide spray that the householders sometimes buy. In Sao Felipe, Bahia, where we had an opportunity to demolish two houses of one family $2\frac{1}{2}$ years apart, we retrieved over 500 P. megistus on each demolition (Minter, 1978).

It is best to burn the old house to destroy the bugs, but this is rarely done. If the house is simply abandoned, the bugs will eventually leave as blood meal sources become insufficient. Adult bugs may fly out; houses demolished months after vacating have few adults. Bugs can also walk many meters (Gilks *et al.*, 1977). In some areas the vacated house is used for chickens, encouraging an increase in the population of vectors that poses a threat to the new household.

In endemic areas, it is impressive to see what little importance the residents of infested houses usually ascribe to these dangerous vectors. They will kill them when they can, but triatomids are a nuisance like bedbugs or cockroaches. Occasionally, people complain after benzene hexachloride (BHC) spraying that the bedbugs have become more of a nuisance than the reduviid bugs. Sometimes during surveys the family will assist the bug catcher with jokes and laughter, catching bugs with their bare hands.

This attitude is difficult to understand unless it is realized that these people have no concept of Chagas' disease and many remain skeptical of what they are told even after discussion. Chagas himself was informed by the local people of the bug nuisance in Lassance, not about the existence of Chagas' disease (Chagas Filho, 1979). The effects are so subtle and long-term that it is not surprising that people do not understand the facts, but a knowledge and awareness of the significance of the bugs is important to encourage collaboration in control programs. In a recent inquiry in Mambai (Bizerra *et al.*, 1981), it was found by the research group after 7 years work in the area that the majority of people had heard of Chagas' disease and many knew that it attacked the heart, but opinions about the way the bug transmitted the disease and how it could be controlled were still primitive.

The remoteness of endemic areas is directly linked to this problem since more services become available when a road is passable throughout the year. Piped water and electricity come to town, and school teachers are contracted by the local administration. If they are very lucky they might even be able to attract a doctor; of course, not to live but to at least hold several clinics a week. These changes, which are occurring all over rural Brasil, affect the level of information about Chagas' disease in the local community. Diffusion of information, from the small town where these services are available to the surrounding rural area where *T. cruzi* transmission is more prevalent, is slow but sure. As such economic development often occurs at the same time as insecticide spraying, it is difficult to assess the relative effect of the two measures on controlling Chagas' disease (Prata, 1980).

Certainly many householders, when they are alerted to the dangers of domestic transmission, take steps to control the problem at home (see Section VII.). However, there are always people who for various reasons are irresponsible and do nothing, and their infested houses act as foci of bug dissemination to the community. Studying maps of bug distribution in houses for 4 years, it is noticeable that in a row of houses some will always escape infestation while others remain permanently infested, although all the houses are of the same basic construction. The author believes that the activity of the residents in killing bugs is responsible in part for this difference. Occasionally, one can see in field work an example of the importance of this human activity; two examples are cited from São Felipe, Bahia: (a) A family of three, all with positive xenodiagnosis, lived in a heavily infested house. The wife was totally blind with cataracts and although she could cook and clean by touch she could not kill bugs until removal of her cataracts improved the situation. (b) A partially paralyzed girl with a lack of coordination because of cerebral atrophy and positive xenodiagnosis spent her time lying on a pallet by a wall, and in the wall was an exceptionally large colony of well-fed *P. megistus.*

Population movements are important at both the national and the local level. People coming from endemic areas and settling in favelas on the periphery of large cities may bring *Trypanosoma cruzi* in their blood and *Triatoma infestans* in their baggage (Barretto, 1967; Dias and Dias, 1979). A progressive urbanization by people in search of work is a feature of South American societies today (Da Silva *et al.,* 1979).

The habit of receiving visitors also has sinister implications in a Chagas' area. In Sao Felipe our attention was drawn to this by the case of acute Chagas' disease in a 9-year-old girl who was sharing a bed with a 14-year-old visitor with a marked megaesophagus and a positive xenodiagnosis. In this area families with few resources frequently receive visitors (Miles, 1976). In Mambai there is a positive correlation between the frequency of visitors and bug presence (Marsden *et al.,* 1982). Reduviidism without *T. cruzi* infection occurs frequently in households, but only one infected visitor can initiate a domestic transmission cycle.

VII. Control of Domestic Transmission

Since bug vectors important in the domestic environment are present over such a wide area of the Americas, the control of Chagas' disease is a concern to the Ministries of Health of the afflicted countries. Although every country in South America regards Chagas' disease as an important endemic problem, national control programs have been most extensive in Brasil, Argentina, and Venezuela where the number of people infected is in the millions. A recent nationwide serological survey in Brasil demonstrated that in some states over 20% of people examined had positive serology, and it was estimated that approximately 6 million people are infected (Camargo, 1979).

The first coordinated national program in Brasil was initiated in 1950 (Pinotti,

1954). The infrastructure of the national malaria service was utilized and by December, 1952 over 200,000 houses had been sprayed, following field trials of the value of Gammexane (benzene hexachloride, BHC, or hexachlorocyclohexane, HCH) in killing domestic bugs (Dias, 1945; Dias and Pellegrino, 1948; Romana and Abalos, 1948). Dias and Dias (1979) and Prata (1980) have described the various phases of the Brasilian control program, which began well but eventually was hampered by lack of funds.

Nevertheless, great strides have been made in the control of Chagas' disease in Brasil, and in many areas particularly in the south the occurrence of triatomids in houses has decreased. The State of São Paulo mounted its own control program in 1965; because it is wealthy, it has been possible to control active transmission to man (Rocha e Silva *et al.*, 1979b). At the same time, housing and asphalting of roads progressed rapidly, which also have had an effect on domestic bug infestations in this state. Spray campaigns in designated areas have three phases which are defined in ministerial procedures (Ministerio de Saude, 1980).

The first phase is preparatory; after financial support is secured, personnel are recruited and transportation arranged; the area is mapped and each house located and examined for bugs. At the same time community leaders are contacted about the objectives of the program, and householders are informed about the attack phase.

The second, or attack, phase is carefully programmed by calculating the number of houses that can be sprayed daily in a given locale. For houses within a reasonable distance a team of two spray applicators, a driver and a supervisor, will spray 16 houses in a day, treating all communities where domestic bugs have been detected. In this so-called massive attack phase, all houses and outhouses in these communities whether infected or not are sprayed with a water-miscible suspension of BHC containing at least 30% gamma isomer. Using a Hudson backpack sprayer, delivery is calculated at not less than 500 mg of gammexane/m^2. On the day of the spraying, all movable furniture is put in the yard and wall hangings (clothes, pictures, umbrellas, etc.) are removed. Small plastic bags contain a weighted quantity of BHC which on dilution with water in the buckets provided gives the correct concentration of insecticide. The backpack spray apparatus is charged with this mixture and the insecticide applied evenly over all internal and external walls of the house and the inside of the roof, the quantity of insecticide used depending on the size of the house. All outhouses and furniture are treated in the same manner. The specifications of the spray apparatus are critical, especially that of the nozzle which must deliver a uniform spray (Paulini and Fromm, 1962).

Unless one has actively participated in a spraying program, it is difficult to imagine the amount of work involved. Homes frequently have to be visited on foot since there is no vehicle access, and the spray team often must sleep in one of the houses visited. Water may be at a distance and the utilization of a tin hat to scoop water into the bucket explained to the author why the SUCAM (Superintendencia da Campanha Contra Malaria) spray teams of Brasil use a headgear more appropriate to World War II. Morale must be high; the campaign is conducted like a military operation with a chain of command from the field team to the regional center of the Ministry of Health. Frequent visits are made to the field site by supervisors, and it is often necessary to rotate personnel in the field to achieve optimum results.

After the spraying, the householder is informed of the nature of residual insecticide activity and warned not to wash or paint the walls; the unpleasant smell of BHC will diminish in 24 hr. This insecticide is relatively safe, and serious toxic effects are rare. However, because chickens and cats may die of insecticide ingestion it is best to keep them out of the house for a few days.

The overall cost of spraying a house in Mambai, Goias in 1980 (expenditures including documents, apparatus, insecticide, gasoline, etc.) was approximately US $5. Over 80% of this sum was spent on salary supplements for the spray personnel; basic salaries are fixed at a national level, but a daily field allowance which is several times the basic salary is an inducement to field workers. Sherlock (1979b) has reported similar costs for various insecticides. As this represents only one spray application in a program requiring multiple applications and does not allow for either the costs of the preparatory and followup phases or administrative costs, it is evident that spray control programs are expensive.

BHC causes an impressive initial mortality and the householder may collect hundreds of dead bugs after a spray application. However, contact with the insecticide is necessary for killing, and although BHC can kill for up to 60 days after application, wall penetration may be poor (Szumlewiecz, 1953). Recently fed bugs resting deep in wall cracks may escape the insecticide effect, and fertile eggs thus situated will also escape (Dias, 1965). From studies based on dismantling infested experimental huts after BHC spraying, a 90% kill of all stages of bugs can be expected in the hot season (Szumlewiecz, 1954).

The duration of effective activity of BHC on the wall will depend on climate, wall particle size, and the nature of the wall surface (Romeiro e Aguilar, 1954; Fomm and Gandini, 1971). Usually, rapid killing can be demonstrated in those bugs coming into direct contact with the sprayed surface for 2 to 3 months. Several different recommendations have been made regarding the frequency of spraying; the two most common are repeat sprayings at 3 or 6 months (Dias *et al.*, 1952). This repeat spraying is usually selective in that only houses in which evidence of bug infestation was found are resprayed, with the objective of killing the residual population that has resisted the initial application (Pedreira de Freitas, 1963).

After the attack phase, there is a third phase of vigilance or follow-up. In routine spraying operations, as De Brito (1968) points out, it is this phase that is

often incomplete. However, there are many experimental programs in the literature in which such follow-up has been carried out over a period of years. These
show a marked reduction in bugs in houses assessed either by manual capture
(Dias *et al.*, 1952; Pedreira de Freitas, 1968) or by house demolition (Pellegrino
and Brener, 1951; Bustamante and Gusmao, 1954). The time required for spraying depends on the number of houses with persistent infestations. The Brasilian
Ministry recommends that when house infestations have dropped below 5% the
area should enter the vigilance phase. Field trials have suggested that two insecticide applications properly spaced could eradicate *Triatoma infestans* from the
domestic environment. *Panstrongylus megistus* is a more difficult problem; two
applications a year for several years reduced *P. megistus* infestations in houses in
Sao Felipe from 32 to 5% (Sherlock and Muniz, 1974). Two widely spaced
applications of BHC (several years apart) reduced the prevalence of domestic *T.
infestans* in houses but reinfestation increased as the study progressed (Fomm *et
al.*, 1971).

BHC has been given particular attention because it is the insecticide used in
the national campaign in Brasil and Argentina. It had also been used with success
in Peru, Chile, and other countries. In Venezuela, Dieldrin (hexachlorodimeth-
anolnaphthalene) is used against *Rhodnius prolixus*. BHC proved to be better
than Dieldrin for *T. infestans* in one field trial (Bustamante *et al.*, 1957); BHC is
cheap and of lower toxicity, and has higher initial and delayed activity against
this species.

Many new insecticides have reached the stage of field trials; their relative
merits have been reviewed by Rocha and Silva (1979), Sherlock (1979), Marconi
et al. (1980), and Tonn (1980). Other than the organochlorine compounds
(DDT, BHC, Dieldrin), organophosphorus compounds have been widely tested,
and in Argentina malathion has been used as an alternative to BHC (Martinez *et
al.*, 1975; Cichero, 1978). In general, organophosphorus derivatives, because
they are less stable and more toxic than organochlorines, have not replaced them.
Carbamates (Baygon, Bendiocarb) and pyrethroids (Decamethrin, Permethrin)
are expensive but have a long residual activity. In a recent field trial of a single
application of decamethrin, 0.1 g/m^2 controlled *T. infestans* for 9 months
(Pinchin *et al.*, 1980). Although BHC is still the insecticide used in most national
programs, some experts feel that the larger scale use of organochlorine compounds is diminishing in favor of some of the alternatives mentioned here (Marconi *et al.*, 1980).

In 1971, the so-called third generation insecticides (juvenile hormone analogs)
seemed a bright prospect (Marsden, 1971). Although their early promise has not
been fulfilled, they could be useful in houses where residual infections persist
because of their long residual activity (Gilbert, 1976). An interesting approach
with both these compounds and certain insecticides is their incorporation within a
plastic matrix [*e.g.*, poly(vinyl chloride)] which permits their slow release over

many months. Field trials of such insecticide formulations show that further technical development is necessary (Pinchin *et al.*, 1978a; 1978b). Precocene antihormones have been shown to induce aldultoids of *R. prolixus* even at the first stage (Tarrant and Cupp, 1978).

Although Triatominae have many natural enemies it has not proved possible to use any of these as a method of control (Barrett, 1976). Small wasps (*e.g.*, *Telenomus* spp.) parasitizing eggs, have been most often studied. In many areas of Brasil a significant percentage of eggs can be found with the neat hole formed by the exit of the newly emerged adult wasp. *Telenomus* is therefore present in balance in the ecosystem, and this balance will be only temporarily disturbed by manipulation of the population. In one house in Mambai many examples of the reduviid *Cosmoclopius* were found in a demolished house (Marsden *et al.*, 1979). Since then we have frequently found this predatory reduviid in vegetation but never again in such numbers in a house. We need to know much more about such predators before their value can be assessed. Another possibility for biological control is pathogenic fungi which have been observed to kill bugs in some laboratory colonies; results have been inconsistent. Sterile male release also has not been successful. The latest suggestion is the nematode *Neoaplectana carpocapsae* that can be sprayed on the walls; it invades the bug hemocoele with lethal results (Minter and Oswald, 1980). This is still being developed and has not been field tested.

It is in the vigilance phase that the participation of the householder is most important. In the preparatory and the attack phases he also has his role; permitting his house to be examined, his belongings to be put in the yard for spraying, and his domestic life to be disturbed with the smell of insecticide and other inconveniences. If, however, he does not get the message that it is his vigilance that will summon the spray team again, then all is lost for, however well organized the vigilance team, they will take time to reach his house and it will cost money. If he shows no interest, the door may be shut against them.

In Mambai, Goias, we were dismayed to find that the people had no idea what vigilance entailed (Bizerra *et al.*, 1981). Accordingly, we visited each house where evidence of bugs had been found. A notice about the dangers of Chagas' disease was read to the family members and another affixed to the wall indicating that any bug found should be sent to a central collecting point. A selfsealing plastic bag with the owner's name and address was provided for this purpose. One method of assessing the success of this spraying program uses two cardboard boxes designed by Gomez Nunez (1965) affixed to the wall over the main beds. These boxes act as part of the wall and are colonized by bugs through the open areas of the box adjacent to the wall; several studies have shown that these are a more sensitive way of assessing light infestations than manual capture (Schofield, 1978). The box, which is filled with folded paper, is taken from the wall by extracting nails from two side panels. These fold over the holes by which the bugs gained entry, and the box is sealed to be examined in the laboratory for bugs, cast skins, eggs, or feces.

The principal objective of the Mambai program is to assess the effectiveness of two spaced BHC applications in controlling transmission by *T. infestans*. However, it will be interesting to see how the Gomez Nunez trap, manual capture, and householder notification compare in identifying residual infestations. Once the presence of bugs is confirmed, the house will be resprayed. After 5 years, a serological survey of children under 5 years old will assess the efficacy of control; this will be repeated at 5-year intervals examining children under 10 and under 15 years successively. Studies at Bambui, Minas Gerais State, where insecticide has been used since 1948, showed that serological conversion of uninfected individuals decreased with time (Dias, 1979b). It is at that point when residual infection is confirmed that a house improvement scheme, which could take the form of wall plastering, would appear most valuable.

Community participation in the vigilance phase and replastering have been described in the literature. Dias and Garcia (1978) have described a health education program in Bambui in which local administrators assisted the people with notification of domestic infestations of bugs after a spraying program. Well-intentioned and successful as the program proved to be, it is somewhat artificial because the area under study had far more resources in terms of motivated personnel and contacts with public health authorities than is normally the case. The very remoteness of many endemic foci makes such programs difficult to maintain. The best plan is to utilize a community leader as was done for malaria surveillance in Brasil. The Ministry regulations for the Chagas' control program in Brasil envisage establishing information posts in all affected localities with more than 25 houses that have reached the vigilance phase. The local person responsible for vigilance would be equipped with forceps to send bugs (in pill boxes) to a central collecting point. There are always examples of noncollaboration; for example, house spraying may not be permitted because a woman is pregnant or the tenants cannot stand the inconvenience. Only careful propaganda beforehand can minimize such refusals.

Studies in Mambai suggest that the majority of householders were disposed to measures that would combat bugs; they buy insecticides for domestic application and have shown a marked increase in wall plastering over a 4-year period. In the year in which the ministry spraying program commenced, two local private spraying enterprises were operative in the area (information about insecticides used and charges has been difficult to obtain). Although this activity was on a small scale it does indicate a response. Also the data from two cross-sectional surveys made 4 years apart (1975–1979) before spraying started in 1980 show that although the number of houses infested had risen significantly (from 52 to

74%), bug densities in individual houses remained low suggesting the individual families were combating the problem on a domestic basis (Marsden *et al.*, 1982).

The importance of house improvement as an accessory measure in Chagas' disease control campaigns was recognized many years ago (Di Primio, 1952; Gamboa and Bauer, 1954). Gamboa (1968) reported a successful program in Venezuela in which roofing materials of corrugated iron and asbestos replaced the traditional palm known to be infested with *R. prolixus*. In afflicted areas in that same country the economy has permitted the construction of 120,000 new houses in 20 years but 500,000 more are still needed (Torrealba and Feliciangeli, 1979). A small program of new house construction in Sao Felipe, Bahia, showed that although a few houses were invaded by adults, colonization had not occurred after 2 years (Macedo, 1981). These houses, costing approximately US $1000 each, were constructed of earth and cement blocks. Beds were initially designed as concrete wall ledges, but this was unacceptable to householders who preferred the space beneath wooden beds to store belongings. Certainly, the construction of such houses is a permanent benefit for the individual family but hardly practical in the present economic climate.

Improvement of existing houses is a more practical solution (Schmidt, 1969). De Brito (1968) describes a program in Brasil in which it was determined that a mixture of three parts of sandy soil to two parts of cowdung provides a plaster with lasting qualities. This was applied by hand or machine to 6335 houses in the State of Minas Gerais during a 3-year period (1958–1961), often by the householders themselves. In 1959, it was calculated that in this state alone 463,169 houses were in need of such plastering. Plastering on such a scale is an immense undertaking but this technique is probably the most viable of the house improvement schemes. In Mambai it was readily adopted by the people as a preventive measure although all qualities of plastering existed, and as Latham *et al.* (1980) pointed out, bad plastering is useless as a bug deterrent. The author has the impression that plastering also raises the general domestic level of hygiene; if people plaster the bedrooms they usually also plaster the living room and whitewash the walls. Flowers appear on the table and a degree of house pride is noted. However, even a good plastering job often neglects to close the cracks near the uprights at the top of the wall where bugs can escape into the roof. Although plastering alone will diminish but not permanently eliminate the transmission risk, it has definite value as an adjunct to a control program (Schofield and Marsden, 1982).

Di Primio (1958) has investigated the qualities of mud bricks with additives of lime and cement for the construction of new houses. The appearance of brick- and tile-making near rivers in endemic areas such as has occurred in Mambai augurs well for the future. Yet mud-brick houses, if poorly constructed without plaster, frequently harbor bugs in the cracks between the bricks. The basic need for plaster remains, and there is still a need for research into simple ways of building rural homes which discourage bug colonization (De Raadt, 1976).

Perhaps two kinds of rural houses should be considered in this regard, that of the family intending to stay and that of the transient. The latter group is very large in Brasil (Da Silva *et al.*, 1979), and includes people who clear and plant the land for a time and then move on. If the head of the household has no intention of staying, his interest in house improvement will be limited and will pose a different problem. The transient immigrating to the favela on the borders of a large city is yet another situation. Only by discovering why people are living as they are and permitting bug colonization can reasonable solutions be found. In a study of housing development among rural Indians in Ecuador, it was shown that modern houses were inferior to traditional dwellings in terms of ambient temperature control and floor space. Housing-related health education should be adapted to the environment and the culture of the local people (Kroeger, 1980).

VIII.   A Concluding Perspective

It is evident that much research on the control of Chagas' disease was done in the late 1940s and 1950s in South American countries. Since then national programs against Chagas' disease have faltered in most countries because the areas affected have low priorities in terms of economic development, and money is in short supply.

The nature of the control program will vary with the area under consideration. Epidemiological differences in human transmission demonstrate that basic research assists in the design of control measures. For example, the palm roof replacements in Venezuela against *Rhodnius prolixus* and the spaced BHC spraying against *Triatoma infestans* were based on knowledge of the life cycles.

Certain points in the routine control program still need to be clarified. Is it necessary to spray all houses and outhouses in a locality where domestic infestations have been found or can control of transmission be achieved by an initially selective spraying? (Reis *et al.*, 1969). Is it not possible to transfer more of the activities of the vigilance phase to the householder with the objective of saving funds? What are the most acceptable modifications to existing permanent houses in different countries that will prevent bug colonization? For different vector species different designs of the control program are needed. Relatively few research workers address these important problems. At the International Congress in Rio de Janeiro in 1979 there were more papers given in immunology (78) than in epidemiology, control, vectors, and new insecticides combined (Coura, 1979).

As a result of control measures other problems will arise. The development by *R. prolixus* of resistance to Dieldrin (Tonn, 1980) is a warning that such resistance could occur in other species and on a wider scale. However, the rapid life cycle of *Rhodnius* species suggests that genetically determined resistance would appear more rapidly than in such species as *Triatoma infestans* or *Panstrongylus megistus* (W.H.O., 1975). The important observation of the Sao Paulo group (Rocha e Silva, 1979) that other species may invade the house after eradication of *T. infestans,* which has virtually lost its capacity for colonization of sylvatic biotopes, illustrates that the threat of reinvasion of houses by another species from in the surrounding vegetation must never be ignored. Because it is still the most important domestic vector, it is obviously the primary target for attack. Yet as Romana (1963) pointed out, the spraying program will fail without community participation. A higher priority must be assigned to Chagas' disease control by public health organizations in afflicted countries (Prata, 1980).

Despite much research, specific chemotherapy remains problematic, and prophylaxis by vaccination seems remote. A significant proportion of today's positive seroreactive patients will burden hospital services in the future with persistent cardiac failure, arrhythmias requiring pacemakers, and corrective surgical procedures for megasyndromes. The control of the transmission of Chagas' disease is a most urgent practical measure for it will result in long-term economic benefits in the developing countries of South America.

Acknowledgment

The author would like to acknowledge the help of Professor Aluizio Prata. Ever since he insisted in 1963 that Chagas' disease was a problem worth investigating, he has been an unfailing source of encouragement and wisdom in the tradition of great *tropicalistas.* The author's studies have received financial support from the London School of Hygiene and Tropical Medicine Special Fund, the Wellcome Trust, and The Conselho Nacional de Pesquisas do Brasil (CNPq).

References

Alvarenga, N. J., and Marsden, P. D. (1975). Estudos sobre persistência de infectividade do *Trypanosoma cruzi.* I. Efeito da temperatura sobre a infectividade de flagelados de amostra Peru de *T. cruzi* obtidos de fezes de triatomíneos. *Rev. Soc. Bras. Med. Trop.* **9,** 283–287.
Amato Neto, V., Rojas, J. R. T., Camargo, M. E., and Silva, L. J. (1977). Estudo baseado na pesquisa de anticorpos IgM antitripanossoma no soro, destinado a avaliar a transmissão con-

(1979c). Studies of the domestic ecology of *Triatoma infestans* by means of house demolition. *Rev. Inst. Med. Trop. São Paulo 21,* 13–25.

Marsden, P. D. (1980). Ecologia domiciliar dos principais vetores no Brasil. *J. Bras. Med.* **38,** 17–22.

Marsden, P. D., Virgens, D., Magalhaes, I., Tavares-Neto, J., Ferreira, R., Costa, C. H. N., Castro, C. N., Macedo, V., and Prata, A. R. (1982). Ecologia doméstica do *Triatoma infestans* em Mambai, Goiá, Brasil. *Rev. Inst. Med. Trop. São Paulo* **24,** 364–373.

Martinez, A., Cichero, J. A., Alania, I. R., and Gonzalez, F. F. (1975). Control of *Triatoma infestans* (Klug) with Malathion concentrate. *J. Med. Entomol.* **11,** 653–657.

Martins, A. V. (1968). "Epidemiologia in Doença de Chagas" (R. J. Cançado, ed.), pp. 225–237. Imprensa Oficial do Estado de Minas Gerais, Belo Horizonte.

Maudlin, I. (1976). Inheritance of susceptibility to *Trypanosoma cruzi* infection in *Rhodnius prolixus. Nature (London)* **262,** 214–215.

Mazza, S., Montana, A., Benitez, C., and Janzi, E. Z. (1936). Transmission del *Schizotrypanum cruzi* al nino por leche de la madre con enfermedad de Chagas. *MEPRA* **28,** 41–46.

Mello, D. A. (1980). Aspectos ecológicos do ciclo silvestre do *Trypanosoma cruzi* em região de cerrado (Municipio de Formosa, Estado de Goiás). Thesis, Univ. São Paulo.

Mello, D. A., and Borges, M. M. (1981). Neonatal transmission of *Trypanosoma cruzi* in *Calomys callosus* (Rodentia). *Trans. R. Soc. Trop. Med. Hyg.* **75,** 754–755.

Miles, M. A. (1972). *Trypanosoma cruzi:* milk transmission of infection and immunity from mother to young. *Parasitol.* **68,** 1–9.

Miles, M. A. (1973). *Personal communication.*

Miles, M. A. (1975). Distribution and importance of Triatominae as vectors of *Trypanosoma cruzi. In* "American Trypanosomiasis Research," p. 48–56. *P.A.H.O. Sci. Publ.* **318,** Washington.

Miles, M. A., Patterson, J. W., Marsden, P. D., and Minter, D. M. (1975). A comparison of *Rhodnius prolixus, Triatoma infestans* and *Panstrongylus megistus* in the xenodiagnosis of a chronic *Trypanosoma cruzi* infection in a rhesus monkey (*Macaca mulatta*). *Trans. R. Soc. Trop. Med. Hyg.* **69,** 377–382.

Miles, M. A. (1976). Human behavior and the propagation of Chagas' disease. *Trans. R. Soc. Trop. Med. Hyg.* **70,** 521–522.

Miles, M. A., Souza, A., Povoa, M., Shaw, J. J., Lainson, R., and Toye, P. J. (1978). Isozymic heterogenicity of *Trypanosoma cruzi* in the first autochthonous patients with Chagas' disease in Amazonian Brazil. *Nature (London)* **272,** 819–821.

Miles, M. A. (1979). Transmission cycles and the heterogenicity of *Trypanosoma cruzi. In* "Biology of the Kinetoplastidae" Vol. 2, (W. H. R. Lumsden, and D. A. Evans, eds.). pp. 117–196. Academic Press, London.

Ministério da Saúde (1980). "Manual de Normal técnicas da Campanha de Controle da Doença de Chagas." Centro de Documentação do Ministério da Saúde, Brasilia.

Minter, D. M., Minter, G. E., Marsden, P. D., Miles, M. A., and Macedo, V. (1973). Domestic risk factor—an attempt to assess the risk of infection with *Trypanosoma cruzi* in houses in Brazil. *Trans. R. Soc. Trop. Med. Hyg.* **67,** 290.

Minter, D. M. (1976a). Effects of transmission to man of the presence of domestic animals in infested houses. *In* "American Trypanosomiasis Research," pp. 330–337. *P.A.H.O. Sci. Publ.* **318,** Washington.

Minter, D. M. (1976b). Feeding patterns of some triatomine vectors. *In* "American Trypanosomiasis Research," pp. 33–46. *P.A.H.O. Sci. Publ.* **318,** Washington.

Minter, D. M. (1978). Triatomine bugs and the household ecology of Chagas' disease. *In* "Medical Entomology Centenary Symposium, Proceedings," pp. 85–93. Royal Society of Tropical Medicine and Hygiene, London.

Minter, D. M., and Oswald, W. J. C. (1980). The nematode *Neoaplectana* in the biological control of some trypanosomatid vectors. *Trans. R. Soc. Trop. Med. Hyg.* **74**, 679–680.

Miranda, J. (1952). Medidas estatísticas da preferência do *Triatoma infestans* pelo tipo de habitações no Municipio de Garça, Estado de S. Paulo. *Arq. Fac. Hig. Saude Publica Univ. São Paulo* **17**, 57–59.

Mott, K. E., Muniz, T. M., Lehman, J. S., Hoff, R., Morrow, R. H., Oliveira, T. S., Sherlock, I., and Draper, C. C. (1978). House construction, triatomine distribution and household distribution of seroreactivity to *Trypanosoma cruzi* in a rural community in North East Brazil. *Am. J. Trop. Med. Hyg.* **27**, 1116–1122.

Neal, R. A., and McHardy, N. (1977). Comparison of infectivity of *Trypanosoma cruzi* blood stream trypomastigotes and metacyclic trypomastigotes from *Rhodnius prolixus. Acta Trop.* **34**, 79–85.

Neghme, A., Schenone, H., Reyes, H., Carrasco, J., and Alfaro, E. (1960). Hallazgo de *Triatoma infestans* en vagones de ferrocarril. *Bol. Chil. Parasitol.* **15**, 86–87.

Nussenwieg, V., Biancalana, A., Amato Neto, V., Sonntag, R., Frietas, J. L. P., and Kloetzel, J. (1953). Ação da violeta genciana sobre o *T. cruzi* in vitro: sua importância na esterilização do sangue destinado a transfusão. *Rev. Paul. Med.* **42**, 57–58.

Omerod, W. E. (1970). Pathogenesis and pathology of trypanosomiasis in man. In "The African Trypanosomiases" (H. W. Mulligam, ed.), pp. 587–601. Allen & Unwin, London.

Paulini, E., and Fomm, A. S. (1962). Estudos relativos a fatores ligados ao inseticida e a sua aplicação que influem sobre a eficácia da desinsetização domiciliária. IV. Observações sobre o comportamento de alguns produtos inseticidas no preparo de suspensão e durante a aspersão. *Rev. Bras. Malariol. Doenças Trop.* **14**, 21–28.

Pedreira de Freitas, J. L. (1963). Importância do expurgo seletivo dos domicilios e anexos para a profilaxia da moléstia de Chagas pelo combate aos triatomíneos. *Arq. Hig. Saúde Pública Univ. São Paulo* **26**, 217–272.

Pedreira de Freitas, J. L. (1968). Profilaxia em Doença de Chagas. *In* "Doenca de Chagas" (J. R. Cançado, ed.), pp. 541–559. Imprensa Oficial do Estado de Minas Gerais, Belo Horizonte.

Pellegrino, J., and Brener, Z. (1951). Profilaxia de um foco de Doença de Chagas nas proximidades de Belo Horizonte (Cidade Industrial). *Rev. Assoc. Med. Minas Gerais* **2**, 233–250.

Pessoa, S. B. (1962). Domiciliação dos triatomíneos e epidemiologia da Doença de Chagas. *Arq. Fac. Hig. Saúde Pública Univ. São Paulo* **27**, 161–171.

Pifano, F. (1973). La dinamica epidemiológica de la enfermedad de Chagas en el Valle de los Naranjos, Estado Carabubo, Venezuela. I. Contribución al estudio de los focos naturales silvestres del *Schisotrypanum cruzi* Chagas 1909. *Arch. Venez. Med. Trop. Parasitol. Med.* **5**, 3–29.

Pinchin, R., Oliveira Filho, A. M., Muller, C. A., Figueiredo, M. J., Szumlewicz, A. P., and Gilbert, B. (1978a). Slow release insecticides for triatomine control: activity and persistence. *Rev. Bras. Malariol. Doenças Trop.* **30**, 45–55.

Pinchin, R., Oliveira Filho, A. M., Ayala, C. A. C., and Gilbert, B. (1978b). Slow release insecticides for triatomine control; preliminary field trials. *Rev. Bras. Malariol. Doenças Trop.* **30**, 57–63.

Pinchin, R., Oliveira Filho, A. M., Fanara, D. M., and Gilbert, B. (1980). Ensaio de campo para avaliação das possibilidades de uso da decametrina (OMS 1998) no combate a triatomíneos. *Rev. Bras. Malariol. Doenças Trop.* **32**, 36–41.

Pinotti, M. (1954). Controle da Doença de Chagas no Brasil. *Rev. Bras. Malariol. Doenças Trop.* **6**, 301–310.

Pipkin, A. C. (1969). The transmission of *Trypanosoma cruzi* by arthropod vectors: anterior versus posterior route infection. *Int. Rev. Trop. Med.* **3**, 1–47.

Prata, A. (1980). Perspectivas de controle da Doença de Chagas no Brasil. *J. Bras. Med.* **38**, 53–65.

Rabinovitch, J. E., Leal, J. A., and Feliciangeli, D. P. (1979). Domiciliary biting frequency and blood ingestion of the Chagas' disease vector *Rhodnius prolixus* Stahl (Hemiptera: Reduviidae) in Venezuela. *Trans. R. Soc. Trop. Med. Hyg.* **73**, 272–283.

Rassi, A., and Rezende, J. M. (1976). Prevention of transmission of *T. cruzi* by blood transfusion. *In* "American Trypanosomiasis Research," pp. 273–278. *P.A.H.O. Sci. Publ.* **318**, Washington.

Reis, U. L., Franca, J. B. M., and Rocha e Silva, E. O. (1969). Um critério de menor custo, com subsidio para escolha do método de combate a triatomíneos vetores da Doença de Chagas. *Rev. Saúde Publica* **3**, 31–39.

Rocha e Silva, E. O., Andrade, J. C. R. and Lima, A. R. (1975). Importância dos animais sinantrópicos no controle da endemia chagásica. *Rev. Saúde Pública* **9**, 371–381.

Rocha e Silva, E. O. (1979). Profilaxia in *Trypanosoma cruzi* e Doença de Chagas (Z. Brener, and Z. Andrade, eds.), pp. 425–449. Guanabara Koogan, Rio.

Rocha e Silva, E. O., Ferraz, A. N., and Souza, J. M. P. (1979a). Indices de dejeção das principais espécies de triatomíneos presentes no Estado de São Paulo, Brasil. *An. Congr. Int. Doença Chagas, Abstr.* **138**. Inst. Oswaldo Cruz, Rio.

Rocha e Silva, E. O., Guarita, O. F., and Ishihata, G. K. (1979b). Doença de Chagas: atividades de controle dos transmissores no Estado de São Paulo, Brasil. *Rev. Bras. Malariol. Doenças Trop.* **31**, 99–119.

Rodriguez, D., and Rabinovitch, J. (1980). The effect of density on some population parameters of *Rhodnius prolixus* (Hemiptera, Reduviidae) under laboratory conditions. *J. Med. Entomol.* **17**, 165–171.

Romana, C., and Abalos, J. W. (1948). Accion del Gammexane sobre los triatomidoes. Control domiciliario. *An. Inst. Med. Reg. Tucuman* **2**, 95–106.

Romana C. (1963). "Enfermedad de Chagas," 242 pp. Lopes Libreros, Buenos Aires.

Romeiro, L., and Aguiar, M. (1954). Ação da temperatura sobre alguns insecticidas. *Rev. Bras. Malariol. Doenças Trop.* **6**, 131–143.

Schenone, H., Villarroel, F., and Alfaro, R. (1978). Epidemiologia de la Enfermedad de Chagas en Chile. Condiciones de la vivienda relacionada com a presencia de *Triatoma infestans* y la proporcion de humanos y animales con *Trypanosoma cruzi. Bol. Chil. Parasitol.* **33**, 2–7.

Schmidt, S. (1969). Experiencia de melhoria de habitação cidade satelite de Planaltina—Vila Vicentia Brasília 1967. *Rev. Bras. Malariol. Doenças Trop.* **21**, 201–244.

Schofield, C. J. (1975). The behavioural biology of Triatominae with special reference to intraspecific communication mechanisms. Ph.D. Thesis, pp. 326. Univ. of London, England.

Schofield, C. J. (1978). Comparison of sampling techniques for domestic populations of Triatominae. *Trans. R. Soc. Trop. Med. Hyg.* **72**, 449–455.

Schofield, C. J. (1979). The behavior of Triatominae (Hemiptera: Reduviidae): a review. *Bull. Entomol. Res.* **69**, 363–379.

Schofield, C. J. (1980a). Nutritional status of domestic populations of *Triatoma infestans. Trans. R. Soc. Trop. Med. Hyg.* **74**, 770–778.

Schofield, C. J. (1980b). Density regulation of domestic populations of *Triatoma infestans* in Brazil. *Trans. R. Soc. Trop. Med. Hyg.* **74**, 761–769.

Schofield, C. J., and Marsden, P. D. (1982). Efecto del revoque de las paredes sobre una poblacion domestica de *Triatoma infestans.* (The effect of wall plastering on a domestic population of *Triatoma infestans.*) *Bol. Of. Sanat. Panam.* **93**, 3–8.

Shaw, J. J., Lainson, R., and Frahia, H. (1969). Considerações sobre a epidemiologia dos primeiros casos autoctones de Doenca de Chagas registrados em Belém, Pará, Brasil. *Rev. Saúde Publica* **3**, 153–157.

Sherlock, I. A., and Muniz, T. M. (1974). Observações sobre o combate ao *P. megistus* com BHC em área infestada do Estado da Bahia, Brasil. *Rev. Bras. Malariol. Doenças Trop.* **26**, 93–103.

Sherlock, I. A. (1979a). "Vetores in *Trypanosoma cruzi* e Doença de Chagas" (Z. Brener, and Z. Andrade, eds.), p. 88. Guanabara Koogan, Rio.

Sherlock, I. A. (1979b). Profilaxia da Doença de Chagas. *Rev. Bras. Malariol. Doenças Trop.* **31**, 121–135.

Sherlock, I. A. (1981). *Personal communication.*

Sjogren, R. D., and Ryckman, R. E. (1966). Epizootiology of *Trypanosoma cruzi* in South Western North America. Part VIII. Nocturnal flights of *Triatoma protracta* (Uhler) as indicated by collections at black light traps. *J. Med. Entomol.* **3**, 81–92.

Soares, V. A., and Marsden, P. D. (1979). Estudos sobre a persistência de infectividade do *Trypanosoma cruzi.* II. Persistência de infectividade do T. Cruzi em barbeiros mortos. *Rev. Bras. Pesqui. Med. Biol.* **12**, 367–370.

Soares, V. A., and Marsden, P. D. (1980). Studies of the persistence of infectivity of *Trypanosoma cruzi.* III. Effect of human sweat. *Rev. Bras. Pequi. Med. Biol.* **13**, 53–55.

Soares, V. A., and Marsden, P. D. (1981). *Unpublished observations.*

Soler, C. A., Schenone, H., and Reyes, H. (1969). Problemas derivados de la reparicion de *Triatoma infestans* en viviendas desinsectadas y el concepto de reinfestacion. *Bol. Chil. Parasitol.* **24**, 83–87.

Sullivan, T. D. (1944). Viability of *Trypanosoma cruzi* in citrated blood stored at room temperature. *J. Parasitol.* **30**, 200.

Szumlewicz, A. P. (1953). A ação tóxica dos vapores do Hexachlorociclohexana sobre o *Triatoma infestans. Rev. Bras. Malariol. Doenças Trop.* **5**, 171–181.

Szumlewicz, A. P. (1954). A eficácia do expurgo domiciliário com Hexachlorociclohexana no controle do vetor da Doença de Chagas (a importância de alguns característicos biológicos dos triatomíneos no planejamento do ciclo de aplicação do inseticida). *Rev. Bras. Malariol. Doenças Trop.* **6**, 63–100.

Szumlewicz, A. P. (1969). Estudos sobre *Triatoma infestans,* o principal vetor da Doença de Chagas no Brasil (importância de algumas de suas caracteristicas biologicas no planejamento de esquemas de combate a esse vetor). *Rev. Bras. Malariol. Doenças Trop.* **21**, 117–160.

Szumlewicz, A. P. (1976). Laboratory colonies of Triatominae, biology and population dynamics. *In* "American Trypanosomiasis Research," pp. 63–82. *P.A.H.O. Sci. Publ.* **318**, Washington.

Tarrant, C. A., and Cupp, E. W. (1978). Morphogenetic effects of Precocene II on the immature stages of *Rhodnius prolixus. Trans. R. Soc. Trop. Med. Hyg.* **72**, 666–668.

Teischmann, T., Tanowitz, H., Wittner, M., and Bloom, B. (1978). *Trypanosoma cruzi:* role of the immune response in the natural resistance of inbred strains of mice. *Exp. Parasit.* **45**, 160–168.

Terval, J. R., and Nogueira, J. L. (1970). Perdas fetais em área de alta prevalência de moléstia de Chagas crônica. *Rev. Inst. Med. Trop. São Paulo* **12**, 239–244.

Tonn, R. (1980). Chagas disease vector control programmes: Evaluation and perspectives. *Unpublished document,* TDR/CHA–Ser/WSP/806.

Torno, C. O., Soares, V., Vexenat, A., Cuba, C. C., Barreto, A. C., Alvarenga, N. J., and Marsden, P. D. (1981). A case study of xenodiagnosis. *Rev. Inst. Med. Trop. São Paulo* **23**, 229–232.

Torrealba, J. W., and Feliciangeli, M. D. (1979). Controle de vectores. Experiência en Venezuela. *Int. Congr. Chagas' Disease, Abstr.* **T1–T2**. Inst. Oswaldo Cruz, Rio.

Wallace, F. G. (1979). Biology of the Kinetoplastida of Arthropods. *In* "Biology of the Kinetoplastidae, Vol. 2" (W. H. R. Lumsden, and D. A. Evans, eds.), pp. 213–240. Academic Press, London.

W.H.O. (1975). Resistance of vectors and reservoirs of disease to pesticides. W.H.O. Tech. Rep. Ser. No. 585.

Winslow, D. J. (1964). *Personal communication.*

Zeledon, R. (1974). Epidemiology, modes of transmission and reservoir hosts of Chagas' disease. *In* "Trypanosomiasis and Leishmaniasis with Special Reference to Chagas' Disease", pp. 51–57. Ciba Found. Symp. No. 20, Elsevier, Amsterdam.

Zeledon, R., Solano, G., Burstin, L., and Swartzwelder, J. C. (1975). Epidemiological pattern of Chagas' disease in an endemic area of Costa Rica. *Am. J. Trop. Med. Hyg.* **24,** 214–225.

Zeledon, R., Alvarado, R., and Jiron, L. F. (1977a). Observations on the feeding and defaecation patterns of three triatomine species (Hemiptera: Reduviidae). *Acta Trop.* **34,** 55–77.

Zeledon, R., Alvarenga, N. J., and Shosinsky, K. (1977b). Ecology of *Trypanosoma cruzi* in the insect vector in Chagas' disease. *P.A.H.O. Sci. Publ.* **347,** 59–70. Washington.

Zeledon, R., and Rabinovich, J. E. (1981). Chagas' disease: an ecological appraisal with special emphasis on its insect vectors. *Ann. Rev. Entomol.* **26,** 101–133.

11

Paleoparasitology: On the Origins and Impact of Human–Helminth Relationships

MICHAEL McKINNON KLIKS
Division of Comparative Medicine
John A. Burns School of Medicine
University of Hawaii
Honolulu, Hawaii

"Pathogens must, in general, contribute to homeostasis in the host–parasite communities if they are to maintain themselves."

J. H. Whitlock (1977)

I. Introduction

Helminth parasites have been found in virtually every animal species examined. Humans may act as definitive, intermediate, or paratenic hosts for at least 100 species of helminths. Phylogenetic evidence indicates that many such mammalian host–helminth parasite associations are very ancient; indeed, it is apparent from our contemporary viewpoint that many helminth parasite species coevolved with their hosts. Thus, as new host species arose in response to ecological separation or the availability of new ecological habitats, novel parasites eventually evolved from preexisting or from free-living species to take advantage of the shelter and/or energy resources provided. Other human parasites were acquired as a result of biocultural alterations involving such factors as diet, home range, shelter selection, and religious practices. It is probable that the selective pressure of helminth parasites on individual hosts and on entire demes and populations of hosts has been important in shaping both their ontogenetic and phylogenetic characteristics.

A detailed consideration of the many examples of helminth parasites which may have been a significant impact on early humans is not possible within the confines of this chapter. Herein, I present a general review of some analytical, theoretical, and speculative aspects of host–parasite systems as they may have affected paleolithic humans during the Pliopleistocene geologic period. Only occasional references will be made to particular helminths of man and animals during this, or subsequent, periods.

All known species of parasitic helminths are endoparasites. Alterations of the external environment lead to successions among free-living animal populations and parasites alike. Modifications of the host's internal physiological and biochemical milieux also result in changes in the parasite fauna, adding another dimension to the adaptive responses of helminths. To paraphrase Odum (1971), the human host provides the address, or habitat, at which certain organisms may practice the profession, or trophic niche, of parasitism. Pavlovsky (1966) has referred to the combined populations of all species of parasites in an individual host as the parasitocenose. Taken together, the host(s), its parasites, their niches, and the biotic and abiotic elements of the internal and external environments in which they functionally exist, will be referred to herein as the parasitogeocenose.[1]

---

[1]In the English translation of Pavlovsky referred to herein (1966, p. 246) the term "parasitocenose" appears only in the glossary of English equivalents of Russian terms prepared by N. D. Levine. Nowhere in the main body of text is the term actually applied to a particular example. Sprent (1969a,b) has also utilized parasitocenose in this way and has suggested "parasitome" for all the stages of a particular parasite in a given host individual. Audy (1965), in discussing the host organism as habitat, has used the term "parasite pattern," or "parasite-mix" in much the same way as parasitocenose of Pavlovsky and Sprent. Pavlovsky's terms "pathobiocenose" (1966; 12) and parasitocenose (1966; 246) apparently include only the biotic elements, i.e., the host and the agents of disease which occur within a definite geographic landscape or "biogeocenose" but not the abiotic elements themselves. Esch et al. (1977) have further defined parasite populations (as opposed to host–parasite entities) as: an "infrapopulation" consisting of all individuals (of all stages) of one parasite species within an individual host; a "suprapopulation" being all individuals of all stages of one parasite species within all hosts (definitive, intermediate, paratenic, etc.) present in an ecosystem. Sprent's parasitome would correspond to an infrapopulation as defined by Esch et al. (1977). Thus, an individual host organism may constitute a microcosm of several parasitomes or infrapopulations. A particular parasite suprapopulation will be the combined "poly-stadial" infrapopulations, both in definitive and intermediate hosts of all species (where multiple hosts exist), of a given parasite species. The community consisting of all parasitomes or infrapopulations within an individual host is what Pavlovsky refers to as the parasitocenose for that host. All of these terms are restricted in that they refer to populations of parasites within specified hosts and apparently do not include the hosts themselves or other biotic and abiotic factors of the ecosystems in which they are functionally embedded. An all-inclusive equivalent term would be "pathobiogeocenose" for disease agents in general, or "parasitobiogeocenose" for metazoan parasites in particular. I have chosen to use the slightly less awkward term "parasitogeocenose" to denote particular host–parasite elements *and* the

The intimacy and complexity of these host–parasite associations are such that the functional ecology of one element cannot be understood without fully considering the effects of variables introduced by the others. Biological relationships between helminth parasites and their individual human hosts range from those of harmless commensals to devastating pathogens; from facultative to obligatory associations; from grazers upon bacteria, food contents, and waste products to those feeding directly upon host tissues. In addition, the spatial, temporal, and even cultural point of view of the observer will influence the determination of the status of a given association. Thus, depending upon a wide variety of host factors such as age, nutritional, and immunological status, and parasite factors such as size and sex distribution of the population, the stage of the parasite, and strain differences in virulence, a given species may produce asymptomatic infection or overt disease. Even in the latter case, cultural factors will often determine at which point along a continuum of effects the presence of the parasites causes, for the human host, a "dis-ease." A number of useful texts treating the ecology of helminth parasites are available (Read, 1931; Baer, 1952; Rogers, 1962; Croll, 1966; Fallis, 1971; Kennedy, 1975, 1976; Esch, 1977; Price, 1980).

It is a generally accepted parasitophyletic principle that, the longer the evolutionary association between a given parasite species and a particular host, the greater will be the degree of mutual tolerance the parties have for one another (Sprent, 1962). Consequently, it is assumed that the more pathogenic parasite species have been recently acquired (Cameron, 1958; Dunn, 1968).[2] As the genus *Homo* has evolved relatively rapidly and recently in geological time, the wedding between the host and its accumulating parasites predictably would be less harmonious than those of older, more stable host–parasite relationships.

An additional, functionally related tenet of parasitological dogma is that, in general, the more pathogenic the parasitic organism, particularly among pre-reproductive-aged hosts, the greater the potential selective pressure it will exert upon the population of hosts. Manifestations of the operation of this principle are exemplified in the development of myriad defense strategies against infection and/or resistance to overt disease based on genetic–biochemical and cultural–behavioral accommodations. The theoretical outcome of these interactions at the population and community levels tends toward the establishment of a state of dynamic equilibrium or homeostasis between hosts of increased resistance and

---

matrix of other pertinent biotic and abiotic elements as a functional unit. To encompass all essential elements of every parasite's life cycle in all host species within a particular geographic landscape or ecosystem (biogeocenose of the Soviets) I would suggest the term "parasitosystem."

[2]This principle frequently does not hold for helminths transmitted between predators/scavengers and their prey which act as intermediate hosts. Though such parasitocenoses are probably as old as the relationships between their hosts, the larval stages frequently incapacitate the intermediate host to the parasites' advantage (Holmes and Bethel, 1972).

economy, that of gathering and primitive hunting. The importance of human behavioral patterns and their manifestation as cultural ecology in promoting and/or preventing helminth diseases will also be a primary focus.

II. Sources and Limitations of Evidence

Any attempt to formulate a tentative reconstruction of the antiquity of parasitocenoses involving hominoids must begin with the basic premise that the progenitors of parasitic helminths had already evolved many tens of millions of years before the great radiation of mammals during the Paleocene and Eocene periods that gave rise to primates from the insectivore line. Comparative studies of the helminth fauna of modern hominoid primates provide some clues as to the genera and species that may have infected the hominid line.

Phylogenetic treatments of the origin and distribution of helminths in general can be found in the works of Hyman (1952a,b), Dogiel (1964), Manter (1967), Noble and Noble (1971), and Odening (1974). The origins of host specificity and its relationship to phylogeny among the cestodes and trematodes (platyhelminths) has been discussed by Baer (1955), Stunkard (1962, 1963), Smyth (1964), and Llewellyn (1965), and for nematode groups by Osche (1958, 1963), Inglis (1965, 1971), and Cameron (1952, 1964). Sprent (1969a) provides a thorough review and cogent commentary on adaptation within host–parasitic systems, parasitophyletic rules, and the ontogeny of host immune response to parasitic infections. Systematics and zoogeographic host–parasite records prior to 1961 have been drawn primarily from Yamaguti (1958–1961).

Direct archeological evidence is scarce as few helminthic diseases have left indelible stigmata on ancient skeletal material. Accidents of nature and the contrivances of man have provided the paleoepidemiologist with a few precious well-preserved mummies (Zimmerman and Smith, 1975; El-Najjar *et al.,* 1980), a handful of coprolites (ancient human feces), and the contents of several paleoprivies (Cockburn *et al.,* 1975; Wilke and Hall, 1975; Kliks, 1975; Anon., 1975). Of course, such isolated data do not provide the population denominators necessary for the rigorous epidemiological evaluation characterizing analyses of contemporary disease events.

Additional information concerning knowledge of parasite diseases, the helminths causing them, and the medicines used in their treatment can be gleaned from oral histories that were eventually set down by ancient scribes and chroniclers along the ragged edges between history and prehistory. Few among these valuable treasures of prehistoric events have been carefully studied by modern epidemiologists (Hoeppli, 1959, 1969, 1972). The Old Testament of the Bible (Mollaret, 1966; Callot, 1970; Hulse, 1971), especially Leviticus, the Talmud

(Sussman, 1967), the *Qur'an,* the Moslem *Hadith* (Hoeppli, 1959, 1969), stone inscriptions and cunieform texts from ancient Mesopotamia (Kinnier-Wilson, 1967; Thompson, 1923), the Egyptian papyri (Hoeppli, 1959, 1972), a few Middle American codices (Guerra, 1966; Garcia-Kutzback, 1976), and several early Chinese manuscripts (Read, 1931; Lu Gwei-Djen and Needham, 1967) have been critically examined. These sources alone will continue to provide scholars for generations with important information; furthermore, many of the Vedic texts of India and ancient Arabian and Persian manuscripts have not yet been systematically treated.

Ancient peoples themselves have left a few graphic records of the parasitic diseases besetting them painted on cave walls, molded on ceramics, or carved into stone stelae (Hoeppli, 1969; Gantzer, 1972). Furthermore, ethnoparasitology and ethnopharmacology[3] can provide living dioramas, visualizations of the possible impacts of parasitic disease. Finally, as the late T. A. Cockburn (1963) has so candidly pointed out, in most reconstructions of remote events it is informed, inductive, and deductive speculation that must provide the most fertile source of untestable hypotheses.

Of the 100 or so helminth parasites common in modern human populations, it is probable that only a few infected the australopithecines of the Pliopleistocene period of about 3 to 7 million years ago. These tool-making, bipedal hominids may have been hosts to a wide variety of zoonotic and "australopithic" parasites, but it is unlikely that they had yet acquired the principal pathogens of *Homo sapiens;* it required thousands of millennia of evolution, migration, and the invention/discovery of culture to facilitate the acquisition of these.

III. General Consideration of the Evolution and Life Cycles of Hominoid Parasites

The helminth parasites of various classes of mammals undoubtedly underwent a coevolutionary radiation parallel to, but somewhat more conservative than, that of their host species. For example, it is apparent from the pioneering phylogenetic–taxonomic analyses of some parasitic helminths of primates by Cameron (1929, 1952, 1964), and later by Inglis and Dunn (1964), Inglis (1965, 1971), Dunn (1966, 1970), Chitwood (1970), Orihel (1970), and Brooks and Glen

---

[3]Ethnoparasitology and ethnopharmacology: The study of parasitic diseases and native medicines used to treat them among contemporary preliterate human populations who make their living today much as hunter–gatherers, nomad pastoralists, and shifting agriculturalists did thousands of years ago.

(1982), that as new *families* and *genera* of primate hosts evolved, new *species* of helminths arose to parasitize them from within existing parasite *genera*. Yamashita (1963) has outlined the ecological bases of primate–helminth host–parasite relationships.

It is of considerable significance that among the *genera* of contemporary human helminth parasites not one is restricted to man alone. Furthermore, only a few adult helminths, i.e., the nematodes *Enterobius vermicularis*, *Onchocerca volvulus*, *Wuchereria bancrofti*, *Dipetalonema perstans*, and *Mansonella ozzardi*, and the cestodes *Taenia saginata* and *T. solium*, are now virtually restricted to humans at the *species* level. Yamashita (1963) has pointed out that among 34 genera of helminths parasitic in both *Homo* and at least one other member of the Hominoidea, man is host to 20, *Pan* to 26, *Pongo* to 13 and *Hylobates* to 14. Seven genera (*Trichuris*, *Stronglyoides*, *Oesophagostomum*, *Ascaris*, *Dipetalonema*, *Dirofilaria*, and *Bertiella*) have been reported from all 4 hominoid genera (Dunn, 1966).

As might be expected, modern *Homo* and *Pan* (chimpanzee and gorilla) share more helminth genera between them than either does with the Asiatic apes *Pongo* (orangutan) or *Hylobates* (gibbon), although some provocative discrepancies have recently been noted (Brooks and Glen, 1982). It is not possible to know if the helminth fauna of modern primates corresponds to that of the Pleistocene; however, the similarities and differences among helminth parasites of arboreal and terrestrial apes and contemporary humans may suggest the composition of a plausible autochthonous fauna. Ecological setting and behavioral attributes thereafter determined the direction and form of later parasite successions.

Modern man is the definitive host to many genera of helminth parasites also found in lower mammals, in particular those occurring naturally in canid, felid, rodent, porcine, and herbivore hosts that shared natural habitats with early man and/or became domiciled or have been domesticated. At the species level, as has long been tragically obvious to those who would control or eradicate human helminth diseases, modern man shares definitive host status with a wide variety of domestic and wild animals. It is generally believed that man did not become more than peripherally involved in these animal parasitocenoses until the relatively recent past, that is, since the origin of agriculture and the domestication of animals (Dunn, 1968; Sprent, 1969a; Cockburn, 1977). These diseases, known as zoonoses, have been thoroughly treated by a number of authors (Cameron, 1926, 1958; Audy, 1958; Fiennes, 1967; W.H.O., 1967; Schwabe, 1969; Sprent, 1969a,b; Garnham, 1971). Schwabe (1969) and Sprent (1969b) have presented useful heuristic frameworks for examining and comparing zoonotic diseases by life cycle type.

Significantly, with the very rare exception of several trematodes of piscivorous birds, humans are not definitive hosts for any helminth genera whose usual definitive hosts are not mammals. The ecological basis for this pattern of broad host restriction and specificity at the family and class level, especially among the nematodes, may be related to the fact that adult stages do not multiply within the definitive host, and that their reproductive potential, at least when compared to the protozoa and bacteria, is relatively limited. Although the number of eggs produced by a female *Ascaris lumbricoides* or a taenioid tapeworm may be thousands per day, the numbers of adults within a given host are usually few, and the perils to be overcome in the external environment, or in seeking the appropriate intermediate host, are awesome. Only by means of exquisitely balanced dynamic equilibria between host and parasite behavior do offspring of parasitic helminths succeed in reaching a suitable host.

Borrowing a term from vertebrate ecology, it may be argued that many helminth parasites function as if they have evolved in a *K* (maximum survival of offspring) rather than a *r* (maximum intrinsic rate of increase) selected manner, as has been reviewed by Esch, Hazen, and Aho (1977). That is, compared with many other metazoans, they are relatively conservative in their reproductive potential; larval survival during free-living periods is maximized within a narrow range of conditions; host-finding capacities are finely tuned to a limited number of intermediate and definitive hosts to minimize reproductive wastage; and populations of adults are maintained at or near the equilibrium size.

Numerous examples of adaptive optimization of offspring survival can be cited, such as the "spring rise" and "arrested development" phenomena among livestock strongyles (Schad, 1977), prenatal, intrauterine, and transmammary infection in hookworms (Stone and Smith, 1973), microfilarial periodicity among filarids (Hawking, 1975), and many examples of specific chemotaxis and chemotropism among trematodes and cestodes. Because helminths have exploited the option of *K* selection by evolving biochemically and behaviorally specific definitive host-finding and population-stabilizing mechanisms, their capacity to make the evolutionary leaps required for expansion into novel host niches across class boundaries has been inevitably limited.

An examination of the breadth of host range of the intermediate stages of certain helminths, however, reveals a considerably expanded repertoire of available potential species. Humans, for instance, may act as suitable (although from the parasites' standpoint, inappropriate) intermediate hosts for helminths parasitic as adults in many more genera and families of vertebrates than those groups with which they share definitive host status (Sprent, 1969b). Most of these helminth life cycles involve predator–prey interactions in which a variety of intermediate hosts in what Sprent (1969b) has termed the parasites' "life pyramid" are debilitated and/or consumed along with the parasite by the definitive host. The advantages to the parasite in having its intermediate stages in a wide range of hosts which are potential food items of the definitive host are obvious (Holmes and Bethel, 1972). Early man, as he moved to exploit new habitats and food resources, fortuitously became an intermediate host in many such helminth cycles long before being infected by the adults of those for which he may act as a true definitive host. It is probable, for example, that vulnerable early hominids were themselves prey of large carnivores and other hominids, and may have routinely transmitted toxocariasis, trichinosis, cysticercosis, hydatid disease, and similar helminth diseases of carnivores.

It is clear that most available helminth parasite habitats were occupied, most life cycle variations exploited, and potential human parasitocenoses well established at the time that the australopithecines emerged from their "nidus of Eden," the tropical forests. All that was required to initiate the accumulation of helminth infections by our hypothetical hominid hosts was to "bite into the apple" of broadened environmental and dietary exposure, thereby entering into many more zoonotic parasitogeocenoses.

IV. Heirlooms and Souvenirs: A Probable Helminthofaunal Succession in the Transition from Arboreal Monkeys and Apes to Terrestrial Hominids

The gradual climatic and biotic changes known to have occurred in East Africa during the later Miocene period led to the fragmentation of the earlier, almost continuous cover of dense tropical rain forest and created instead a mosaic ecosystem characterized by many diverse macro- and microenvironments and their marginating border zones or ecotones (Coopens et al., 1976). Over a span of several million years, australopithecine hominids differentiated from pongids and evolved to exploit the new terrestrial habitats consisting primarily of stream courses lined by gallery forest, intervening open savanna grasslands, flat plains surrounding shallow lakes, and deciduous scrub (Clark, 1980). Remnants of vast, closed, and biotypically monotonous rain forests survived of course, but except for a few brief millennia of expansion during interglacial pluvial periods they continued to recede.

The contraction of the forest biome, and the simultaneous development of several new biomes and intervening ecotones characterized by their openness and a richness and diversity of available plant and animal resources, provided the ecological substrates for the relatively rapid evolution of several novel types of terrestrial hominid and pongid primates. The emergence of a variety of closely related hominids as habitats for helminths can also be regarded as having given rise, in turn, to "internal ecotones" within which preexisting parasites could readily speciate.

Sprent (1969a,b) has appropriately termed "heirloom species" those original parasites that have persisted in *Homo* up to the present, and "souvenir species" those that have been acquired during our long trudge to humanity (Fig. 1). Successional changes in the original hominoid fauna accompanying adaptation to a progressively more terrestrial existence were, at first, probably quantitative in nature. I suggest that host species for a time remained both accessible and susceptible to infection by preexisting autochthonous, helminth parasites but that the prevalence and intensity of infection tended to decrease as host exposure time within a particular forest or arboreal biogeocenose diminished. Behavioral or ecological exclusion from, or inclusion in, parasitocenoses doubtlessly preceded phylogenetically determined and biochemically based susceptibility or nonsusceptibility.

For example, several of the filarial nematodes of modern anthropoid primates exhibit differential infection rates among a variety of susceptible hosts that seem to be related to the altitude of the host's principal habitat and the restricted vertical distribution of the required arthropod vectors (Dunn, 1966, 1970). The similar, well-documented vertical stratification of infection rates of several species of malarial parasites among forest animals is clearly related to vector and parasite behavior (Dunn *et al.*, 1968). Although precise field data are not available, a reasonable hypothesis is that primate filarial worms such as *Loa loa, Dipetalonema,* and *Dirofilaria,* having vectors which generally prefer to feed in the middle and upper levels of the forest canopy, would tend toward lessened prevalence and intensity of infection among terrestrial forest and/or savanna-dwelling primates. Conversely, the occurrence of the filarial genera *Wuchereria, Brugia,* and *Onchocerca,* whose vectors feed in more open areas, would be expected to be much more common among terrestrial primates, including humans, than among those that are mainly arboreal.

Such contemporary spatial distribution patterns would represent the end result of evolutionary processes leading eventually to speciation and lessened compatibility between host and parasite. The human heirloom species *Loa loa* is the only filarid of primates naturally occurring in both Old World and New World hosts, which suggests a Miocene origin (Chitwood, 1970). Infection with this worm, which can cause serious pathology in man, may have been very common and quite nonpathogenic in early hominids as it now is in contemporary primates (Nelson, 1965; Fiennes, 1965). In Africa hundreds of millennia of ethological and ecological separation between humans and arboreal primates, and the acquisition of distinct vectors with differing biting habits (Kershaw, 1957; Duke, 1972), apparently have resulted in the establishment of two separate, conspecific worm populations.

In contrast, infections with two other probable heirloom filarial parasites, *Dipetalonema streptocerca* and *D. perstans,* remain quite common and generally asymptomatic both in man and in a variety of primates. It is possible that the catholic host preference and wide-ranging flight behavior of their biting gnat

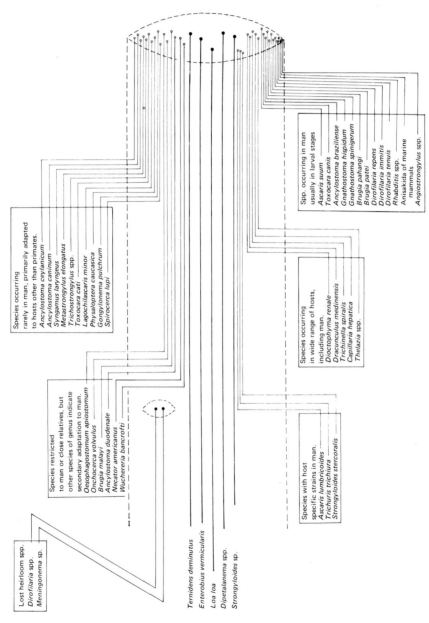

Lost heirloom spp.
Dirofilaria spp.
Meningonema sp.

Species restricted
to man or close relatives, but
other species of genus indicate
secondary adaptation to man.
Oesophagostomum apiostomum
Onchocerca volvulus
Brugia malayi
Ancylostoma duodenale
Necator americanus
Wuchereria bancrofti

Species occurring in man,
rarely in man, primarily adapted
to hosts other than primates.
Ancylostoma ceylanicum
Ancylostoma caninum
Syngamus laryngeus
Metastrongylus elongatus
Trichostrongylus spp.
Toxocara cati
Lagochilascaris minor
Physaloptera caucasica
Gongylonema pulchrum
Spirocerca lupi

Ternidens deminutus
Enterobius vermicularis
Loa loa
Dipetalanema spp.
Strongyloides sp.

Species with host
specific strains in man.
Ascaris lumbricoides
Trichuris trichiura
Strongyloides stercoralis

Species occurring
in wide range of hosts,
including man.
Dioctophyma renale
Dracunculus medinensis
Trichinella spiralis
Capillaria hepatica
Thelazia spp.

Spp. occurring in man
usually in larval stages
Ascaris suum
Toxocara canis
Ancylostoma braziliense
Gnathostoma hispidum
Gnathostoma spinigerum
Brugia pahangi
Brugia patei
Dirofilaria repens
Dirofilaria immitis
Dirofilaria tenuis
Rhabditis spp.
Anisakida of marine
mammals
Angiostrongylus spp.

FIG. 1. Diagram illustrating the heirloom and souvenir components of the parasitocenose, using nematodes occurring in man as examples. Solid lines represent heirloom parasites; hollow lines represent souvenir parasites. Adapted from Sprent (1969a).

vectors have inhibited the course of ecologic succession by continuously infecting human hosts, thereby maintaining the host–parasite equilibrium at a moderately pathological level. As with *Loa loa,* a human-specific strain of *D. perstans* has arisen owing perhaps to long-term isolation of parasite populations among its biting gnat vectors and hominid hosts.

The human filarial worms *Wuchereria bancrofti, Brugia malayi,* and *Onchocerca volvulus* were probably acquired as souvenirs of terrestrial existence. The first two species are closely related and almost certainly evolved as human parasites in Southeast Asia concurrent with the development of primitive agriculture; *O. volvulus* is probably of African origin and is virtually restricted to humans.

Infection with the above-mentioned helminths is rarely directly fatal among contemporary Old World monkeys, apes, and humans and therefore probably exerted little selective pressure on their hosts. However, another recently discovered primate filarid, *Meningonema peruzzii,* whose adult stage normally inhabits the medullary leptomeninges of African cercopithecoid monkeys, is the probable cause of serious disease which occurs rarely in humans (Orihel, 1973) and perhaps in other apes. The arthropod vector of *M. peruzzii* is not yet known, but considering the parasite's frequency in high canopy-dwelling arboreal monkeys, the vector's biting habits are likely to be such that infections in terrestrial primates, including humans, are exceeding rare.

One is tempted to speculate about the effect that *any* central nervous system involvement, however slight, would have had on the nascent intellectual capabilities and thus, population dynamics, of early hominids that were not yet fully terrestrial. The overall effect on the rate and direction of hominid evolution caused by changes in the prevalence and intensity of infection by such hypothetical helminth parasites, and of many others which have completely disappeared cannot be objectively assessed from our temporally narrow window on evolutionary processes.

However, a parallel contemporary example is provided by the dramatic effect of the meningeal nematode of North American cervids, *Paraelaphostrongylus tenuis,* on the population dynamics and distribution of its several hosts. This worm is well tolerated by its host, the whitetail deer, but causes severe neurological disorders in all other host species. The result is greatly increased direct mortality, susceptibility to predation and environmental stresses, and gross interference with normal mating and maternal care of offspring (Anderson and Prestwood, 1979). This striking morbidity and mortality differential is sufficiently great to have caused within a few decades extinctions of moose, elk, mule deer, and woodland caribou, and the subsequent colonization of much of their previous ranges throughout eastern and well into western North America by the whitetail deer. Only local, ecological isolation due to topographical factors has permitted the survival of populations of adversely affected host species. Hypothesizing for the moment the existence of a similar differential central nervous system effect caused by *Meningonema* or a similar helminth that is transmitted only among various forms of arboreal primates, one can readily construct a plausible model for the rapid extinction of those demes of adversely effected host species which were not ecologically isolated from the pathogen by the adaptation of a terrestrial habitat. Persistence of susceptibility to infection would have the effect of continuously reinforcing the survival and reproductive advantage of individuals and populations no longer exposed to the disease and could eventuate the emergence of distinct host species.

Among the probable original hominid helminth parasites that did survive the transition from branch to bush was the ancestral form of the pinworm *Enterobius vermicularis*. These tiny worms, most "human" of all helminths, inhabit the cecum and appendix, from which gravid females migrate to tickle the perianal skin while releasing their sticky and almost immediately infective ova. The gregarious behavior of all hominoids, the fact that young primates defecate in their nests, and the frequency of hand-to-mouth contact are well suited to the requirements of the genus *Enterobius*. No other hosts are required, there is no immunity, and a single individual host can continuously reinfect itself. Cameron (1964) has shown that a given species of *Enterobius* is usually restricted to one genus of primate. Members of the genus occur in both African (cercopithecoid) and South American (ceboid) monkeys, indicating that the genus arose prior to the geological separation of these primate lines (Inglis, 1961, 1971).

The human form, *E. vermicularis,* is most closely related to species normally parasitizing hominoid apes rather than cercopithecoid and ceboid monkeys (Cameron, 1929). Although among the pongids the chimpanzee occasionally has been found naturally infected, the pinworm is the most host-specific of all human nematodes (Chitwood, 1970) and probably evolved concurrently with the emergence of the genus *Homo* from *Australopithecus*. A recent cladistic study by Brooks and Glen (1982) has confirmed the host–parasite coevolution hypothesis of Cameron (1964). Furthermore, their comparison of cladograms of host phylogeny and parasite characters suggests that the genus *Homo* is not as linearly related to the *Pongo–Gorilla–Pan* group as has been previously assumed, but is more closely affiliated with hylobatids (gibbons).

The deceptively delicate eggs of *E. vermicularis* frequently have been found preserved in ancient human feces and mummies (Wei, 1973; Wilke and Hall, 1975). Infection rates apparently reached hyperendemic proportions among the world's most dedicated apartment dwellers, the crowded Pueblo Indians of Canyon del Muertos and of similar sites in the North American Southwest (Fry and Moore, 1969, El Najjar *et al.,* 1980). Pinworm in man was known to the Greeks, the ancient Egyptians, the Persians, the Chinese, and to the Ayurvedic physicians of India (Hoeppli, 1959). The sixteenth century *Florentine Codex* indicates that the Aztecs recognized *Enterobius* as small white worms "common in the folk'' which ''when one sleeps, they come forth'' (Dibble and Anderson, 1963; Book XI: pp. 98–99). Other than restless evenings and occasional anal pruritis caused by scratching during the perianal peregrinations of gravid females, pinworm has virtually no impact on its host.

Helminth species with infective stages (embryonated eggs or free-living larvae) that undergo an obligatory period of development in the soil are referred to as geohelminths.[4] Transmission is direct requiring no intermediates. Host specificity is generally high, and host immunity is usually negligible or ineffective. The population dynamics of such host–parasite relationships tend to resemble those of directed, deterministic processes characterized by being tenaciously endemic in host populations and causing low mortality but significant morbidity (Whitlock 1977). Within a given group of hosts (human or other animal) distributions of the frequency and intensity of such infections tend to be over-dispersed (Crofton, 1971). Thus, although the great majority of hosts will harbor relatively trivial infections, the worm burdens of a few will constitute a disproportionately large portion of the total parasite biomass. The bases of this distribution are environmental (edaphic, meterological), genetic, and behavioral: given a marginally suitable external and internal environment, continuous intense exposure can overcome ''normal'', genetically determined host resistance. It is upon these heavily infected individuals, rather than upon entire populations, that the biogeocenotic forces of selection exert their influence (Bradley, 1974).

The soil-transmitted strongyle nematode genera *Oesophagostromum, Ternidens,* and *Trichostrongylus* probably originated among ruminants in Africa. At the present time they also occur as natural infections in humans, baboons, gorillas, and chimpanzees; *Ternidens* has been reported from primates only. Soil contamination with infective eggs or larval stages from ungulate and primate feces must have been exceedingly common in early man's habitat. When present in large numbers, these worms could have caused serious, even directly fatal, disease among early terrestrial primate populations. *Ternidens* and *Oesophagostomum* have failed to adapt well to modern man's habits and habitats, persisting in humans mainly as remnant species in a few small foci of tropical Africa, including modern hunter–gatherers (Nelson, 1972).

The contemporary nematode occupants of the enteric blood-sucking niche in man belong to the strongyle genera *Ancylostoma* and *Necator,* which are probably derived from hybrids among similar types occurring in canids and felids. It is unlikely the adult stages of either had fully adapted to early man; they are more probably souvenirs of a later pastoral–agricultural period coincidental with the domestication of the dog during the Neolithic. However, as certainly as our ancestors have shared caves with wild pigs, jackals, hyenas, felids, and bears

---

[4]A more accurate term would be ''edaphohelminths'' to indicate development and transmission associated with the soil (Gr., *edaphos*), rather than with the planet earth (Gr., *geo*).

since the earliest times, they must also have suffered from the intensely pruritic dermatitis produced by the invasive migrating third-stage hookworm larvae of animal origin. Such cutaneous experiments in evolution led at some point in time to the establishment of worm ecotypes capable of achieving the visceral migration necessary for reaching sexual maturity in humans. Ancylostomatid-like ova and larvae have been reported from possibly human coprolite material several thousand years old found in Brazil (Ferreira *et al.*, 1980).

Members of the heirloom genus *Strongyloides* appear to be well adapted to the gregarious behavior and promiscuous defecation habits of arboreal primates: three species have been recovered from more than 15 primates (Yamashita, 1963; Chitwood, 1970). Although the nematode is generally considered to be soil-transmitted, actual contact with terrestrial "soil" is not always required. Motile larvae rather than eggs are passed in the host's feces, and these are capable of developing to the infective stage within 24 hr. Infections in an arboreal habitat could occur through contact with contaminated perianal fur, branches, or nesting materials. Heavy infections in young or stressed hosts can be devasting and surely caused sporadic mortality in primate populations from the earliest times. The very delicate structure and small size of *Strongyloides* spp. adult intestinal and larval fecal stages greatly reduces the likelihood of their being recovered in archaeological contexts. However, other rhabditoid nematodes, probably free-living saprophagous types, have been recovered from ancient human coprolites (Dunn and Watkins, 1970; Kliks, 1975; Dusseau and Porter, 1974).

Human ingestion of embryonated eggs of the common ascaridoid nematodes of canids and felids (*Toxocara, Toxascaris*) also can lead to serious disease, particularly in young, prereproductive, and pubescent hosts. Visceral migration of the larval stages stimulates an initial allergic-type immune response. Larvae can accumulate in tissues leading to eventual ocular and central nervous system involvement that would have greatly increased the host's susceptibility to predators in the past.

Available evidence suggests that the most common contemporary soil-transmitted helminths of man, *Ascaris* and *Trichuris,* are human-adapted strains originating in pigs concurrent with the development of sedentary village life in Neolithic times; these will not be discussed further in this chapter.

As most trematode and cestode parasitocenoses require the participation of terrestrial and/or aquatic intermediate hosts, arboreal primates are not now (and probably never were) commonly infected by these helminths (Fiennes, 1967; Dunn, 1970). However, several members of the cestode families Anoplocephalidae (*Bertiella* spp.) and Hymenolepidae (*Hymenolepis* spp.) are common intestinal parasites in both terrestrial and arboreal monkeys and apes, and in man. Significantly, members of both parasite groups are transmitted via the accidental ingestion of small, widely distributed arthropods. These heirloom tapeworms usually are nonpathogenic and quite catholic in their host range among primates.

Among helminth cycles first encountered by early terrestrial hominids in Africa, those of the passively acquired schistosome blood flukes have certainly had the most significant and continuous social and economic impact on individuals, on demes, and later with the advent of irrigated agriculture on entire populations. I suggest that the terrestrial, diurnal, and omnivorous behavior of baboons has been important in facilitating the adaptation of preexisting ungulate schistosome species to early humans in Pleistocene Africa and their later dissemination. The role of contemporary baboons as naturally infected definitive hosts for several human schistosome species has been recognized only recently (Nelson *et al.*, 1962; Wright, 1977).

The many African species of baboons (*Papio, Cyanocephalus, Theropithecus, Mandrillus*) including extinct giant forms were probably the primates most important in effectively preadapting and amplifying those strains of animal schistosomes and other helminths potentially capable of infecting hominids. These diurnally active animals share with humans a gregarious and territorial social nature, a preference for aquatic habitats, omnivorous food habits, and promiscuous defecation patterns (Washburn and DeVore, 1961; Freeland, 1976). Several types of baboon remains frequently occur in Pleistocene deposits associated with australopithecines (Butzer and Issac, 1975). It is not surprising that modern *Homo* and baboons also share at least 20 species of helminth parasites (Stiles and Hassall, 1929; Yamashita, 1963; Fiennes, 1967).

Epidemiological models approximating the complex population dynamics of schistosome infective processes in human and molluscan hosts have been designed by MacDonald (1965) and Hairston (1965) with recent qualitative improvements by May (1977). Successful infection of susceptible definitive hosts involves several random behavioral elements related to exposure to water that contains appropriate infective stages in sufficient numbers. As schistosomes have separate sexes, a further stochastic parameter involves the probability of worms of both sexes effectively pairing within the host. Climatic conditions suitable for snail hosts, the population densities of appropriate snail phenotypes, their tolerance for the infection, and their effective life span are a few of the subtle deterministic biological factors regulating these parasitocenoses. Acquired immunity and/or natural resistance in humans appears to regulate the intensity of infection but does not result in the elimination of all the worms. Concomitant immunity may also limit worm burdens among susceptible hosts, but behavioral factors have resulted in humans becoming involved in preexisting schistosome cycles from the earliest times to the present (Nelson, 1972; Desowitz, 1980).

In summary, to make a general inference based on the available paleoecological and zoogeographic data and modern host–parasite records, early terrestrial hominids may have escaped from continuous exposure to certain parasitocenoses restricted to the arboreal forest biome. Other helminths with less environmentally or host-restricted cycles made the transition and were also functional in the emerging mosaic of savanna, lacustrine, and riverine habitats into which the terrestrial australopithecines rapidly radiated. A few of these parasites have persisted as heirloom species in modern man. However, the terrestrial habitats were already occupied by a great variety of carnivores and herbivores and their helminths, and among these there were many more potential hominid parasites to be gained as souvenirs than had been lost.

V. Human Inventions and Interventions in the Adaptive Evolution of Helminth Parasites

As gatherers of plant foods, scavengers, and occasional predators upon invertebrates and small vertebrates, the earliest terrestrial hominids probably contributed little to the population dynamics of preexisting mammalian helminth parasitocenoses. The invention of wood implements and later, stone tools, greatly increased hominid impact on the biotic community. Use of tools in the collection and preparation of food also brought hominids into intimate contact with a wide variety of heretofore inaccesible habitats and animals and their parasites. Accumulating knowledge of plant and animal resources eventually led to the continuous predation upon herd-forming artiodactylids, to nomad pastoralism, and finally to animal and plant domestication. Primitive agriculture and animal husbandry made possible the development of villages and eventually cities, concentrating large numbers of human and animal hosts and their now shared helminths.

The collective intelligence of "civilized" humans made possible the collation of empirical (and only recently, experimental) knowledge concerning disease origins and processes. When applied as rules of hygiene, dietary proscriptions, or therapeutic regimens, this increase in information content altered the structure of the ecosystem as a whole. Over the short term, the resulting successions in the biotic community have been generally favorable to man and his domesticates. However, man's inventions, and by means of them, his interventions in the "natural order," have resulted in a continuously changing helminth fauna. These processes are continuing and were also evident during historical times as local introductions and extinctions (i.e., filariasis in North America), as oscillations (i.e., schistosomiasis in Africa), and in the origins (i.e., angiostrongyliasis and anisakiasis) of helminth–human interaction.

References

Allison, A. C. (1975). Interactions of genetic predisposition, acquired immunity and environmental factors in susceptibility to disease. *In* "Man-Made Lakes and Human Health" (N. F. Stanley, and M. P. Alpers, eds.), pp. 407–427. Academic Press, New York.

Anderson, R. N., and May, R. N. (1978). Regulation and stability of host parasite population interactions. I. Regulator processes. *J. Anim. Ecol.* **47**, 219–247.

Anderson, R. C., and Prestwood, A. K. (1979). Lungworms. *In* "The Diseases of the White-tailed Deer" (F. Hayes, ed.). U.S. Dept. Interior, U.S. Wildlife Serv., Washington, D.C.

Anon. (1975). "Helminths in archaeological and pre-historic deposits: Annotated Bibliography No. 9. (1910–1975)." Commonwealth Institute of Helminthology. St. Albans, Herts.

Audy, J. R. (1958). The localization of diseases with special reference to the zoonoses. *Trans. R. Soc. Trop. Med. Hyg.* **52**, 308–334.

Audy, J. R. (1965). Types of human influences on natural foci of disease. *In* "Theoretical Questions of Natural Foci of Diseases, Proceedings of a Symposium" (B. Rosicky, and K. Heyberger, eds.), pp. 245–253. Czechoslovak Acad. of Sci., Prague.

Baer, J. G. (1952). "Ecology of Animal Parasites." Univ. of Illinois, Urbana.

Basset, A., Lariviere, M., and Basset, M. (1974). Formes cliniques et epidemiologie de l'onchocercose au Senegal. *Int. J. Dermatol.* **13**, 135–138.

Bradley, D. J. (1972). Regulation of parasite populations: A general theory of the epidemiology and control of parasitic infections. *Trans. R. Soc. Trop. Med. Hyg.* **66**, 697–708.

Bradley, D. J. (1974). Stability in host–parasite systems. *In* "Ecological Stability" (M. B. Usher, and M. H. Williamson, eds.), pp. 71–87. Chapman & Hall, London.

Brooks, D. R., and Glen, D. R. (1982). Pinworms and primates: a case study in evolution. *Proc. Helminthol. Soc. Wash.* **49**, 76–85.

Butzer, K. W., and Issac, G. L. (eds.) (1975). "After the Australopithecines: Stratigraphy, Ecology and Culture in the Middle Pleistocene." Aldine, New York.

Callot, J. (1970). La peste des Philistins n'est pas non plus la Bilharziose. *Presse Med.* **78**, 615–618.

Cameron, T. W. M. (1926). The helminth parasites of animals and human disease. *Proc. R. Soc. Med.* (Comp. Med.) **20**, 547–556.

Cameron, T. W. M. (1929). The species of *Enterobius* Leach, in primates. *J. Helminthol.* **7**, 161–182.

Cameron, T. W. M. (1952). Parasitism, evolution, and phylogeny. *Endeavor* **Oct.**, 193–199.

Cameron, T. W. M. (1958). Parasites of animals and human disease. *In* "Animal Disease and Human Health" (O. V. St. Whitelock, ed.). *Ann. N.Y. Acad. Sci.* **70**, 564–573.

Cameron, T. W. M. (1964). Host specificity and the evolution of helminth parasites. *Adv. Parasitol.* **2**, 1–34.

Chitwood, M. B. (1970). Comparative relationship of some parasites of man and Old and New World subhuman primates. *Lab. Anim. Care* **26**, 389–394.

Ciba Foundation (1974). "Parasites in the Immunized Host: Mechanisms of Survival," Symp. 25 (N. S.). Elsevier, Amsterdam.

Clark, J. E. (1980). Early human occupation of African savanna environments. *In* "Human Ecology in Savanna Environments" (D. R. Harris, ed.), pp. 44–71. Academic Press, London.

Cockburn, T. A. (1963). "The Evolution and Eradication of Infectious Diseases." John Hopkins Univ. Press, Baltimore, Maryland.

Cockburn, T. A. (1977). Where did our infectious disease come from? The evolution of infectious disease. *In* "Health and Disease in Tribal Societies," Ciba Found. Symp. 49 (P. Hugh-Jones, ed.), pp. 103–114. Elsevier/North Holland, Amsterdam.

Cockburn, T. A., Barraco, R. A., Rayman, T. A., and Peck, W. H. (1975). Autopsy of an Egyptian mummy. *Science* **187** (4182), 1155–1160.

Cohen, S., and Sadun, E. H., eds. (1976). "The Immunology of Parasitic Infections." Blackwell, Oxford.

Coppens, Y., Howell, F. C., Isaac, G. L., and Leakey, R. E. F., eds. (1976). "Earliest Man and Environments in the Lake Rudolf Basin." Univ. of Chicago Press, Chicago, Illinois.

Croll, N. A. (1966). "Ecology of Parasites." Heinemann, London.

Crofton, H. D. (1971). A quantitative approach to parasitism. *Parasitology* **62**, 197–193.

Damian, R. J. (1964). Molecular mimicry: antigen sharing by parasite and host and its consequences. *Am. Nat.* **98**, 129–149.

Desowitz, R. S. (1980). Epidemiological–ecological interactions in savanna environments. *In* "Human Ecology in Savanna Environments" (D. R. Harris, ed.), pp. 457–477. Academic Press, London.

Desowitz, R. S. (1981). "New Guinea Tapeworms and Jewish Grandmothers." Norton, New York.

Dibble, L. E., and Anderson, A. J. O. (1963). "General History of the Things of New Spain (Florentine Codex)." Monograph, School of American Research, Univ. of Utah; Museum of New Mexico, Santa Fe.

Dineen, J. K. (1963). Immunological aspects of parasitism. *Nature* **197**, 268–269.

Dogiel, V. A. (1964). "General Parasitology." Oliver & Boyd, Edinburgh.

Duke, B. O. L. (1972). Behavioral aspects of the life cycle of *Loa*. *In* "Behavioral Aspects of Parasite Transmission" (E. U. Canning, and C. A. Wright, eds.), pp. 97–107. Linnean Soc. Academic Press, London.

Dunn, F. L. (1966). Patterns of parasitism in primates. *Folia Primatol.* **4**, 329–345.

Dunn, F. L. (1968). Epidemiologic factors: health and disease in hunter-gatherers. *In* "Man The Hunter" (R.B. Lee, and I. Devore, eds.), pp. 221–228. Aldine, Chicago.

Dunn, F. L. (1970). Natural infection in primates: Helminths and problems in primate phylogeny, ecology and behavior. *Lab. Anim. Care* **20**, 383–388.

Dunn, F. L., Lim, B. L., and Tap, L. F. (1968). Endoparasite patterns in mammals of the Malayan rain forest. *Ecology* **49**, 1179–1184.

Dunn, F. L., and Watkins, R. (1970). Parasitological examination of prehistoric human coprolites from Lovelock Cave, Nevada. *Contribution* **10**, 176–185. Archaeol. Res. Facility, Univ. of California, Berkeley.

Dusseau, E. M., and Porter, R. J. (1974). The search for animal parasites in paleo-feces from Upper Salts Cave. *In* "Archaeology of the Mammoth Cave Area" (P. J. Watson, ed.), p. 59. Academic Press, New York.

El-Najjar, M., Bentez, J., Fry, G., Lynn, G. E., Ortner, D. J., Reyman, T. A., and Small, P. A. (1980). Autopsies on two Native American mummies. *Am. J. Phys. Anthropol.* **53**, 197–202.

Esch, G. W., ed. (1977). "Regulation of Parasite Populations." Academic Press, New York.

Esch, G. W., Hazen, T. C., and Aho, J. M. (1977). Parasitism and *r* and *K*-selection. *In* "Regulation of Parasite Populations" (G. W. Esch, ed.), pp. 9–62. Academic Press, New York.

Fallis, A. M. (ed.) (1971). "Ecology and Physiology of Parasites." Hilger, London.

Fenner, F. (1971). Infectious disease and social change: Part 2. *Med. J. Aust.* **1**, 1099–1102.

Ferriera, L. F., de Araujo, A. J., and Confalonieri, U. E. C. (1980). The finding of eggs and larvae of parasitic helminths in archaeological material from Unai, Minas Gerais, Brazil. *Trans. R. Soc. Trop. Med. Hyg.* **74**, 789–799.

Fiennes, F. (1967). "Zoonoses of Primates." Cornell Univ. Press, Ithaca, New York.

Freeland, W. J. (1976). Pathogens and the evolution of primate sociality. *Biotropica* **8**, 12–24.

Fry, G. F., and Moore, J. G. (1969). *Enterobius vermicularis:* 10,000-year-old human infection. *Science* **166**, 1620.

Gantzer, J. (1972). Die Gesichts verstümmelungen auf den Keramiken der Mochica-Kultur (Facial multilations on ceramics of the Mochica culture). *Med. Welt* **23**, 137–141.

Garcia-Kultzback, A. (1976). Medicine among the ancient Maya. *South. Med. J.* **69**, 938–940.

Garnham, P. C. C. (1971). "Progress in Parasitology." Univ. of London, Athlone Press, London.

Guerra, F. (1966). Aztec Medicine. *Med. Hist.* **10,** 315–338.

Hairston, N. C. (1965). On the mathematical analysis of schistosome populations. *Bull. W.H.O.* **33,** 45–62.

Haldane, J. B. S. (1957). Natural selection in man. *Acta Genet. Stat. Med.* **6,** 321–332.

Hawking, F. (1975). Circadian and other rhythms of parasites. *Adv. Parasitol.* **13,** 123–182.

Hoeppli, R. (1956). The knowledge of parasites and parasitic infections from ancient times to the 17th century. *Exp. Parasitol.* **5,** 398.

Hoeppli, R. (1959). "Parasites and Parasitic Infections in Early Medicine and Science." Univ. of Malaya Press, Singapore.

Hoeppli, R. (1969). "Parasitic Disease in Africa and the Western Hemisphere." Verlag für Recht und Geselschalt, Basel.

Hoeppli, R. (1972). Haematuria parasitaria and urinary calculi: early indications from Africa. *Acta Trop.* **29,** 205–217.

Holmes, J. C., and Bethel, W. M. (1972). Modification of intermediate host behavior by parasites. *In* "Behavioral Aspects of Parasite Transmission" (E. U. Canning, and C. A. Wright, eds.), pp. 123–151. Linnean Soc. Academic Press, London.

Hulse, E. V. (1971). Joshua's curse and the abandonment of ancient Jericho: schistosomiasis as possible medical explanation. *Med. Hist.* **15,** 376–386.

Hyman, L. H. (1951a). "The Invertebrates. I. Platyhelminthes and Rhynchocoela. The Acoelomate Bilateria." McGraw Hill, New York.

Hyman, L. H. (1951b). "The Invertebrates, III. Acanthocephala, Aschelminthes, and Entoprocta. The Pseudocoelomate Bilateria." McGraw-Hill, New York.

Inglis, W. G. (1961). The oxyurid parasites (Nematoda) of primates. *Proc. Zool. Soc. London* **136,** 103–122.

Inglis, W. G. (1965). Patterns of evolution in parasitic nematodes. *In* "Evolution of Parasites," *Symp. Br. Soc. Parasitol. 3rd* (A. E. R. Taylor, ed.), pp. 79–124. Blackwell, Oxford.

Inglis, W. G. (1971). Speciation in parasitic nematodes. *Adv. Parasitol.* **9,** 185–223.

Inglis, W. G., and Dunn, F. L. (1964). Some parasites (Nematoda) from neotropical primates. *Z. Parasitenkd* **24,** 83–87.

Kennedy, C. R. (1975). "Ecological Animal Parasitology." Wiley, New York.

Kennedy, C. R., ed. (1976). "Ecological Aspects of Parasitism." North-Holland Publ., Amsterdam.

Kershaw, W. E. (1957). The population dynamics of the filariae of man with particular reference to *Loa loa* and *Onchocerca volvulus. In* "Biological Aspects of the Transmission of Disease" (C. Horton-Smith, ed.), pp. 141–145. Oliver & Boyd, Edinburgh.

Kinnier-Wilson, J. V. (1967). Organic diseases of ancient Mesopotamia. *In* "Diseases in Antiquity" (D. Brothwell, and A. T. Sandison, eds.), pp. 191–208. Thomas, Springfield, Illinois.

Kliks, M. (1975). Paleoepidemiological studies on Great Basin coprolites: Estimation of dietary fiber intake and evaluation of the ingestion of anthelmintic plant substances. *Occasional paper.* Archeol. Res. Facility, Univ. of California, Berkeley.

Llewellyn, J. (1965). The evolution of parasitic platyhelminths. *In* "Evolution of parasites," *Symp. Br. Soc. Parasitol. 3rd* (A. E. R. Taylor, ed.), pp. 47–77. Blackwell, Oxford.

Lu Gwei-Djen, and Needham, J. (1967). Records of diseases in ancient China. *In* "Diseases in Antiquity" (D. Brothwell, and A. T. Sandison, eds.), pp. 222–237. Thomas, Springfield, Illinois.

Luzzatto, L. (1979). Genetics of red cells and susceptibility to malaria. *Blood* **54,** 961–976.

MacDonald, G. (1965). The dynamics of helminth infections with special reference to schistosomes. *Trans. R. Soc. Trop. Med. Hyg.* **59,** 489–506.

McNeil, W. H. (1976). "Plagues and Peoples." Anchor, Garden City, New York.

Manter, H. W. (1967). Some aspects of the geographical distribution of parasites. *J. Parasitol.* **53**, 3–9.

May, R. M. (1977). Togetherness among schistosomes: Its effects on the dynamics of the infection. *Math. Biosci.* **35**, 301–343.

May, R. M., and Anderson, R. M. (1978). Regulation and stability of host–parasite population interactions. II. Destabilizing processes. *J. Anim. Ecol.* **47**, 749–767.

Mollaret, H. H. (1969). L'arche d'alliance et la maladie de Phillistins. Dysenterie, peste, ou parasitose? *Presse Med.* **77**, 2111–2114.

Nelson, G. S. (1965). Filarial infections as zoonoses. *J. Helminthol.* **39**, 229–250.

Nelson, G. S. (1972). Human behavior in the transmission of parasitic diseases. *In* "Behavioral Aspects of Parasite Transmission" (E. U. Canning, and C. A. Wright, eds.), pp. 109–122. Linnean Soc. Academic Press, London.

Nelson, G. S., Teesdale, C., and Highton, R. B. (1962). The role of animals as reservoirs of bilharziasis in Africa. *In* "Bilharziasis," *Ciba Found. Symp.* (G. E. W. Wolstenhome, and M. O'Connor, eds.), pp. 127–156. Little, Brown, Boston.

Noble, E. R., and Noble, G. A. (1971). "Parasitology: The Biology of Animal Parasites." Lea & Febiger, Philadelphia, Pennsylvania.

Odening, K. (1974). Ontogenese and Lebenszyklus bei Helminthen und ihre Widerspiegelung in der Wirtsklassifikation. *Zool. Anz.* **192**, 43–55.

Odum, E. P. (1971). "Fundamentals of Ecology" 3rd ed. Saunders, Philadelphia, Pennsylvania.

Orihel, T. (1970). The helminth parasites of nonhuman primates and man. *Lab. Anim. Care* **20**, 395–401.

Orihel, T. C. (1973). Cerebral filariasis in Rhodesia—a zoonotic infection? *Am. J. Trop. Med. Hyg.* **22**, 596–599.

Osche, G. (1958). Beitrag zur Morphologie, Okologie und Phylogenie der Ascaroidea (Nematoda). Parallelen in der Evolution von Parasit und Wirt. *Z. Parasitenk.* **18**, 479–572.

Osche, G. (1963). Morphological, biological, and ecological considerations in the phylogeny of parasitic Nematodes. *In* "The Lower Metazoa, Comparative Biology and Phylogeny" (E. C. Dougherty, ed.), pp. 283–302. Univ. of California Press, Berkeley.

Pavlovsky, E. N. (1966). "Natural Nidality of Transmissable Diseases" (N. D. Levine, ed.). Univ. of Illinois Press, Urbana.

Price, P. W. (1980). "Evolution and Biology of Parasites." Princeton Univ. Press, Princeton, New Jersey.

Read, B. (1931). Treatment of worm diseases with Chinese drugs. *In* "Pen Ts'ao Kang Mu," with notes. *Nat. Med. J. China* **17**, 644–654.

Rogers, W. P. (1962). "The Nature of Parasitism." Academic Press, New York.

Schad, G. A. (1977). The role of arrested development in the regulation of nematode populations. *In* "Regulation of Parasite Populations" (G. W. Esch, ed.), pp. 111–169. Academic Press, New York.

Schwabe, C. E. (1969). "Veterinary Medicine and Human Health." Williams & Wilkins, Baltimore, Maryland.

Smithers, S. R. (1976). Immunity to trematode infections with special reference to schistosomiasis and fascioliasis. *In* "Immunology of Parasitic Infections" (S. Cohen, and E. H. Sadun, eds.), pp. 296–332. Blackwell, Oxford.

Smyth, J. D. (1964). Genetical aspects of speciation in trematodes and cestodes: some speculations. *Int. Congr. Parasitol, 1st, Rome* **1**, 473–475.

Sprent, J. F. A. (1962). Parasitism, immunity and evolution. *In* "The Evolution of Living Organisms" (G. S. Leeper, ed.), pp. 149–165. Melbourne Univ. Press, Melbourne.

Sprent, J. F. A. (1969a). Evolutionary aspects of immunity of zooparasitic infections. *In* "Immunity to Parasitic Animals" (G. J. Jackson, ed.), pp. 3–62. Appleton, New York.

Sprent, J. F. A. (1969b). Helminth "zoonoses": an analysis. *Helminthol. Abstr.* **38,** 333–351.

Stanley, N. F., and Alpers, M. P., eds. (1975). "Man-Made Lakes and Human Health." Academic Press, London.

Stiles, C. W., and Hassal, A. (1929). Key-catalog of parasites reported for primates (monkeys-lemurs) with their possible public health importance and key-catalog of primates from which parasites are reported by C. W. Stiles, and Nolan, M. B. *Hyg. Lab. Bull.* **152.** U.S. Govt. Printing Office, Washington, D.C.

Stone, W., and Smith, F. W. (1973). Infection of mammalian hosts by milk-borne nematode larvae: A review. *Exp. Parasitol.* **34,** 306–312.

Stunkard, H. W. (1962). The organization, ontogeny and orientation of the Cestoda. *Q. Rev. Biol.* **37,** 23–44.

Stunkard, H. W. (1963). Systematics, taxonomy and nomenclature of the Trematoda. *Q. Rev. Biol.* **38,** 221–233.

Sussman, M. (1967). Disease in the Bible and the Talmud. *In* "Diseases in Antiquity" (D. Brothwell, and A. T. Sandison, eds.), pp. 209–221. Thomas, Springfield, Illinois.

Thompson, R. C. (1923). "Assyrian Medical Texts." Mifford, Oxford.

Washburn, S. L., and DeVore, I. (1961). Social life of baboons and early man. *In* "Social Life of Early Man" (S. L. Washburn, ed.), pp. 91–105. Aldine, Chicago.

Wei, O. (1973). Internal organs of a 2100 year-old female corpse. *Lancet* **2,** 1198.

Wells, C. (1978). Disease and evolution. *Biol. Hum. Affairs* **43,** 1–13.

Whitlock, J. H. (1977). "The Population Biology of Disease." Div. Biol. Sci., New York State College Vet. Med. Cornell University, Ithaca, New York.

Whitlock, J. H., Crofton, H. D., and Georgi, J. R. (1972). Characteristics of parasite populations in endemic trichostrongyloidosis. *Parasitology* **64,** 413–427.

Wilke, P. J., and Hall, H. J. (1975). Analysis of ancient feces: A descriptive bibliography. *Occasional paper.* Arch. Res. Facility, Univ. of California, Berkeley.

W.H.O. (1967). Joint FAO/WHO Expert Committee on Zoonoses. 3rd report. *W.H.O. Tech. Rep. Ser.* **378.**

Wright, C. A. (1977). The ecology of African schistosomiasis. *In* "Human Ecology in the Tropics" (J. P. Garlick, and W. J. Keay, eds.), pp. 127–143. Halstead, New York.

Yamaguti, S. (1958–1961). "Systema Helminthum" Vol. *I, II, III, IV.* Wiley (Interscience), New York.

Yamashita, J. (1963). Ecological relationships between parasites and primates. I. Helminth parasites and primates. *Primates* **4,** 1–96.

Zimmerman, M. R., and Smith, G. S. (1975). A probable case of accidental inhumation of 1600 years ago. *Bull. N.Y. Acad. Med.* **2,** 828–837.

Brucellosis in Nigeria: Epidemiology and Practical Problems of Control

OLANIPEKUN K. ALAUSA

Department of Epidemiology and Community Health
University of Ilorin
Ilorin, Kwara, Nigeria

I. Introduction

A. The World of Zoonoses

Zoonoses are those diseases and infections that are naturally transmitted between vertebrate animals and man (W.H.O., 1958). Since the dawn of history the diseases of man have been compared with those of animals. It was not, however, until the discovery of the pathogenic properties of certain bacteria and other lower organisms that similarities between several communicable diseases of man and animals were properly assessed. Until the beginning of the present century, the animal origin of only a small number of human diseases had been recognized (rabies, cowpox, anthrax, and a few zooparasitic infections). At the present time, far more than 100 zoonoses are known. In fact, it has become evident that the animal world is a reservoir for the agents of numerous human diseases (W.H.O., 1959), and there is ample reason to believe that most of the present infectious diseases of the human race have originated in animals. The pathogenic organisms adapted themselves to the environment of the human body as either parasites or commensals. The effects produced in both man and animals are mainly deter- mined by the invasive capacities of the pathogen and the host's resistance to it. Zoonoses are among the commonest hazards to man, especially so in the tropical and subtropical areas where arthropod vectors may play a significant role in their transmission.

B. Important Historical Aspects of Brucellosis as a Zoonosis

The term *brucellosis* is applied to an infectious disease occurring in many species of animals and man and attributable to infection with bacterial organisms of the genus *Brucella,* the first member of which was discovered by Sir David Bruce in 1886 (Bruce, 1887). Brucellosis is a zoonosis, primarily an infectious disease of domestic animals which, under special circumstances, may readily be transmitted to man through contact, ingestion, inhalation, and accidental inocu- lation (W.H.O., 1971). The animals that are known to serve commonly as sources of human infection are cattle, goats, sheep, and swine.

Brucellosis has been present in hoofed animals since ancient times. The fos- silized remains of animals in certain regions show bone changes consistent with those observed in brucellosis. The European bison, the Persian hillgoat, and the Maltese goat have been suffering from brucellosis for a long time (Van der Hoeden, 1964). The first clinical report of the disease in man is ascribed to Hippocrates, as early as the fifth century B.C. Later, diseases resembling bru- cellosis were frequently reported in the Mediterranean area. Brucellosis reached Spain in the fifteenth century and was brought to the New World by the Span- iards. Malta acquired importance as a focus for the spread of brucellosis during the Crimean War, when the disease was differentiated specifically from other febrile ailments in the area.

The relationship of the disease in animals to human infection was first recog- nized in 1906 when Themistocles Zammit, a Maltese physician and member of the British Mediterranean Fever Commission, showed that man acquired "Malta fever" by drinking infected goat's milk; this observation was an outstanding landmark in the epidemiology of brucellosis. The first practical method in the prevention and control of human brucellosis was demonstrated in 1908 when the ban of the consumption of unboiled goat milk among the troops stationed in Malta led to a remarkable drop in the number of cases and deaths among the military population.

C. Global Geographical Distribution of Brucellosis

The distribution of brucellosis in man and animals is practically worldwide, and available official statistics as well as the literature indicate that human cases have been reported in Europe, North America, Asia, South America, and Africa, including Kenya and Nigeria (Mediterranean Fever Commission, 1905–1907; Spink, 1956; Dalrymple-Champneys, 1960; W.H.O., 1964; Roy *et al.*, 1965; Cox, 1966; W.H.O., 1973; Esuruoso, 1974a; Alausa, 1977). Bovine brucellosis caused by *B. abortus* has the widest distribution and has occurred in nearly every country of the world (W.H.O., 1971).

The epidemiological pattern of brucellosis among the populations of different countries usually depends on the predominant type of farm animals that serve as reservoirs and sources of human infection. Spread of infection from man to man very rarely occurs. By contrast, infection of animals is an important factor in the ecology of *Brucella,* because infected animals readily infect one another. However, man's role in the spread of infection among animals is still an important one; by domesticating the animals and herding them together he provides conditions which, although age-old, are unnatural and greatly increase the ease with which *Brucella* spp. survive both inside and outside their hosts. Thus, man's risk of infection is closely related to the endemicity of animal infection, the methods of animal husbandry, human food habits, the standards of hygiene, and economic activities involving animals which are known to serve as sources of human infection. Contact with aborting and infected animals, consumption of infected milk, milk products, and meat, exposure to aerosols of infective dust, and handling wool or infected animals in the slaughterhouse all increase human risk. This is the case in tropical African countries with developing livestock industries where herding of animals still remains largely traditional and unscientific. The geographical and epidemiological picture of brucellosis therefore varies from area to area in different parts of the world, and local factors have to be studied carefully in planning control and eradication programs.

The incidence and prevalence of brucellosis in man and animals is difficult to determine in any particular locality, and therefore is not known accurately in many parts of the world. As in tuberculosis, the reported cases may bear very little relation to the real incidence/prevalence of infection (Wilson and Miles, 1964). Brucellosis is unfamiliar to practitioners in many countries, particularly in West Africa (Alausa, 1979b). Not all countries require physicians to report cases of brucellosis (undulant fever), and veterinarians do not report cases of infectious abortion to public health authorities. Therefore, data on incidence and/or prevalence may be deceptive. In most developed and economically advanced countries where epidemiological surveillance is observed and cases are reported to the public health authorities, the incidence/prevalence of brucellosis may appear high, but in developing and economically poor countries without facilities for surveillance, few or no cases may be reported although infection may be rife.

D. Worldwide Socioeconomic Significance of Brucellosis

Brucellosis is of particular importance among the zoonoses, not only because of its direct impact on man's health but also because of the economic losses and reductions in animal protein supplies for which it is responsible. The gravity of brucellosis in terms of human illness, physical incapacity, and loss of manpower, in addition to economic loss, remains a matter of major concern in many parts of the world. This realization led to the formation of the Joint F.A.O./W.H.O. Expert Committee on Brucellosis which meets periodically to discuss and review current problems in human and animal populations. In many countries brucellosis contributes substantially to a low standard of living and the World Health Assembly (W.H.O., 1969), recognizing this fact, requested both F.A.O. and W.H.O. to assist member countries in assessing, in a more analytical and systematic manner, the economic losses caused by brucellosis and the cost of services combating it. W.H.O. therefore has drawn up guidelines for such studies which are required whenever funds are requested from national and international sources (W.H.O., 1971; Guidelines, 1972).

II. Description of Nigeria and Information on Livestock Activities

A. General Information and Demographic Characteristics

Nigeria is the largest country in West Africa. It lies between latitude 4° 21' and 14° north of the equator and between longitude 2° 20' and 14° 30'; thus, it is situated entirely within the tropics. It occupies an area of approximately 92 million ha, extending from the southern coastline northward for over 1040 km; from the western border to the east is 1120 km at the widest part. Figure 1 is a map of Africa showing the geographical boundaries of Nigeria and its size relative to other countries in West Africa. Its population of over 80 million (unofficial 1973 census figure) is by far the largest in Africa; approximately 70%

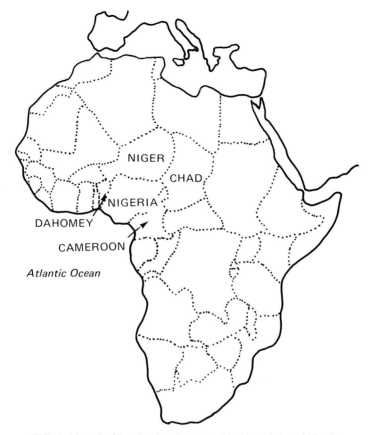

FIG. 1. Map of Africa showing the geographical boundaries of Nigeria.

of the population live in rural areas that lack basic and infrastructural social amenities. Nigeria operates under a federal system of government, with 19 states and a federal capital in Lagos.

Specific demographic and health data are not readily available in Nigeria since there is no national registration of births, diseases (except internationally reportable and epidemic diseases), and deaths in most parts of the country. Thus vital statistics and similar specific data are usually estimated. The demographic characteristics of Nigeria, as "estimated" by the W.H.O. African Region (W.H.O., 1976) are summarized as follows

1. Population density, between 90 and 150 inhabitants/km² (in the northern states, with a high nomadic population, it can be less than 50 inhabitants/km²)
2. Crude birth rate, 49.6/1000 population
3. Crude death rate, 24.9/1000 population

4. Infant mortality rate, not available (probably about 150 per 1000 live births)
5. Population growth rate, approximately 2.5%
6. Population under 15 years, approximately 40%
7. Life expectancy at birth, about 52 years
8. Literacy rate, 20 to 40% (lower in the north than south)
9. Per capita gross national product (G.N.P.) US $500 (grossly unevenly distributed)

Medical and health facilities in Nigeria are mainly hospital based in urban areas, with emphasis on curative rather than on preventive services. The remote agricultural rural areas, where the majority of the population lives, are deprived of health services. These people, who are mainly peasant farmers, rely heavily on traditional methods of medicine. In 1980, the total number of registered physicians in Nigeria was just over 5000; during this same year, there were fewer than 500 veterinary doctors working in the whole country.

B. Information on Economic and Livestock Activities in Nigeria

All the various governments of the federation emphasize the development of industrial enterprises but recognize fundamentally that agriculture is a significant aspect of the country's overall socioeconomic development. Thus agricultural products and crude petroleum constitute the basis of the country's economy and foreign capital.

Cattle, sheep, and goats form a considerable part of the internal economy of the northern states of Nigeria where the number of cattle per population is highest. Over 90% of the estimated 8.5 million head of cattle in Nigeria belonged to the Fulani nomads of the northern states (Sanwo, 1975). Some of these nomadic Fulani herd their cattle, which number over 1 million annually, through marked animal tracks and by roads down from the north to feed the great centers of population in the more southernly parts of the country. The hides and skins from these animals represent one of the country's major exports, bringing in over 30 million Nigerian naira (US $62 million) each year.

Nigeria still imports a considerable number of cattle from neighboring northern countries, notably the Republics of Niger and Chad. In 1974 alone, about 300,000 cattle entered Nigeria from Niger and Chad through marked routes between the Nigerian northern borders and these neighboring countries without observing any international health regulations. As incomes continue to rise in Nigeria, the demand for meat and therefore for livestock production and importation increases. Beef is the animal protein most readily available to the majority of Nigerians.

Although Nigeria has embarked on development of her livestock industry, its management still remains largely with nomadic herdsmen who have an extensive grazing system moving with their cattle from one place to another at 6- to 9-month intervals. Therefore, the growth rate and productivity of breeding animals are low due mainly to reproductive diseases in dairy and beef cattle. The country's herd population growth rate is estimated at about 1.5%/year, whereas the human population growth is estimated at about 2.5%/year (Sanwo, 1975; W.H.O., 1976). Most of the settled herds in Nigeria are privately owned with little or no veterinary supervision.

Generally, the Fulani-raised cattle are sold to butchers at lower prices than are government-raised animals. Therefore, livestock dealers buy cattle from the nomadic Fulanis at low, reasonable prices and resell them to butchers at higher prices. However, according to the Fulani tradition cattle from nomadic herds are normally sold only under certain conditions, the important ones being (1) when there is high and favorable calf production and (2) when money is needed for an "essential" or urgent expenditure, including family maintenance, marriages, or holy pilgrimages to Saudi Arabia. Thus, when the calf production is reduced or depleted for whatever reason, the Fulani nomadic herdsmen will retain their remaining cattle. The Fulanis measure economic achievement as the total number of cattle they own at a particular time rather than their cash value; they prefer to withdraw all their savings from the bank than to reduce the number of their cattle. The Fulanis also prefer to consume large quantities of raw milk (which may be infected with *Brucella abortus* organisms) rather than to slaughter and eat their own cattle.

There are very few meat-packing facilities in the country, and the surroundings of most of the local council-managed abattoirs are dirty, lacking good environmental sanitation. The butchers and meat sellers often wear torn clothes exposing parts of their bodies. In addition, animals are privately slaughtered on a large scale in Nigeria, particularly during ceremonies (marriages, funerals, birthday parties) and religious festivals. Retail distribution of meat products takes place under deplorable sanitary conditions in public markets and streets, very often without previous inspection by public health authorities. These situations obviously encourage direct spread of *Brucella abortus* from infected animals to abattoir workers, meat vendors, and consumers.

III. Epidemiology of Brucellosis in Nigeria

A. Infection of Animals with *Brucella abortus* (Bovine Brucellosis)

Within the past two decades, observations on nomadic herds of cattle and flocks of sheep and goats in the northern states of Nigeria, and on many government-owned, settled cattle herds in different parts of the country, have revealed that bovine brucellosis is widespread in Nigeria; there is a pattern of low and high infection rates in specific areas (Esuruoso, 1965; Adams and McKay, 1966; Banerjee and Bhatty, 1970; Esuruoso and Hill, 1971; Esuruoso and Van Blake, 1972; Esuruoso, 1974a). The infection rate was as high as 60% among breeding cows and heifers investigated in the western states of Nigeria (Esuruoso, 1974a), but only 4.27% of 2550 goats sampled in different parts of the country had *B. abortus* agglutinin titers of 50 I.U. or more (Falade *et al.*, 1976).

In other parts of the country, especially in the northern states, the infection rates in the various herds have been generally low; 0–20% of animals examined showed serological evidence of infection. Among the reasons that were given for the apparent difference in infection rates between cattle in the two areas of the country were (1) that the cattle in nomadic herds in the north are constantly moving and are therefore not likely to accumulate infection or spread it to each other as effectively as settled herds in the west and (2) that nomadic herding in the intense savanna heat of the north probably imposes a natural limit on the rate of *B. abortus* infection of cattle. However, the nomadic animals do come together in relatively small areas at certain seasons when watering places and grazing area are restricted and herds have to converge for survival. During this period, high infection rates as were observed in the settled herds in the south may occur (Fig. 2).

Cattle traded in and from the northern states, and those from across the Nigerian borders from the Republics of Chad and Niger, also showed serological evidence of infection (Esuruoso, 1974b). This clearly indicates that brucellosis in Nigeria cannot be considered as only a national problem.

Epidemiological investigations of bovine brucellosis in western Nigeria have also revealed high rates of infertility and abortions among cattle under various management regimes (nomadic or settled herds). For instance, an abortion rate of 42% was reported among pregnant cows on one farm estate, where serological evidence of bovine brucellosis remained at 50% (Esuruoso, 1974b). Periodically, outbreaks of active bovine brucellosis occur in which a very large herd is involved, resulting in heavy economic loss to the farmers and severe social disruption to the immediate human community (Alausa, 1979a).

The high prevalence of brucellosis among range cattle in many states of Nigeria can cause abortion and affect the fertility rate resulting in heavy economic loss to the livestock industry in the country.

B. Epidemiology of Human Brucellosis

In Nigeria many more people are choosing livestock farming because of the government's financial incentives to farmers to increase food production for the

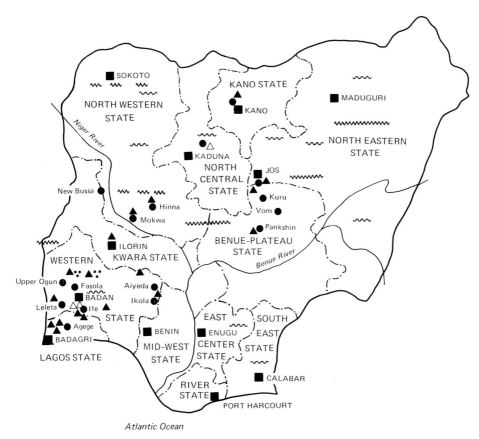

FIG. 2. Distribution of bovine brucellosis in Nigeria (Esuruoso, 1974b). —·— = state boundaries, ■ = state capitals, ● = locations of herds and slaughter houses recently sampled for brucellosis, ▲ = locations of herds with brucellosis reactors, △ = locations of slaughtered cattle with brucellosis reactors, ∴ = locations of cattle where *Brucella abortus* has been isolated, ⁓ = sources of trace cattle found to be reactors at slaughter, ∿ = areas where brucellosis has been reported (Adams and McKay, 1966; Banerjee and Bhatty, 1970; Esuruoso and Hill, 1971; Esuruoso and Van Blake, 1972).

increasing human population. Thus, larger numbers of people are being exposed to risks of *B. abortus* infection, and many of them have no immediate or direct access to effective medical care.

Extensive epidemiological studies have revealed a significantly higher prevalence of infection among those persons who are occupationally exposed, including herdsmen, abattoir workers, and veterinarians, than among the occupationally nonexposed population, including blood donors and normal pregnant women (Alausa and Osoba, 1975; Alausa and Awoseyi, 1976; Alausa, 1977;

Alausa, 1979a). Of 1192 people who were regarded as nonexposed to risk of *B. abortus* infection in western Nigeria, only 11.4% were found to have significant titers of *Brucella abortus* agglutinin (of 100 I.U. or more), whereas 31.8% out of 569 known to be occupationally exposed to risk of infection had a significant titer of *B. abortus* agglutinin ($p < .001$) (Table I) (Alausa and Awoseyi, 1976; Alausa, 1977).

The prevalence and the level of human *B. abortus* infection have been found to be significantly higher among the northern population than in the people living in the western states of the country. Among the occupationally nonexposed groups, 21.3% of the 178 northerners examined had antibody titers of 100 I.U. or more; among the occupationally exposed groups, 70.4% of the 71 northerners examined had high antibody titers (100 I.U. or more). The differences in the infection rates among the corresponding groups in western and northern states were statistically significant ($p < .001$) (Alausa, 1977) (Table II).

Although the number of cattle per person is highest in northern states of the country, animals in settled herds in western states have higher rates of bovine brucellosis than do the nomadic herds of northern states. Nevertheless, among the human populations in Nigeria the northerners showed higher *Brucella* infection rates than the people living in the western states. Therefore, consideration of the prevalence and level of human infection caused by *B. abortus* in Nigeria should be based upon the following important factors:

1. The geographical location of the livestock farm; whether the farm is located in the north or south of the country (Alausa, 1977).
2. The number of cattle per human population (Alausa, 1977).

TABLE I

Seroepidemiological Evaluation of *Brucella abortus* Antibodies in Western Nigeria

	Antibody Titer (I.U.)						
	<25	25	50	100	200	>400	Total
Group A: Cross-section of healthy population:							
Blood donors, UCH Ibadan (479), Antenatal Women (713)	563	250	243	104	28	4	1192
(%)	(47.2)	(21)	(20.4)	(8.7)	(2.4)	(0.3)	(100)
Group B: Occupationally exposed population:							
Abattoir workers, veterinarians, dairy farmers, and herdsmen around Ibadan, Fashola, and Igbo-Ora	196	78	114	102	47	32	569
(%)	(34.5)	(13.7)	(20)	(17.9)	(8.3)	(5.6)	(100)
Total	759	328	357	206	75	36	1761
(%)	(43.1)	(18.6)	(20.3)	(11.7)	(4.3)	(2.0)	(100)

TABLE II

Seroepidemiological Evaluation of *Brucella abortus* Antibodies in Northern Nigeria

	Antibody Titer (I.U.)						
	<25	25	50	100	200	>400	Total
Group A: Cross-section of healthy population:							
blood donors at A.B.U., Zaria	60	43	37	23	10	5	178
(%)	(33.7)	(24.2)	(20.8)	(12.9)	(5.6)	(2.8)	(100)
Group B: Occupationally exposed population:							
herdsmen around Jos, Kaduna, Zaria, Kano	2	3	16	28	13	9	71
(%)	(2.8)	(4.2)	(22.5)	(39.4)	(18.3)	(12.7)	(100)
Total	62	46	53	51	23	14	249
(%)	(24.9)	(18.5)	(21.3)	(20.5)	(9.2)	(5.6)	(100)

3. The rate of active infection in the cattle herd (Alausa and Awoseyi, 1975) and the level of human exposure (Fig. 3) and occupational contact with infected animals (Alausa, 1977, 1980).
4. The system of animal husbandry whether nomadic or settled herds (human infection in areas of nomadic animal husbandry is common) (Abdussalam and Fein, 1975).

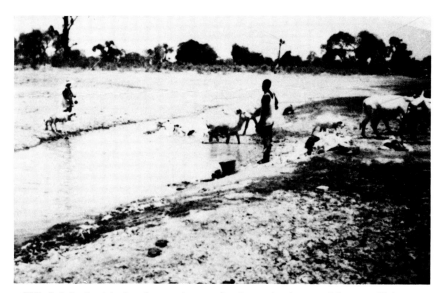

FIG. 3. Irrigation lake in a farm settlement, showing cattle, sheep, and farmers utilizing water from the same source.

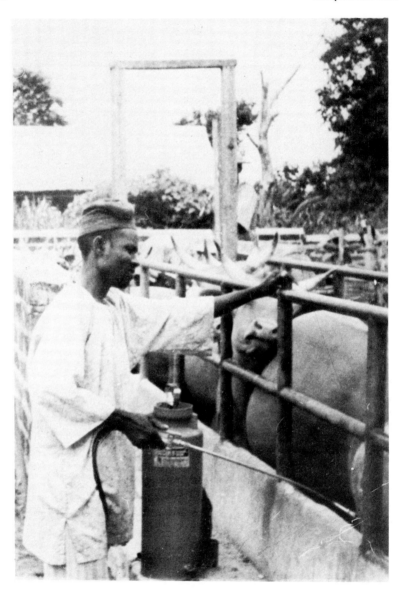

FIG. 4. Livestock worker without protective clothing applying disinfectant to cows in a settled herd.

5. Imported bovine infection from neighboring countries: cattle imported from the Republics of Niger, Chad, and Guinea were found to show serological evidence of *B. abortus* infection (Esuruoso, 1974b).

The important identifiable sources of *B. abortus* infections of man in Nigeria include

1. Direct transmission from infected animals through abraded skin, nasopharyngeal mucosa, and the conjunctivae among the traditional livestock farmers and abattoir workers as a result of poor personal hygiene, unsanitary workplace environmental conditions, and unscientific livestock management (Fig. 4); aerosol infection through the mucous membrane of the respiratory tract.
2. Ingestion of infected milk, especially on the farms, or eating of half-roasted meat (barbecued), which is a popular menu at social gatherings among elite urbanites.

C. Important Clinical Considerations of Human Brucellosis in Nigeria

Although the rate of infection among occupationally exposed individuals is high in Nigeria, the prevalence and incidence of active and clinical brucellosis is very low. Thus, most of the people showing serological evidence of brucellosis in the country have subclinical infection. In a longitudinal survey between 1973 and 1976 among 326 people from different occupational groups, including veterinary staff, meat vendors, and dairy farmers in Ibadan (capital of a western state of Nigeria), 11 were found with high *Brucella*-saline-agglutinating (S.A.T.) titers of 400 I.U. and higher, using the laboratory method described by Kerr *et al.* (1968). All 11 people were symptom-free when their initial blood samples were collected in 1973, and subsequently in 1974 and 1975. In addition, *B. abortus* agglutination tests in the presence of 2-mercaptoethanol (2-ME test) were negative for the same 11 people (Alausa and Osoba, 1977). The 2-ME test distinguishes between the two immunoglobulins, IgG and IgM, responsible for agglutination in the saline agglutination test (S.A.T.). The addition of 2-ME destroys the agglutinating activity of IgM (Anderson *et al.*, 1964). Agglutination in the presence of 2-ME is therefore due to IgG and is indicative of active *Brucella* infection (Reddin *et al.*, 1965; Kerr *et al.*, 1966; Wilkinson, 1966; Kerr *et al.*, 1968; Elberg, 1973). Although these 11 individuals showed no clinical evidence of active brucellosis during the 2-year period of follow-up, the levels of their anti-*Brucella* antibodies (by the S.A.T. test) remained high at 400 I.U. and higher throughout the study (Alausa, 1977b).

Abbatoir and similar workers who are repeatedly exposed to *B. abortus* are known to suffer from active infection only rarely (Henderson and Hill, 1972). This might be attributed to the biological behaviour of *B. abortus,* which has a high degree of infectivity but a low level of pathogenicity in man (Christie, 1974). As *B. abortus* is the most common species encountered in Nigeria, this explains why the rate of active *B. abortus* infection among the occupationally exposed human population is low.

Protection against many bacterial and viral diseases by natural active immunity resulting from subclinical infection is well known. Subclinical *Brucella* infection, giving rise to antibody formation in different groups of people occupationally or accidentally exposed to *B. abortus,* has also been reported by many workers in Europe and America (Henderson and Hill, 1972).

The presence of subclinical infection with varying levels of humoral antibody to *B. abortus* among those who have been in contact with infected cattle should therefore always be kept in mind by physicians if misdiagnosis of some fatal disease[1] simulating brucellosis is to be avoided. This needs to be particularly reemphasized in tropical areas where many diseases can simulate acute brucellosis. Therefore, a positive S.A.T. antibody should not be accepted as the only reason for making a diagnosis of brucellosis in a patient occupationally exposed to *B. abortus* in Nigeria.

Occasionally, large-scale outbreaks of active bovine brucellosis that could spread to the occupationally exposed human population may result in a sudden increase in the incidence of acute human brucellosis in a particular geographical area. Such an outbreak was encountered and investigated in 1976 in Ibarapa Division of Oyo State of Nigeria when 11 nomadic herds consisting of 782 animals were found with acute bovine brucellosis; 89 (51.4%) of the total 173 herdsmen involved had acute brucellosis. In addition, 12 (23.5%) of the 51 abattoir workers in the area contracted acute brucellosis (Alausa, 1979a). Ecological, cultural, and socioeconomic factors contributed immensely to the causation, propagation, epidemiological investigation, and eventual control of the episode.

IV. Prevention and Control of Brucellosis in Nigeria

Human brucellosis is mainly an occupational disease in Nigeria, and therefore realistic control measures should be along the following three major lines.

---

[1]The important differential diagnosis of brucellosis in tropical countries includes (at least) malaria, typhoid fever, pulmonary tuberculosis, hepatic cirrhosis, Hodgkins' disease, sarcoidosis, rheumatic fever, subacute bacterial endocarditis, appendicitis, and psychoneurosis.

A. Limitation and Control of Infection in Animal Reservoirs

This can be achieved through the establishment of a State–Federal Joint Brucellosis Control Program, similar to the initial control program in the United States in 1934 (Busch and Parker, 1972). The Federal Government of Nigeria should be responsible for the interstate and international control regulations against importation of infected animals into the country and for movement of animals between States. The various state governments in Nigeria should be responsible for the control program within their respective jurisdictions.

Because the ideal approach to prevention of human infection, requiring complete eradication of infection in animals through the slaughter policy, is presently impracticable in Nigeria, a selective vaccination program for beef cattle in settled herds should be introduced because of the present high prevalence of brucellosis in the animal population in different parts of the country. Vaccination of nomadic herds will however still present some difficulties.

B. Control of Contaminated Environment and Animal Products

This requires that scientific farming should be encouraged, modern meat-packing houses be built, and health education of livestock farmers and meat handlers be intensified in different parts of the country. Good sanitation and proper hygiene should be maintained on the farms and in meat houses. Personnel should wear coveralls, gloves, and goggles to prevent direct infection through abraded skin and the conjunctivae. Raw milk should be avoided until regular screening services can be provided on the farms.

C. Prevention and Elimination of Human Infection

This can be realistically approached at present in Nigeria through (1) careful control of working conditions and periodic screening of livestock farmers and handlers and (2) early diagnosis and treatment of active cases of human brucellosis. Thus, one of the important aspects of any brucellosis control program in Nigeria is the provision of adequate facilities for the early diagnosis of the infection in different parts of the country. This would probably involve the establishment of industrial or occupational health services, which would need support by many peripheral public health laboratories. These essential social services, at present very scarce in Nigeria, are located mainly in urban centers.

Vaccination of exposed people as a method of controlling brucellosis, suggested by Versilova (1965) and practiced in the Soviet Union, is not considered suitable in the Nigerian situation despite prevailing poor standards of beef and dairy farming management and a high probability of occupational human infection. Apart from the well-known disadvantages associated with human vaccination (Christie, 1974; Spink *et al.*, 1962; Pappagianis *et al.*, 1966), the vaccine is usually indicated for occupational groups exposed to infection with *B. melitensis* (W.H.O., 1971). In Nigeria, human *Brucella* infection is largely caused by *B. abortus* which is recognized to be of low pathogenicity for man.

References

Abdussalm, M., and Fein, D. A. (1975). Brucellosis as a world problem. International symposium on brucellosis (II), Rabat, 1975. *Dev. Biol. Stand.* **31**, 9. (S. Karger, Basel, 1976).

Adams, J. W., and McKay, J. (1966). Bovine brucellosis survey in Northern Nigeria. *Nature (London)* **212**, 217.

Alausa, O. K. (1977). Brucellosis: epidemiology and practical problems of control in Nigeria. *Public Health* **91**, 141.

Alausa, O. K. (1979a). The investigation and control of a large-scale community outbreak of brucellosis in Nigeria. *Public Health* **93**, 185.

Alausa, O. K. (1979b). Human brucellosis in Nigeria: clinical aspects and its importance as an occupational disease. *Ghana Med. J.* **18**, 3.

Alausa, O. K. (1980). Incidence and seasonal prevalence among an occupationally-exposed population to brucellosis. *Trop. Geogr. Med.* **32**, 12.

Alausa, K. O., and Awoseyi, A. (1976). Brucellosis: the situation in western Nigeria. *Trop. Geogr. Med.* **28**, 54.

Alausa, K. O., and Osoba, A. O. (1975). Brucella seroreactivity in Western Nigeria (an epidemiological study). *Trans. R. Soc. Trop. Med. Hyg.* **69**, 259.

Alausa, O., and Osoba, A. O. (1977). Subclinical human *Brucella* infection in Ibadan, Nigeria. *Ghana Med. J.* **16**, 251.

Anderson, R. K., Jenness, R., Brumfield, H. P., and Gough, P. (1964). *Brucella*-agglutinating antibodies: relationship of mercaptoethanol. *Science* **143**, 1334.

Banerjee, A. K., and Bhatty, M. A. (1970). A survey of bovine brucellosis in northern Nigeria (a preliminary communication). *Bull. Epizoot. Dis. Afr.* **18**, 333.

Bruce, D. (1887). Note on the discovery of a micro-organism in Malta Fever. *Practitioner* **39**, 161.

Busch, L. A., and Parker, R. L. (1972). Brucellosis in the United States. *J. Infect. Dis.* **125**, 239.

Christie, A. B. (1974). Brucellosis. *In* "Infectious Diseases: Epidemiology and Clinical Practice," 2nd ed., p. 842. Livingstone, London.

Cox, P. (1966). Brucellosis: a survey in south Karamoja. *East Afr. Med. J.* **43**, 43.

Dalrymple-Champneys, W. (1960). "Brucella Infection and Undulant Fever in Man", pp. 1–196. Oxford Univ. Press, London.

Elberg, S. S. (1973). Immunity to brucella infection. *Medicine (Baltimore)* **62**, 239.

Esuruoso, G. O. (1965). Brucellosis in moor plantation dairy. *In* "Ministry of Agriculture and Natural Resources, Western Region of Nigeria—Official Report."

Esuruoso, G. O. (1974a). Bovine brucellosis in two southern states of Nigeria. II. The incidence and implications of infection in range cattle. *Bull. Epizoot. Dis. Afr.* **22**, 35.

Esuruoso, G. O. (1974b). Bovine brucellosis in Nigeria. *Vet. Rec.* **95**, 54.

Esuruoso, G. O., and Hill, D. H. (1971). Sero-epidemiological survey of bovine brucellosis in the dairy herds of western state of Nigeria. *Niger. Agric. J.* **8**, 147.

Esuruoso, G. O., and Van Blake, H. E. (1972). Bovine brucellosis in two southern states of Nigeria. I. An investigation of selected herds. *Bull. Epizoot. Dis. Afr.* **20**, 269.

Falade, S., Sellers, K. C., and Ojo, M. O. (1976). A serological survey of caprine brucellosis in Nigeria. *Bull. Epizoot. Afr.* **4**, 335.

Guidelines (1972). Preparation and evaluation of bovine brucellosis programs and criteria and principles for the analysis of bovine brucellosis programs. Proc. Inter-American Meet. on Foot-and-Mouth Disease and Zoonoses Control, 4th. *PAHO Sci. Publ.* **236**, 96.

Henderson, R. J., and Hill, D. M. (1972). Subclinical brucella infections in man. *Br. Med. J.* **3**, 154.

Kerr, W. R., Coghlan, J. D., Payne, D. J. H., and Robertson, L. (1966). The laboratory diagnosis of chronic brucellosis. *Lancet* **2**, 1181.

Kerr, W., McCaughey, W. J., Coghlan, J., Payne, D., Quaife, R., Robertson, L., and Farrell, I. (1968). Techniques and interpretations in the serological diagnosis of brucellosis in Man. *J. Med. Microbiol.* **1**, 181.

Mediterranean Fever Commission (1905–07). Reports of the Commission Appointed by the Admiralty, the War Office, and the Civil Government of Malta, for the Investigations of Mediterranean Fever, under the Supervision of an Advisory Committee of the Royal Society. Harrison, London.

Pappagianis, D., Elberg, S. S., and Cough, D. (1966). Immunization against brucella infection: effects of graded dose of viable attenuated *Brucella melitensis* in humans. *Am. J. Epidemiol.* **84**, 21.

Reddin, J. L., Anderson, R. K., Jenness, R., and Spink, W. W. (1965). Significance of 7S and macroglobulin agglutinins in human brucellosis. *N. Engl. J. Med.* **272**, 1263.

Roy, P. B., Mehta, N. R., Asnomi, K. G., Shah, H. H., and Maharjan, B. K. (1965). Serological study of brucellosis in man and cattle in Jammagar. *Indian J. Med. Res.* **9**, 822.

Sanwo, P. (1975). Causes of cattle shortage. *Daily Times of Nigeria.* July 26, 1975 p. 19.

Spink, W. W. (1956). *In* "The Nature of Brucellosis," 464 pp. Minnesota Univ. Press, Minneapolis.

Spink, W. W., Hall, J. W., Finstad, J., and Mallet, E. (1962). Immunization with viable *Brucella* organisms. Result of a safety test in humans. *Bull W.H.O.* **26**, 409.

Van der Hoeden, J. (1964). "Zoonoses." Elsevier, London.

Versilova, P. A. (1965). Ways of prophylaxis of brucellosis among the population of U.S.S.R. *Indian J. Pathol. Bacteriol.* **8**, 1.

Wilkinson, P. C. (1966). Immunoglobulin. Patterns of antibodies against *Brucella* in man and animals. *J. Immunol.* **96**, 457.

Wilson, G. S., and Miles, A. A. (1964). *In* "Topley and Wilson's Principles of Bacteriology and Immunity," 5th ed., p. 2039. Arnold, London.

World Health Organization (1958). Joint FAO/WHO Expert Committee on Brucellosis (3rd Report). *W.H.O. Tech. Rep. Ser.* **148**. Geneva.

World Health Organization (1959). Immunological and Haematological Surveys: Report of a Study Group. *W.H.O. Tech. Rep. Ser.* **181**. Geneva.

World Health Organization (1964). Joint FAO/WHO Expert Committee on Brucellosis (4th Report). *W.H.O. Tech. Rep. Ser.* **289**. Geneva.

World Health Organization (1969). Resolution W.H.A. 22. 35. *W.H.O. Off. Rec.* **176**, 16. Geneva.

World Health Organization (1971). Joint FAO/WHO Expert Committee on Brucellosis (5th Report). *W.H.O. Tech. Rep. Ser.* **464.** Geneva.

World Health Organization (1973). Brucellosis in man (officially reported cases). *In* ''World Health Statistics Report, **26:** Abstr., Int. Symp. on Brucellosis (II), Rabat, 1975''. *Dev. Biol. Stand.* **31,** 16.

World Health Organization (1976). The role of auxiliary veterinary personnel in surveillance. *Wkly. Epidemiol. Rec.* **51,** 77.

13

Epidemiological Patterns in Directly Transmitted Human Infections

A. D. M. SMITH

Department of Zoology
University of Adelaide
Adelaide, South Australia, Australia

I. Introduction

The importance of behavioral factors in determining patterns of transmission in directly transmitted human diseases within small communities has long been established (Bailey, 1957). Studies on the pattern of disease spread through individual households have been of primary importance in the measurement of basic epidemiological parameters such as the latent and infective periods of specific infections (Hope Simpson, 1952; Bailey, 1954). Mathematical models of simple epidemics, incorporating behavioral assumptions about the nature and frequency of contact between individuals, have been of great value in such studies (Becker, 1979).

The importance of behavioral and sociocultural factors in determining patterns of disease transmission at larger spatial scales is less well established. Such studies as there are have tended to focus on island communities (Bartlett, 1957;

Black, 1966) and on isolated hunter–gatherer societies (Black, 1980; McNeill, 1980). Nevertheless, behavioral factors clearly must be important in determining regional and national patterns in disease incidence and transmission. Moreover, for a number of the directly transmitted diseases, but especially for the common childhood diseases (such as measles, whooping cough, diphtheria, and scarlet fever), compulsory notifications coupled with high levels of incidence and national recording at relatively fine spatial scales provide a good data base from which to explore some of the behavioral factors underlying disease transmission.

Section II of this chapter provides an introduction to the theoretical background employed in the analyses described in later sections. Specifically, the behavioral assumptions underlying models of disease transmission are discussed in detail. The main analysis, in Section III, is concerned with the epidemiological patterns to be found in the common childhood viral and bacterial diseases, particularly measles, and of the possible behavioral factors underlying them. The implications of these analyses for the control of such diseases by vaccination are investigated in Section IV, and Section V outlines the general conclusions on the importance of behavioral factors in understanding the dynamics of directly transmitted human infections.

II. Theoretical Background

A. Disease Transmission

An important factor in the epidemiology of all infectious diseases is the rate at which new cases of infection are acquired by individuals in the host population. In theoretical models that seek to explain observed patterns of disease incidence within one or more host populations, it is the transmission term that describes the rate at which susceptible individuals in the population acquire infection. Since the early theoretical work of Ross (1911) and Kermack and McKendrick (1927), it has invariably been assumed that the transmission term in models for directly transmitted infectious diseases is of the form βXY, where X and Y represent, respectively, the number (or the density) of susceptible and infectious individuals in the population and where β is some "transmission coefficient."

There are a number of key behavioral assumptions underlying this form of the transmission term. One of the most important assumptions is that the population is "closed," that is, there is no immigration of infectious individuals. The population is also assumed to be homogeneous and freely mixing, so that there is a constant probability of "contact" between any two individuals in the population in any given period of time. Thus the actual rate of contact for any one individual with other individuals would be directly proportional to population size (or density). If population size is denoted by the symbol N, then the net contact rate for any individual will be of the form $\beta'N$ where β' is a constant that will be some function of the characteristic behavior of individuals in such a freely mixing population.

Considering now the rate of contact of any individual with the infected individuals in the population, the individual contact rate $\beta'N$ must be modified to take into account the proportion of individuals in the population which are infectious at any given moment. Assuming that the population size is reasonably large, the individual contact rate with infectious individuals is $\beta'NY/N$, that is, $\beta'Y$. Thus, the contact rate between susceptible and infectious individuals in the population must be the product of the individual contact rate with infecteds and the total number (or density) of susceptibles, and the net contact rate between susceptible and infectious individuals will be $\beta'XY$. Because only a proportion β'' of such contacts will actually result in the infection being transmitted to susceptible individuals, the net transmission rate of infection within the population (equivalent to the rate of loss of susceptible individuals that become infected) will be of the form $\beta'\beta''XY$. Note that the constant β'' will also presumably be a function of some overall behavioral characteristic of the population. Setting $\beta = \beta'\beta''$, the transmission term is given by βXY. Thus, β represents some "effective" rate of contact between individuals in a freely mixing population, and will be some complex function of social and behavioral characteristics of the individuals in such a population.

B. A Simple Model

The transmission term is only one component, albeit an important one, in models that seek to describe the dynamics of directly transmitted diseases in human populations. A considerable variety of mathematical models have been developed for the analysis of such diseases (Bailey, 1975). There has been a recent renewed interest in the use of simple deterministic models, composed of first-order differential equations, for the analysis of endemic and recurrent epidemic phenomena (Dietz, 1975; Dietz, 1976; Anderson and May, 1982). The development of this approach and the assumptions underlying it are outlined below as a basis for the analysis and interpretation of observed epidemiological patterns in later sections of this chapter.

It is assumed first of all that population size N is constant. This assumption seems reasonable even in situations where the population size is changing, so long as the time scale of the change is long compared with the epidemiological time scales of interest. For the population size to be constant, the net input of susceptible individuals into the population due to births must equal the net

son, 1982). The case $\alpha = 1$ would correspond to the assumption of a freely mixing population, whereas $\alpha = 0$ would represent a situation in which the number of contacts per unit of time for an individual was a fixed constant (β'), independent of population size. The overall transmission term produced as a result of this change would be of the form $\beta XYN^{\alpha-1}$. This yields the usual transmission term βXY when $\alpha = 1$; for $\alpha = 0$ the transmission term will be $\beta XY/N$, with the rate of disease transmission being proportional to the prevalence of infection, Y/N, rather than its overall incidence Y. This seems to be the case for sexually transmitted diseases (Yorke $et\ al.$, 1978).

The effect of replacing the transmission terms βXY in Eqs. (1) and (2) by the form $\beta XYN^{\alpha-1}$ is now considered. The expression for the basic reproductive rate of the disease is modified to

$$R_0 = \beta\sigma N^{\alpha}/[(\mu+\sigma)\ (\mu+\gamma)] \tag{7}$$

Clearly, as α decreases from one toward zero, the value of R_0 will depend less and less on population size.

The more general form of Eq. (7) can be used to explore the relationship between R_0 and N where age prevalence data are available over a range of population sizes. Equation (7) can be transformed using natural logarithms to yield the expression

$$\ln R_0 = \ln\{\beta\sigma/[(\mu+\sigma)\ (\mu+\gamma)]\} + \alpha\ln N \tag{8}$$

which is a linear regression of the form

$$\langle y = a + bx \rangle$$

where $y = \ln R_0$, $x = \ln N$, $a = \ln\{\beta\sigma/[(\mu+\sigma)\ (\mu+\gamma)]\}$, and $b = \alpha$. Given a series of observed values for R_0 over a range of population sizes N together with estimates of the parameters μ, σ, and γ, it should be possible to estimate the values of α and β using standard regression techniques. Estimates of these parameters for a number of common childhood diseases are derived in Section III.

III. Childhood Viral and Bacterial Diseases

In contrast with the sexually transmitted diseases, most of the common childhood viral and bacterial diseases are characterized by the development of life-long immunity following recovery from infection. Models of the type outlined in Section II can be used to analyze the endemic and recurrent epidemic behavior of such diseases. In this section (III), such models are used to investigate the relationship between the basic reproductive rate of a disease R_0 and the size of the community in which the disease is found. The spatial variation in R_0 is also examined, together with spatial and temporal patterns of incidence of measles in England and Wales. Some possible behavioral and social factors underlying such patterns are discussed.

A. Effects of Community Size

The relationship between disease transmission and community size has been of continuing interest to epidemiologists. Early theoretical studies by Kermack and McKendrick (1927) showed the existence of a "threshold theorem," effectively a critical threshold density below which a disease could not persist in a population. Bartlett (1956, 1957, 1960) used stochastic models to investigate the critical community size for measles, taking into account the periodic incidence of the disease (recurrent epidemic behavior) and the probability of "fadeout." The critical community size for measles in the United States appeared to be about 200,000. Black (1966) investigated the critical community size for measles epidemics in insular populations, and Fenner (1980) reviewed the effects of sociocultural development on disease persistence for a wide range of infectious diseases. He concluded that viral diseases such as measles, smallpox, and rubella could not have existed in paleolithic hunter–gatherer societies, and that only those viral diseases marked by latency and recurrent infectivity, such as herpes simplex and chickenpox-zoster, could have persisted in such small communities.

Community size can affect other aspects of disease transmission besides persistence. Griffiths (1974) has shown that the mean age at attack of measles was lower in conurbations than in rural areas of England and Wales during the period 1956–1969. Anderson and May (1982) have estimated the value of R_0, the basic reproductive rate, for a number of directly transmitted infectious diseases in a variety of geographical locations and over a series of time spans from the early part of the twentieth century to the present. Estimates for R_0 are generally higher in urban than in rural settings, and there is a clear trend toward increasing values of R_0 over time, possibly associated with increasing levels of urbanization.

Where age-prevalence data are available for communities over a series of known size ranges, they may be used to calculate the mean age at infection A and hence R_0, and so explore the relationship between the intrinsic reproductive rate of a disease and community size. Equation (7), based on the dynamic model [Eqs. (1–4)] and the general form of the transmission term (Section II,C), serves as a theoretical basis for exploring this relationship. Estimates of the parameters α and β of Eq. (7) can be obtained using the linearized form [Eq. (8)] and standard least squares regression. Two sets of data are analyzed here. The first set is for measles, whooping cough, scarlet fever, and diphtheria in New York

TABLE IA

The Average Age at First Infection A as a Function of Community Size
in New York State in the Years 1918–1919[a]

	Mean age at infection A (years)			
Community size	Measles	Whooping cough	Scarlet fever	Diphtheria
200,000–50,000	9.0	6.3	10.5	10.6
50,000–10,000	9.0	5.7	10.2	11.5
10,000– 2,500	10.7	6.9	11.2	12.5
Under 2,500	12.9	8.2	12.3	14.2

[a]Data from Fales (1928).

State in the years 1918–1919 (Fales, 1928). The mean ages at infection for these diseases over a range of community sizes are shown in Table IA. The records of the Registrar General for England and Wales also provide age-specific prevalence data for a number of notifiable diseases over a broadly similar range of community sizes. Values for the mean age at infection A and for the basic reproductive rate R_0 were calculated for measles for the years 1950–1955, and are shown in Table IB.

The relationship between $\ln R_0$ and $\ln N$ for both sets of data is shown in Fig. 2. There are insufficient data points for each disease to establish clearly whether the relationship is, indeed, linear, and the New York State data suggest at least at the upper end of the range a curvilinear relationship with community size.

Least squares estimates for the parameters α and β are given in Table II. The most notable feature of these results is the very low values for the estimates of α. This indicates that the effect of community size on the mean age at infection and

TABLE IB

The Average Age at Infection A and the Basic Reproductive Rate R_0 for
Measles in England and Wales in the Years 1950–1955[a]

	Measles	
Community size	Mean age at infection A	Basic reproductive rate R_0
Urban, 100,000+	3.9	18.7
Urban, 50,000–100,000	4.2	17.5
Urban, 50,000–[b]	4.5	16.5
Rural	5.0	15.0

[a]Data from Registrar General's Statistical Reviews for England and Wales.
[b]50,000 or less.

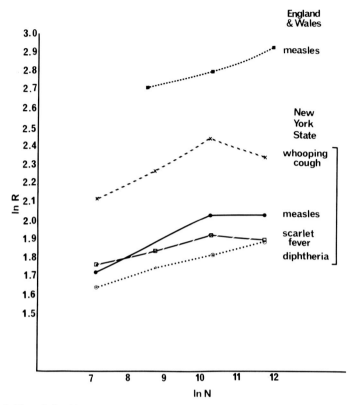

FIG. 2. The relationship between the intrinsic reproductive rate of a disease (R_0) and community size (N), plotted on a natural log–log scale and based on the data shown in Tables IA and IB.

TABLE II

Estimates of the Parameters α and β of Eq. (7)
in the Text Using Data from Tables IA and IB

Source	$\hat{\alpha}$[a]	$\hat{\beta}$[a]
New York State 1918–1919		
Measles	0.07	199
Whooping cough	0.06	95
Scarlet fever	0.03	100
Diphtheria	0.05	76
England and Wales 1950–1955		
Measles	0.06	507

[a]Estimated parameters.

on the basic reproductive rate of these diseases is relatively slight, a conclusion which seems apparent from inspection of the untransformed data in Table I. Certainly the estimated values are far from $\alpha = 1$, the assumption inherent in the conventional form βXY of the transmission term. The results correspond much more closely to a model in which disease transmission is independent of community size. A more detailed interpretation of these results is given in Section III,C.

Two other aspects of the results are worth noting. The first is that the values of α for all the diseases are roughly the same order of magnitude, as might be expected in diseases for which the modes of transmission are similar. The second aspect is that the value for β for measles is much higher in England and Wales in 1950–1955 than in New York State in 1918–1919. This might indicate some change in the infectivity of the disease over time. It might also be explained by differences in the mixing rates within the respective populations, although whether these differences are characteristic of the geographic location or of the time cannot be distinguished.

B. Patterns in Space and Time

Long periods of compulsory notifications combined with high levels of incidence and their recording at fine spatial scales have resulted in a number of common childhood infectious diseases providing suitable case examples for the study of spatial and temporal dynamic processes. The study of spatial diffusion of successive epidemic waves of measles in an island community provides a recent example (Cliff et al., 1981). This section will examine some spatial and temporal patterns in measles in England and Wales, moving from the national through the regional to the more local scales.

1. THE NATIONAL PATTERN

A widely observed feature of measles epidemiology is a characteristic 2- or 3-year cycle in disease incidence. Yorke et al. (1979) and Dietz (1976) have examined some possible causes underlying such cyclic behavior, and Anderson and May (1982) have shown the relationship between the period of the cycle and the intrinsic reproductive rate of the disease. The incidence of measles for England and Wales in the period 1950–1973 is shown in Fig. 3. The 2-year cycle, with alternating years of high and low incidence, is clearly evident until 1967. A national program of immunization against measles was instituted in 1968 and the clear 2-year cycle in incidence prior to this date is no longer apparent. It can also be seen that the immunization program, while substantially reducing the incidence of the disease, has by no means eradicated it.

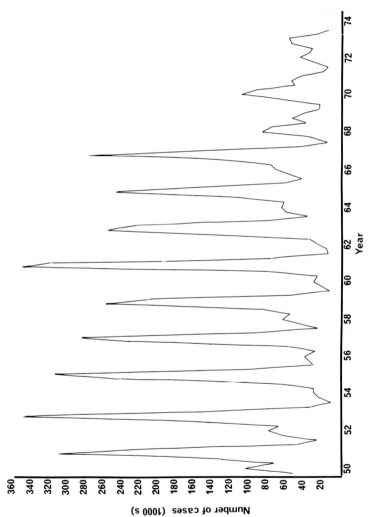

FIG. 3. The incidence of measles in England and Wales in the years 1950–1973, based on quarterly returns of the Registrar General for England and Wales.

Apart from the clear 2-year cycle in its incidence, measles also exhibits a characteristic seasonal pattern. The factors underlying this seasonality have been explored by Yorke and London (1973) and London and Yorke (1973), and the implications of seasonality for the longer term dynamics by Dietz (1976) and Yorke et al. (1979). An analysis of weekly records for England and Wales by Fine and Clarkson (1982) has revealed some new and interesting features in this seasonal pattern. They examined weekly incidence from 1950 to 1979 and also calculated changes in the "transmission parameter" (closely corresponding to β) over time. Their examination revealed a remarkably stable pattern in which the lowest incidence occurs in Weeks 36 to 39 of each year, and in which there is a series of three peaks in transmission which seem to correspond to periods of return to school after holidays. With the mean age at infection for measles at about 4 to 5 years, schools seem to play a major role in disease transmission. The seasonal patterns were found to persist across years of both high and low incidence in the regular 2-year cycles prior to the start of the immunization program, and despite the loss of the clear biennial cycle in incidence since the onset of widespread vaccination, the timing of the annual minimum in measles incidence and the approximate association in the pattern of transmission with the timing of the school year has been maintained.

2. REGIONAL VARIATIONS

The effects of community size on the basic reproductive rate of measles in England and Wales were explored in Section III,A. The results indicated that values for R_0 were generally higher in urban than in rural areas. The same data source also permits an examination of regional variations in R_0 in England and Wales over the same period of time (Fig. 4).

The first point to note is that the regional range in variation of R_0 from 15.0 to 19.7 is greater than is expected from urban–rural differences, where the range was from 15.0 to 18.7. Moreover, the value of R_0 for Wales II (for example) with no large urban centers is higher than that for the London and South Eastern region, which is dominated by the London conurbation. The second point to note is that with the exception of southern Wales (Wales I) there is a fairly distinct latitudinal gradient in values of R_0, with higher values occurring in the North.

The reasons for these regional variations in the basic reproductive rate of measles remain open to speculation, but social or behavioral causes cannot be discounted. Some correlation of North-South differences with social conditions seems probable, as conditions are generally poorer in the North. The discrepancy in the trend of southern Wales, a depressed industrial region, tends to support this speculation. Social conditions might affect disease transmission through features such as average family size or patterns of social contact within a local

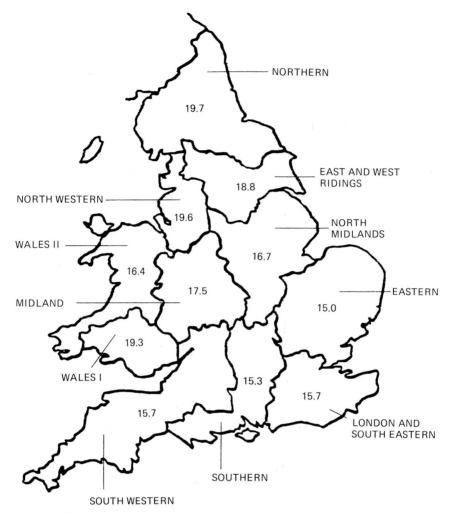

FIG. 4. The intrinsic reproductive rate (R_0) for measles for each standard region in England and Wales, averaged over the years 1950–1955.

community. Northerners are generally considered to be more "gregarious" than persons from the South, though it is uncertain whether this is true also of the children who represent the portion of the population most at risk from the disease. In any case, social factors such as these would be very difficult to quantify.

Apart from the intrinsic reproductive rate, patterns in the incidence of measles over time can also be examined regionally. Figure 5 shows the quarterly inci-

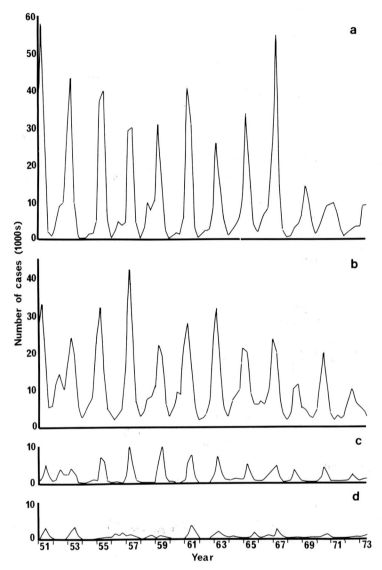

FIG. 5. The incidence of measles 1951–1973 by quarters in (a) Greater London, (b) Lancashire, (c) Northumberland, and (d) Cornwall.

dence of measles from 1950 to 1973 for four counties, chosen from four different regions, and representing a gradient from wholly urban through mixed urban and rural to rural areas. The biennial cycle in incidence shows clearly for Greater London (Fig. 5a) and the overall pattern is very similar to that for the whole of England and Wales (Fig. 3). The pattern for Lancashire (Fig. 5b) in the North Western region is very similar to that for Greater London and for the whole country. The pattern for this county is determined by the two large urban centers, Liverpool and Manchester, which provide most of the cases. Northumberland (Fig. 5c) in the Northern region is mainly a rural county, although Newcastle provides one major urban population center. Here the pattern of incidence is erratic from 1950 to 1954 but settles down to a biennial cycle which peaks slightly ahead of the national cycle in 1955 and 1957 but lags behind it in 1959 and 1961. The final pattern shown is for Cornwall (Fig. 5d), a county isolated at the end of a peninsula in the Southwestern region and containing no large urban centers. The pattern here is quite erratic and peaks in incidence, where they do correspond roughly to peaks in the national pattern of incidence, generally lag behind them.

3. LOCAL PATTERNS

A number of recent geographic studies of epidemic diffusion have focused on patterns in outbreak of measles in the southwest of England (Haggett, 1976; Murray and Cliff, 1977; Cliff and Ord, 1978; Haggett, 1978; Cliff and Haggett, 1979). These studies have been based on an analysis of weekly records of measles incidence at the local district level and have generally covered the period from September 1966 to December 1970. Attempts have been made to model the local and regional spread of the disease over this period, using autoregressive and moving-average models, Kalman filter models, and process-based models of both the Hamer–Soper type (Soper, 1929) and the chain binomial form (Bailey, 1957).

No clear picture of spatial diffusion of measles has emerged from these studies. At the local level, patterns of incidence in measles show a great deal of stochastic variation with frequent periods of fadeout of the disease outside the major urban centers. Analysis reveals a strong contagious element in the spatial spread of the disease, with new outbreaks occurring close to existing ones, but this is scarcely surprising. There is also evidence for the spread of outbreaks of measles from the high density urban areas that serve as the main reservoirs for disease persistence. However, there is no clear evidence of hierarchical spread through the urban-size system. Modeling focused on attempts to predict the timing of new outbreaks of disease, and the process-based models were found to be more useful in this respect.

C. Discussion

This section has examined some epidemiological patterns associated with childhood viral and bacterial infections. In particular, the dynamics of measles in England and Wales have been discussed. The basic reproductive rate R_0 of this disease has been examined for its regional variation and its possible correlation with community size, and patterns in the incidence of measles over time have been studied at a series of spatial scales. These different aspects of measles epidemiology are now drawn together and discussed in the light of the behavioral assumptions underlying disease transmission.

The relationship between the basic reproductive rate of a disease R_0 and community size was explored in Section III,A using Eq. (7), which was derived from the model described in Eqs. (1–4), but using the generalized form of the transmission term $\beta XYN^{\alpha-1}$. The estimated value of α for measles in England and Wales (and indeed for the other childhood diseases in the United States) was found to be much closer to zero than to unity. This result might be interpreted as indicating the inappropriateness of models using the more usual form βXY for the transmission term, since these correspond to the case $\alpha = 1$. However, a quite different interpretation of the results arises from consideration of one of the original assumptions underlying both models.

The key assumption, in this case, is that the population is closed. It seems very unlikely that this assumption would be met by any community or subset of the population within England and Wales. It is conceivable, however, that England and Wales as a whole might effectively act as such a closed unit, with inputs from Scotland and from outside the United Kingdom having little impact on the overall dynamics of transmission within the unit. Viewed in this way, the results of the analysis of the relationship between R_0 and community size within England and Wales can be seen as confirming the essential homogeneity of England and Wales as an epidemiological unit. If this hypothesis is correct, then rather than expecting to find $\alpha = 1$ throughout a series of communities within England and Wales, one would expect to find $\alpha = 0$, with any subunit of the population having an identical value of R_0 to the population of England and Wales as a whole.

This view of England and Wales as an epidemiological unit is, in general, reinforced by the other results. The clear biennial cycle in measles incidence for England and Wales prior to the immunization program, together with the observation that in general nearly synchronous cycles occur between widely separated regions (at least those dominated by large urban centers), tend to reinforce the view that, at least with respect to the transmission of measles, England and Wales can be treated as a unit. Fine and Clarkson (1982) point out that the clear biennial cycle in measles also occurred in France, but 1 year out of phase with the cycle in England and Wales. However, the cycle is not generally apparent in the United States, although individual cities do show the 2-year cycles in incidence.

The picture which seems to emerge, then, is one in which England and Wales together do seem to fulfill the assumptions inherent in the basic model [Eqs. (1–4)] representing a closed, freely mixing population. This does not mean, of course, that the behavioral assumption of an equal chance of contact between any two individuals in the populations is actually met. It simply means that the level of general mixing in the population as a whole tends to integrate patterns of contact at local levels to produce a situation in which the assumptions of the simple model are nearly met at the national level. Thus, any local differences which may be due to community size or other factors tend to be swamped by the overall dynamics of the disease in the population.

This picture is, of course, not quite accurate. Some regional differences do persist and these may well be attributable to social or behavioral factors. Similar factors may underlie the complex patterns which emerge from scrutiny at the finer spatial scales. Clearly, the results obtained at the broader spatial scale do not negate the importance of behavioral factors in producing the observed epidemiological patterns (as in the correlation of seasonal patterns in measles incidence with social behavior determined by the timing of school holidays) or in accounting for the apparent homogeneity of the whole population with respect to measles transmission. The important point to note is that differences in epidemiological patterns, which may be detectable at local or even regional levels, do not invalidate the application of the simple sort of model outlined in Section II,A to the transmission of measles at the national level.

IV. Implications for Control

The discovery of vaccines which induce long-lasting immunity to a number of viral and bacterial infections has led to the development of large-scale programs of immunization against such diseases. A crucial factor in determining the success of such programs is the proportion of the population which must be immunized in order to eradicate the disease, or, looked at another way, the level of herd immunity which will prevent the disease from successfully establishing itself in a given population.

The relationship between the basic reproductive rate of a disease R_0 and the proportion p of the population which must be vaccinated soon after birth in order to achieve disease eradication is now well understood (Dietz, 1975; Dietz, 1976; Anderson and May, 1982). This relationship is of the form $p > 1 - 1/R_0$ and is independent of any particular model on which calculation of R_0 might be based.

Anderson and May (1982) have shown that this relationship implies that a vaccination coverage of about 94% would be required to eradicate measles from England and Wales, and that this coverage rises with the average age at which vaccination is administered.

It was suggested in Section III that England and Wales can be treated as a single epidemiological unit with respect to measles transmission, and that models of the type described in Eqs. (1–4) are appropriate for the analysis of measles dynamics at this scale of aggregation. Nevertheless, analyses in Section III showed that certain variations in R_0 do occur, both regionally and with respect to levels of urbanization. The question must be asked, Do such variations in R_0 warrant a modification in the overall national immunization program to allow for these regional and urban–rural differences?

Quite simply, they do not. The values of R_0, both regionally and with respect to community type, are shown in Table III together with the vaccination coverage required to eradicate measles for each value of R_0. The regional range in required vaccination coverage is 93.3–94.9% and the range is even smaller where based on the type of community. Since the current vaccination coverage for measles in England and Wales is at only about half this level, these differences do not appear to be at all significant, and no special regional or urban

TABLE III

The Value of R_0 and the Percentage Vaccination Cover
Required to Eradicate Measles for England and Wales
1950–1955, by Region and as a Function of Community Size

Region and size of community	R_0	Percentage vaccination cover
Region		
Northern	19.7	94.9
North Western	19.6	94.9
East and West Ridings	18.8	94.7
Midland	17.5	94.3
North Midland	16.7	94.0
Eastern	15.0	93.3
South Western	15.7	93.6
Southern	15.3	93.5
London and South Eastern	15.7	93.6
Wales I	19.3	94.8
Wales II	16.4	93.9
Size		
Urban, 100,000	18.7	94.7
Urban, 50,000–100,000	17.5	94.3
Urban, 50,000 or less	16.5	93.9
Rural	15.0	93.3

policy seems necessary. This does not, of course, preclude the necessity for such policies with respect to vaccination against other sorts of disease, or for the same disease in other countries.

Behavioral factors can play an important role in quite another way in determining the vaccination coverage required for disease eradication. These can operate through the practice of isolating infective individuals as soon as clinical symptoms of the disease are diagnosed. It can be seen from Eqs. (5) and (7) that the size of R_0 is directly proportional to the term $1/(\mu + \gamma)$, which represents the average period of infectiousness of the disease in an individual. Reducing the effective length of this infective period can result in a substantial reduction in R_0 and hence in the level of vaccination coverage required.

V. Discussion

A key factor in the analysis of behavioral factors in disease transmission is the need to identify the appropriate population unit of epidemiological study. The importance of this can be seen from the analysis of measles at the different spatial scales, where attempts to establish the relationship between the basic reproductive rate R_0 of the disease and community size were confounded by the fact that the values of R_0 in individual communities were dominated by the national pattern because of the general level of mixing and migration of individuals between communities. Although behavioral patterns clearly underlie this homogenizing effect, in this case such factors have been uncovered by a study of patterns in the disease rather than having been used to understand such patterns. Nevertheless, such integrative effects are clearly important for highly infectious diseases.

Another interesting feature of the analysis is the way in which regularity in the national patterns develops from marked irregularity at finer spatial scales. Regular patterns do seem to reemerge at the level of the individual household or institution, but these are judged on a much shorter time scale. However, different aspects of behavior would appear to underlie disease transmission at different spatial scales.

Although behavioral factors undoubtedly underlie patterns in disease transmission for the common childhood infections, understanding of the nature of such factors may not be of great practical importance for such diseases. First, although the expression for the basic reproductive rate of these diseases [Eq. (5)] incorporates the behavioral component through the parameter β, a direct measure of this parameter is not required in order to estimate R_0. Second, the observed regional and urban–rural differences in R_0 for measles in England and Wales do not appear to warrant any major modifications to the national immunization program, at least in terms of the vaccination coverage required for disease eradication. Finally, it is doubtful whether changes in behavioral practices or in social organization in order to influence the transmission of childhood diseases would be either practical or acceptable, as they would require changes on such a scale as to totally alter the structure of Western societies as they exist today.

Acknowledgment

I am indebted to Roy Anderson for helpful discussions and for commenting on the manuscript. The work was supported by a contract to the Imperial College Centre for Environmental Technology from the U.K. Department of the Environment to investigate "The Stability and Resilience of Environmental Systems: The Implications for Environmental Management."

References

Anderson, R. M. (1982). Transmission dynamics and control of infectious disease agents. *In* "Population biology of infectious diseases" (R. M. Anderson, and R. M. May, eds.). Springer-Verlag, Berlin.

Anderson, R. M., and May, R. M. (1982). Directly transmitted infectious diseases: control by vaccination. *Science* **215,** 1053–1060.

Bailey, N. T. J. (1954). A statistical method of estimating the periods of incubation and infection of an infectious disease. *Nature (London)* **174,** 139–140.

Bailey, N. T. J. (1957). "The mathematical theory of epidemics." Griffin, London.

Bailey, N. T. J. (1975). "The mathematical theory of infectious diseases and its applications." Griffin, London.

Bartlett, M. S. (1956). Determining the stochastic models for recurrent epidemics. *In* "Mathematics, statistics and probability," pp. 81–109. *Proc. Berkeley Symp. Mathematics,* 3rd, **4:** Statistics and probability.

Bartlett, M. S. (1957). Measles periodicity and community size. *J. R. Stat. Soc. Ser. A* **120,** 48–70.

Bartlett, M. S. (1960). The critical community size for measles in the United States. *J. R. Stat. Soc. Ser. A* **123,** 37–44.

Becker, N. G. (1979). The uses of epidemic models. *Biometrics* **35,** 295–305.

Black, F. L. (1966). Measles endemicity in insular populations: critical community size and its evolutionary implication. *J. Theor. Biol.* **11,** 207–211.

Black, F. L. (1980). Modern isolated pre-agricultural populations as a source of information on prehistoric epidemic patterns. *In* "Changing disease patterns and human behavior" (N. F. Stanley, and R. A. Joshe, eds.), pp. 37–54. Academic Press, London.

Cliff, A. D., and Haggett, P. (1979). Geographical aspects of epidemic diffusion in closed communities. *In* "Statistical applications in the spatial sciences" (N. Wrigley, ed.), pp. 5–44. Pion, London.

Cliff, A. D., and Ord, J. K. (1978). Forecasting the progress of an epidemic. *In* "Towards the dynamic analysis of spatial systems" (R. L. Martin, N. J. Thrift, and R. J. Bennett, eds.), pp. 191–204. Pion, London.

Cliff, A. D., Haggett, P., Ord, J. K., and Versey, G. R. (1981). "Spatial diffusion. An historical geography of epidemics in an island community." Cambridge Univ. Press, London.

Dietz, K. (1975). Transmission and control of arbovirus diseases. *In* "Epidemiology" (D. Ludwig, and K. L. Cooke, eds.), pp. 104–121. *SIAM–SIMS Conf. Ser.* **21.** Society for Industrial Applied Mathematics, Philadelphia.

Dietz, K. (1976). The incidence of infectious diseases under the influence of seasonal fluctuations. *In* "Mathematical models in medicine" (J. Berger, W. Buhler, R. Repges, and P. Tautu, eds.), pp. 1–15. Lecture Notes in Biomathematics, Vol. 11. Springer-Verlag: Berlin.

Fales, W. T. (1928). The age distribution of whooping cough, measles, chicken pox, scarlet fever and diphtheria in various areas of the United States. *Am. J. Hyg.* **8,** 759–799.

Fenner, F. (1980). Sociocultural change and environmental diseases. *In* "Changing disease patterns and human behaviour" (N. F. Stanley, and R. A. Joshe, eds.), pp. 7–26. Academic Press, London.

Fine, P. E. M., and Clarkson, J. A. (1982). Measles in England and Wales—I. An analysis of factors underlying seasonal patterns. *Int. J. Epidemiol.* **11,** 5–14.

Great Britain, Registrar General (1950–1974). Statistical review of England and Wales. H. M. Stationary Office, London.

Griffiths, D. A. (1974). A catalytic model of infection for measles. *Appl. Stat.* **23,** 330–339.

Haggett, P. (1976). Hybridizing alternative models of an epidemic diffusion process. *Econ. Geogr.* **52,** 136–146.

Haggett, P. (1978). Regional and local components in elementary space-time models. *In* "Timing space and spacing time" (T. Carlstein, D. Parkes, and N. Thrift, eds.), pp. 19–34. Arnold, London.

Hope Simpson, R. E. (1952). Infectiousness of communicable diseases in the household. *Lancet* **2,** 549–554.

Kermack, W. O., and McKendrick, A. G. (1927). A contribution to the mathematical theory of epidemics. *Proc. R. Soc. Ser. A* **115,** 700–721.

London, W. P., and Yorke, J. A. (1973). Recurrent outbreaks of measles, chicken pox and mumps. 1. Seasonal variation in contact rates. *Am. J. Epidemiol.* **98,** 453–468.

McNeill, W. H. (1980). Migration patterns and infection in traditional societies. *In* "Changing disease patterns and human behaviour" (N. F. Stanley, and R. A. Joshe, eds.), pp. 27–36. Academic Press, London.

Muench, H. (1959). "Catalytic models in epidemiology." Harvard Univ. Press, Cambridge, Massachusetts.

Murray, G. D., and Cliff, A. D. (1977). A stochastic model for measles epidemics in a multi-regional setting. *Inst. Br. Geogr. Publ., New Series* **2,** 158–174.

Ross, R. (1911). "The prevention of malaria," 2nd ed., Murray, London.

Soper, H. E. (1929). Interpretation of periodicity in disease prevalence. *J. R. Stat. Soc. Ser. A* **92,** 34–61.

Yorke, J. A., and London, W. P. (1973). Recurrent outbreaks of measles, chicken pox and mumps. 2. Systematic difference in contact rate and stochastic effect. *Am. J. Epidemiol.* **98,** 469–482.

Yorke, J. A., Hethcote, H. W., and Nold, A. (1978). Dynamics and control of the transmission of gonorrhea. *J. Sex. Transm. Dis.* **5,** 51–56.

Yorke, J. A., Nathanson, N., Pianingiani, G., and Martin, J. (1979). Seasonality and the requirements for perpetuation and eradication of viruses. *Am. J. Epidemiol.* **109,** 103–123.

Index